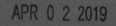

# THE END OF THE BEGINNING

# THE END OF
# THE BEGINNING

*Cancer, Immunity, and the*
*Future of a Cure*

## MICHAEL S. KINCH

PEGASUS BOOKS
NEW YORK LONDON

THE END OF THE BEGINNING

Pegasus Books Ltd.
148 W. 37th Street, 13th Floor
New York, NY 10018

Copyright © 2019 Michael S. Kinch

First Pegasus Books edition April 2019

Interior design by Maria Fernandez

Library of Congress Cataloging-in-Publication Data is available.

ISBN: 978-1-64313-025-5

10 9 8 7 6 5 4 3 2 1

Printed in the United States of America
Distributed by W. W. Norton & Company, Inc.
www.pegasusbooks.us

*This book is dedicated to the memories and families of*
*Harold Noe, Thomas Noe, William Zellner, and all the victims of cancer*
*hoping the beginning of the end is near...*

# CONTENTS

# Introduction

I t was the same campus, the same sunny day, and almost the exact same parking spot I had occupied just a few weeks before. However, the circumstances could not have been more different. On my previous trip, I was an invited guest, hosted by a former colleague to present the highlights from the cutting-edge oncology research we were conducting at a biotechnology company just a few miles up the road from the National Institutes of Health (NIH) Bethesda, Maryland, campus where I was currently standing. The name of the company was MedImmune, a conflation of two words meant to reflect a focus on developing novel ways of unleashing the power of the immune system to promote medicine. While the company had already made a name for itself in infectious diseases, I had been tasked with building a portfolio of products to target cancer. The company was largely focusing its efforts to unharness the power of monoclonal antibodies, the guided missiles of the immune system that can be as specific and destructive as the most advanced smart bombs that were used in the second Gulf War just two years before.

I had been recruited from Purdue University, where my academic work as a professor had led to the discovery of ways monoclonal antibodies could be created and deployed to seek out and destroy metastatic cells. These rogue killers comprise the most invasive and deadly tumor cells and tend to elude both the surgeon's knife and chemotherapy. My tenure at Purdue had been granted just a year or two earlier and I was happily obsessed with understanding the processes behind metastasis. Nonetheless, throughout these halcyon academic years, I had always been gripped with a passion to apply research to alleviate human suffering in "the real world," which was quite distinct from trying to cure experimental mouse tumors, the mainstay of academic research.

Nineteen ninety-eight was a pivotal year, though this was not clear to me at the time. I was in my third year as an assistant professor at Purdue and had published a scientific manuscript detailing a project initiated while transitioning from my postdoctoral studies at the Lineberger Cancer Center at the University of North Carolina to my start at Purdue. We had identified a type of cellular behavior distinguishing benign cells from their malignant counterparts and I hoped these differences might provide a new opportunity for targeting cancer.

I have been extraordinarily lucky to be in the right place and time at key points. Working in 1995 with colleagues at Chapel Hill and at nearby Glaxo Pharmaceuticals (located down the road in Research Triangle Park, North Carolina), we innovated a novel approach to create monoclonal antibodies to characterize or, if we were very lucky, actually convey some use in targeting metastatic cancer. Our rationale back in 1995 was based upon emerging evidence for a new approach using monoclonal antibodies as a much-needed alternative to conventional chemical toxins. Only one monoclonal antibody had ever been approved for cancer at the time.

The drug Rituxan® (rituximab), as we will see, had been developed by a start-up biotechnology company in San Diego (IDEC Pharmaceuticals) and marketed by another biotechnology company located outside San Francisco (Genentech). Rituximab had overcome all the hurdles necessary to be approved by the Food and Drug Administration (FDA) in 1997 and it was to be used in the battle against a type of blood cancer known as a *lymphoma*. Early sales of the drug were promising but not overwhelming. The reason for the lag in sales was in part because monoclonal antibody drugs were not very familiar to most physicians (or even many scientists). However, this drug would go on to log peak annual revenues of more than $7.3 billion in 2015 alone and become the twelfth-highest selling drug in history (undoubtedly fated to move even higher because antibody drug sales are not as susceptible to generic competition as more conventional medicines are).

Looking back to 1998, the commercial view of monoclonal antibody therapeutics was not terribly optimistic. For one thing, the nascent field was considered, by many industry experts, to be unrealistic based on economics alone. Such views were justified based on the high costs needed to manufacture these large molecules, which might cost hundreds of dollars per dose (as compared with pennies for many conventional medicines). Moreover, key patents filed by early biotechnology pioneers meant a substantial portion of revenues—as much as one-third for some medicines—would have to be surrendered to competitors. To break even, some antibody drug companies contemplated asking prices of up to $10,000 for a single course of treatment—an outrageous proposition at the time.

Ten thousand dollars today seems almost like a bargain, when insurance companies are, with increasing frequency, asked to spend hundreds of thousands or even millions of dollars on some medicines. However, this price tag seemed utterly absurd to many in the late 1990s. Hence, many conventional pharmaceutical companies focused on standard medicines comprised of small and less complex molecules (think of aspirin). In contrast, monoclonal antibodies were large and unwieldy beasts (e.g., a thousand times larger than aspirin). To manufacture a single antibody requires the precise arrangement of four large proteins, each situated in just the right way, to ensure an antibody drug is stable, safe, and efficacious.

This complex construction could not be performed in the massive fermentation tanks used to manufacture small molecules but instead required something with far greater sophistication: the honed skills of human or other mammalian cells. Yes, these cells actually served as the factories, and the technology needed to engineer the production of proteins in these tiny workshops had only been enabled in the 1970s and 1980s. All the antibody drugs described herein were produced by cells obtained from discarded human or animal tissues and then modified using genetic engineering to produce the antibody of interest.

The high costs of growing the antibody-producing cells, purifying their protein products, and ensuring the resultant drug remained viable accounted for for the bulk of the expense of monoclonal antibody drugs. These costs were compounded by an enormous amount of intellectual property (patents and royalties) that drastically increased the cost of manufacturing antibodies. Consequently, there were few biotechnology companies, or more accurately, investors, willing to take the plunge into such a risky enterprise. In my years as an academic, I spoke with representatives from many conventional pharmaceutical companies and most indicated their unease with utilizing monoclonal antibodies for any indication, and certainly not for cancer.

Cancer at the time was a relative backwater in drug development. I vividly recall one conversation with a pharmaceutical company executive, who stated cancer would likely forever remain so as "there had never been a single blockbuster" in the field (*blockbuster* being an industry vernacular for a drug generating a billion dollars in annual revenue). The "real money," she continued, was in a drug a person would need to take every day for the rest of their life (such as a medication for hypertension or high cholesterol). One problem with oncology was that treatment tended to be short-term (weeks or months) and if you were effective, therapy may never be needed again. The alternative was the patient would expire from the disease. Either way, the patient would not take the medicine for very long. Given the crass connotations, I recall being quite shaken and can recall the details of this conversation as if it occurred yesterday. Simply put, there was not much interest in cancer or antibodies in the 1990s world of pharmaceuticals.

One exception was MedImmune.

The firm was originally founded in 1988 by an entrepreneurial pair of physicians, Wayne Hockmeyer and Franklin Top, who had retired from leadership roles at the Walter Reed Medical Center. Founded as Molecular Vaccines, Inc., in May 1987 (the name was changed to MedImmune in October 1990), the company had opened its doors in a small research laboratory in an utterly nondescript building on Firstfield Road in Gaithersburg, Maryland, lodged between a sleepy post office and a row of apartment buildings that were not aging terribly well.

Hockmeyer and Top had partnered with a venture capitalist to build upon research they had begun at Walter Reed years before. A lead project had sought to develop antisera to prevent respiratory syncytial virus (RSV) infection in premature infants. RSV causes cold-like symptoms in most children and adults every year or so. Although a simple infection to you and me, this same virus can cause irreparable lung damage and frequent death in premature infants. The risk from RSV persists for a year or two as the lungs are particularly vulnerable and slower to develop and heal in these frail babies. The first serum-based RSV therapies to be deployed by MedImmune were indistinguishable in many ways to the antisera deployed to treat diphtheria and rabies as pioneered by Louis Pasteur and Robert Koch more than a century before. However, the two former army men, Hockmeyer and his former commanding officer, Top, were not content to focus only upon these sera-derived therapeutics, but had plans to utilize the newly developed power of monoclonal antibody technology.

Within a decade, MedImmune had overcome many adversities to gain an FDA approval both for their antisera (known as RespiGam®) and the monoclonal antibody product destined to replace it: Synagis®. As the latter product closed in on a $1 billion in annual sales with the start of a new millennium, the company had already begun to expand its pipeline to include vaccine technologies to prevent infection by human papilloma virus (a subject addressed later in this book), and were actively exploring both antibody and vaccine technologies for use against an array of infectious diseases. The key in biotechnology, as in investigative reporting, is to follow the money. In this regard, the biotech community, unlike their more staid pharmaceutical cousins, had begun to believe the money led to oncology.

This paradigm shift in the private sector view of cancer had begun at about the same time as my troubling conversation with the pharmaceutical executive about the reluctance of the industry to embrace oncology. In 1998, a drug named Taxol® reached the blockbuster milestone of grossing more than $1 billion in annual revenues, the first cancer drug to reach this landmark. In that same year, a pioneering company of the biotechnology sector with the name of Genentech gained an FDA approval for a second monoclonal antibody for cancer, a drug known as *trastuzumab* (Herceptin®). Trastuzumab was targeted at the highly organized community of breast cancer patients, who helped advocate and advertise the advantages of Herceptin over more traditional breast cancer treatment therapies. You could feel a seismic shift as this motivated and well-informed breast cancer community was suddenly filled with hope. The success of trastuzumab triggered an overdue deluge of investment targeted to develop new breast cancer medicines.

Beyond breast cancer, the concerns about the relatively small market of individuals requiring oncology drugs were offset by the recognition that a cure for cancer, even a partial cure that extended life by a few years, could command high prices. Adjusting their mindset, biotechnology and pharmaceutical corporate executives were suddenly driven by the expectation that a new blockbuster could arise from medicines delivering large sums per patient, even if this came from a small number of people treated for a short time. In other words, small populations could generate profits if the outcome could justify a high price. This approach to generate prodigious earnings from a small population would soon dominate the biopharmaceutical industry, displacing the concept of more widely used and lifelong products that yielded lower revenues per patient, but were prescribed year after year.

As MedImmune was becoming one of the first biotechnology companies to achieve profitability based on revenues derived from their infectious disease products, I hoped the monoclonal antibodies I had developed in North Carolina might serve as a scientific tool. My primary focus, following the work I had started at UNC, would be on a basic scientific question about cancer cell behavior. The goal for these antibodies was to help train new graduate students in how to conduct research. Each student would be assigned a random antibody (there were more than six hundred) to learn the basic techniques provided by antibodies in the laboratory. If one of these young students happened to stumble upon something with these antibodies, then we could take an opportunities approach to pursue it further.

Everything changed when my first student, and then my second, began obtaining exciting results with these antibodies. Their findings revealed unexpected potential for identifying and potentially targeting metastatic cells. Consequently, these side projects soon dominated my laboratory at Purdue. Their discoveries would ultimately determine many of our young family's life choices, including where we lived and our sources of employment, for most of the next decade, redirecting the careers and personal lives of myself and my wife, Kelly (also a cancer researcher). Unbeknownst to us, we were in the middle of an extraordinary burst in the enterprise of biotechnology in general and cancer immunology in particular.

By the beginning of the new millennium, my research had become obsessed with a molecule functionally altered and overexpressed on cancer cells. This protein, known as *EphA2*, normally was restricted to the developing embryo and was mostly turned off (or found at very low levels) in benign cells. In its normal function, EphA2 served to decrease cell growth and invasiveness. In contrast, our laboratory had demonstrated cancer cells found a way to reprogram EphA2 to promote tumor cell growth and favor metastasis. Our work culminated in the description of a vicious cycle whereby the malevolent behavior of the EphA2 protein caused it to accumulate within malignant cells, thereby further enhancing the aggressiveness of tumor cells and in turn increasing the levels of EphA2. The cause and effect of EphA2 and disease progression would continue to spiral up to the point where the tumors had become killers dependent upon EphA2. Most importantly, we had uncovered a means by which carefully selected EphA2 monoclonal antibodies (made specially for this purpose) could override this process and essentially short-circuit tumor cells, selectively killing them while sparing benign cells.

As word began to spread about our work in an obscure laboratory in one of many Big Ten schools and in the midst of agrarian Indiana, I began receiving invitations to speak about our work at other universities, as well as an occasional biotechnology company. Returning from a whirlwind trip to the West Coast on a red-eye flight in the early summer of 2001, I stopped by my office to check the mail and ask about my students, with the goal of returning home to catch up on some much-needed sleep. Within seconds after stepping into my office, the phone rang. I was tempted to ignore the call, but fate intervened and I answered.

The caller was the new president of Purdue, Martin Jischke, asking if I could take some time to meet with an alumnus. I was informed this gentleman had founded a biotechnology company, which also happened to work on monoclonal antibodies. Having never spoken with the president, it would have been challenging (and perhaps career-ending) to decline. Nonetheless, my overwhelming sense of exhaustion forced me to try and beg off the meeting. I asked the name of the alumnus. "Wayne Hockmeyer" was the reply. I had never heard of him and so asked what company he had founded. The answer, "MedImmune," was vaguely familiar and I struggled to remember why (being notorious for an awful memory). President Jischke then indicated MedImmune had recently launched a drug called Synagis®, which prevented infection from a virus called RSV. That fact jogged my memory and forced a concession that a much-desired nap was not destined to be part of my immediate future. I immediately agreed to meet with him.

The reason for my sudden change in heart was in part because our elder child, Sarah, had developed RSV-triggered asthma as an infant. This entailed months of increasing familiarity with albuterol dispensed by nebulizers, which would ease her breathing during asthmatic events. Sarah, by this time, was a toddler and her asthma bouts were happily becoming a distant memory. More contemporary concerns arose for our son, only six months old at the time. Always a rather energetic child (even *in utero*), Grant had kicked his mother so hard he tore a hole in the amniotic sac, which caused him to stop progressing at roughly thirty-three weeks of gestational development. He was born prematurely a week later and while not the smallest preemie in the neonatal intensive care unit, his older sister Sarah's prior history with RSV caused his pediatrician to prescribe Synagis. My wife and I, who both worked with monoclonal antibodies, were amused by the fact our son was one of the rare few who was receiving such medicines (though our insurance company was surely less thrilled by the prospect of covering the shots, which cost roughly $800 per month). Thus, the utterance of the name Synagis by the Purdue president had been sufficient to convince me to meet with Dr. Hockmeyer.

Though I was undoubtedly not at top form (still bleary-eyed from the flight and un-showered), the meeting went surprisingly well. Hockmeyer and I discussed shared interests in monoclonal antibodies. This prompted a generous offer from him to visit MedImmune at its Gaithersburg, Maryland, headquarters. A few weeks later, I found myself giving a seminar in the boardroom of a relatively small, but extraordinarily dynamic organization. I had flown in to give a talk at noon and, as is the custom, met with a few people in the morning. My flight itinerary meant I only had two or three hours before I would have to leave to catch the return plane, particularly given returning to Dulles airport required negotiating the Capital Beltway, a ring road notorious for unbearable delays. As my talk was meant to last but an hour, this was not a major worry. The interest by the dozen or so people during the seminar was infectious and the discussion lasted more than two hours. As the talk concluded, the sustained adrenaline rush and nervous drinking of an endless cup of water meant my bladder was nearing the point of embarrassment and I excused myself ever so briefly. Upon returning, I found the room had quickly cleared out except for the chief executive officer, David Mott, who I had learned had recently taken the helm from Hockmeyer. David is quite direct and got straight to the point: MedImmune was interested in starting an oncology program and wanted me to lead it. I was humbled and dumbfounded. Here I was, a confirmed academic, being asked to sacrifice tenure and jump into a risky biotechnology venture. Compounding this, I had also just been offered a very attractive opportunity at the University of Virginia.

I returned to Indiana and excitedly discussed with Kelly the adventures from my visit to Maryland. We agonized about this sudden new opportunity, which represented an apples-to-oranges comparison with the options provided by academia. In a detailed and enlightening conversation, my wife made me realize the depths of my own ignorance, which is one of her more extraordinary and occasionally annoying talents. Although a switch to the private sector would mean giving up tenure, she could sense (more than even I) the opportunity at MedImmune would fulfill a wish to apply science to medicine, which has always been a passion. We both loved Charlottesville and I had secretly dreamed of working at "Mr. Jefferson's School" even before I had ever seen the place (as the reader will soon see, I am more than a bit of a history nerd). Yet, even as a graduate student studying basic biology, I self-identified as a cancer researcher.

An early motivation for becoming a cancer researcher had been spawned two decades before, when I lost both grandfathers to the disease. During high school, my maternal grandfather, Harold, had been diagnosed with colon cancer on the day after Thanksgiving in 1982 and had died thirteen months later, after an agonizing struggle that ravaged his formerly muscular frame and reduced him to a virtual skeleton as he lay on his deathbed. This disease had figuratively metastasized throughout our close-knit family and tainted our views of the holiday season for many years to come.

What we didn't know at the time was this same disease was also metastasizing through the family as well. By my senior year in college, an uncle was diagnosed with pancreatic cancer and, like many stricken with this particularly horrible disease, would succumb within months. Furthermore, my paternal grandfather perished within a year from the complications of fighting both colon and prostate cancer.

These family tragedies would ultimately help shape my professional life as a youthful passion for science matured into a desire to even the score with a disease that had taken such a personal toll. By the time my paternal grandfather died from cancer, I was already working toward my doctorate in immunology at the Duke University Medical Center in Durham, North Carolina, determined to apply this learning to cancer. As we have already seen, I would later perform postdoctoral studies at the University of North Carolina, which later led to the EphA2 story.

Just minutes after midnight on September 11, 2001, my wife and I landed at National Airport in Washington, D.C. Arriving at the hotel early in the morning, our plan had been to tour Gaithersburg with a realtor later in the day and on September 12 discuss potential positions at MedImmune. The planned agenda was obviously undermined by the horrific events of the day and, had I possessed any common sense, we would have politely declined a job offer in a town where planes crashed into buildings and instead opted for a safe and happy life in quaint Charlottesville, Virginia. Having never been burdened with such sense, we accepted the position at MedImmune and soon began growing a pipeline of cancer programs, mostly based around monoclonal antibodies.

One follower of our work at MedImmune was a former colleague of mine from Chapel Hill, Geoff Clark, who happened to work down the road at the National Cancer Institute (NCI). During the summer of 2004, Geoff asked me to give a seminar at NCI in Bethesda and I found myself discussing EphA2, MedImmune, and the pipeline of innovative products we were intent upon developing. It was like many other seminars but more memorable to me given the location on the NCI campus in Bethesda, a storied locale with a rich history in the war against cancer.

A couple of months later, I was back at NCI. Only this time, I did not enter through the front doors as an invited guest to expound about the scientific progress of the day but through the side door marked, "Patients Only." For this visit, I was accompanied by my mother and, after being processed, we were given wristbands and sent up to the Medical Genetics Branch. Our visit had been triggered by a recent diagnosis of a close family member, who had been experiencing discomfort in his lower abdomen for much of the past year. As alluded to above, his father had died from pancreatic cancer.

At the age of forty-one, a persistent stomachache in this otherwise healthy young man was diagnosed as invasive colon cancer. Thankfully, the disease responded nicely to chemotherapy, which included another pioneering monoclonal antibody Avastin®, which had been approved by the FDA just weeks before his diagnosis. Given the early onset of the disease, his doctors recommended an early form of genetic testing, which revealed a condition known as *hereditary nonpolyposis colorectal cancer* (or HNPCC). Also known as *Lynch Syndrome*, this genetic change is described by many online cancer-based webpages as an "autosomal dominant indication with high penetrance."

My mother had called me on the night of diagnosis to ask me to explain exactly what that particular quagmire of words meant. Upon hearing this diagnosis, my mouth went dry as I tried to choke out an explanation. Though my heart and brain were both racing, I explained the diagnosis meant my cousin had inherited a bad copy of a gene from one of his parents and therefore had a high (basically 100%) likelihood of developing cancer. I then reassured her I would do a little more research on Lynch Syndrome and call her back.

As the bile rose in my throat, my thoughts began to resemble the gyrations of a Whirling Dervish. Though from my perspective I was a paragon of composure, it took Kelly a mere split second to reinforce the fact I am not destined to play professional poker (though I tend to be quite popular at neighborhood poker games for some unknown reason). The panic on my face and in my voice were palpable.

I decided to calmly consult my textbook on cancer. The "bible of cancer" had been compiled by Vincent T. DeVita, Theodore S. Lawrence, and Steven A. Rosenberg. This thick two-volume set had a section on the subject of Lynch Syndrome, which confirmed patients with the gene mutation almost invariably develop either colon or endometrial cancer. The good news was we knew our family member was recovering nicely (and would continue to do so). Nonetheless, the swirling sensation in my head continued as I found myself trying to calmly explain to my mother that we might want to confirm the exact wording of the diagnosis, but without explaining why and thereby causing undue panic. Within a day, I was staring, mouth agape, at a faxed page of a pathology report verifying the genetic changes and cementing the diagnosis.

Almost immediately, I began calling in every favor ever owed to me. Within a few hours, I had managed to book a colonoscopy and an appointment with the head of the NCI medical genetics program focused on HNPCC. Lynch Syndrome patients are of interest to the NCI, in part because they offer a means to study the science, medicine, and sociological impact of a current or impending cancer diagnosis (the cancer can take decades to develop). In return, NCI offers counseling about treatment options and reproductive decision-making. Our first step was to discuss the situation with a counselor.

After flying my mother to Washington, we met with the head of the program, who interviewed us extensively to gain more information about our family and personal health histories. We entered the meeting under the assumption that my mother's father, whose death from colon cancer at the age of seventy-one, had inspired my interest in cancer research, represented yet another victim of Lynch Syndrome. Moreover, we assumed my grandfather had likewise passed down the gene to my uncle, who had died of pancreatic cancer, and to his children, one of whose diagnosis with colon cancer had triggered this visit to NCI.

These assumptions were overturned when the genetic counselor learned my aunt (by marriage, who also happened to be her best friend from childhood onward) had been diagnosed with cervical cancer many years before. This fact was new to me as well. The genetic counselor explained that past cases of endometrial cancer were frequently misdiagnosed as cervical cancer. Consistent with this, my mother recalled my aunt's mother had likewise been diagnosed with cervical cancer. These facts suddenly and decisively favored a likelihood the genetic component of the disease had passed from the maternal lineage and not the paternal lineage I shared with this relative.

Although selfishly reassuring to our side of the family, we were in a quandary. Do we reveal this putative lineage or remain silent? The genetic counselor was adamant we were both ethically and legally obligated to remain silent. The rationale behind this mandate is that such information may be unwanted by others. In other words, it would be selfish (and illegal) for us to reveal something with a potential impact that could affect another person's life or decisions unless they indicated their desire to discuss it. Although frustrating, we remained silent and the years passed.

Almost a decade later, I had moved to Yale University and was sitting in my living room when the phone rang. The caller was a cousin of my relative (from the other side of the family), who confided he had just been diagnosed with HNPCC following a bout of colon cancer at forty years of age. He had not been aware our shared relative also had this disease until hours before and, knowing my professional background, was calling to ask about the scientific and medical implications of this diagnosis. Thankfully, the story ends well for all the affected individuals, who have resumed happy and healthy lives, having conquered their cancers. Indeed, such outcomes are likely to become even more routine, as we will explore throughout *The End of the Beginning*.

The title of this book parrots a line from a famous speech given by arguably the greatest speaker, who has blessed the English language. In his "Bright Gleam of Victory" speech, Prime Minister of the United Kingdom Winston S. Churchill delivered a victory serenade. Events in North Africa had finally given the nation a reason to celebrate following the successful conclusion of the Second Battle of El Alamein, in which an offensive by General Bernard Law Montgomery's Eighth Army chased Erwin Rommel's Afrika Corps westward out of Egypt and through the Libyan desert. Once combined with the United States Army driving eastward from its beachheads near Algiers, the joining of American and British forces had forever expelled the Nazis from the African shores and would soon facilitate the later invasion and capitulation of Sicily and Italy. In a celebratory speech to Parliament on November 10, 1942, Churchill was nonetheless pragmatic enough to counsel, "This is not the end. This is not even the beginning of the end. But it is the end of the beginning."

This insight is an apt way to summarize extraordinary advances made in the treatment of cancer in the past few years. A remarkable series of events has allowed us to witness the potential to prevent or utterly eradicate some forms of the disease and, for even the most cautious doctors and patients, to seriously contemplate a cure—a much hoped for but rarely achieved goal of cancer therapy.

The newfound juxtaposition of "cancer" and "cure" in the same sentence may be attributable to our ability to harness the extraordinary power of the human immune system and redirect it to combat cancer. The breakthroughs made in the war against cancer are not entirely different from the achievements attained by Churchill's armies in the deserts of Egypt. As we will see, these successes may have even more relevant parallels to another desert war, which occurred in the Iraqi desert in the latter years of 20th century.

One goal of *The End of the Beginning* is to convey the extraordinary success toward developing cures for cancer, particularly over the past quarter century. To achieve a goal viewed by most as insurmountable just a decade ago, it is necessary to convey an understanding of the history of cancer and the evolution of our understanding of its dynamic interplay with the immune system. In doing so, we will meet the various personalities and weapons used to target elusive tumor cells and the accumulation of breakthrough science facilitating the rapid translation into lifesaving technologies that have begun to dramatically increase the quality and quantity of life for cancer patients, including many lifelong cures.

While dramatic improvements are being made by harnessing the immune system to target cancer, these are not without risk, and we will also touch upon some of the risks these new technologies entail. For many, the risks associated with immune therapies outweigh the benefits. As with the discovery of gunpowder, the airplane, or the power of the atom, understanding is vital to anticipating and preventing the potential for abuse and misuse.

In developing the story, I reach back into my own personal history, not because my own work was particularly impactful but because I happened to be in the right place at the right time to serve as a witness to many of the events described herein. It seems appropriate to fill in some of the gaps with my biography to allow the reader to assess whether I have any credibility in doing so.

I presently serve as an associate vice chancellor and professor at Washington University in St. Louis, a top-five medical school among whose specialties are immunology and cancer research. As we will see, Washington University has helped lead the fight to find new ways to recruit the body's immune system in the fight against cancer. In this context, I have been actively engaged in the science and application of cancer research and drug development.

Since earning a doctorate in immunology from the Duke University Medical Center, I have split my career equally between the biopharmaceutical industry and academia, most recently leading drug development at Yale University before joining Washington University in 2014. My responsibilities have included leadership in two of the world's leading biomedical research centers that share the responsibility of analyzing and supporting drug and vaccine research and development.

Prior to Yale, I lived in suburban Washington, D.C., amidst a thriving biotechnology community. My experiences there included helping to guide a medium-sized biotechnology company by the name of MedImmune into a large biotechnology juggernaut. As detailed above, I was tasked at Med-Immune with developing a team and a pipeline of products devoted to the eradication of cancer by targeting the body's immune defenses. I joined MedImmune in 2001 as a team of one. Within five years, we had built a team of more than forty scientists and a portfolio of twenty-one programs. These projects included an overview of the vaccines being deployed to eliminate cervical cancer from the world, as well as the development of cancer-specific smart bombs in the form of armed and unarmed monoclonal antibodies, all of which are profiled in this book.

Over the course of the past two decades, the arsenal of medicines available to treat cancer have improved dramatically. Prior to the development of immune-based therapies, patient care had been made possible for the first time with the introduction of chemotherapies using obnoxious substances. As a brief summary of this era, using the same words I used to teach cancer biology at the Purdue campus of the Indiana University School of Medicine, "the goal of cancer therapy is to kill the tumor just before you kill the patient."

These conventional therapies were sometimes effective but always legendarily brutal, often causing an increase in quantity of life only at the expense of a lowered quality of life. Following substantial progress in discovering new chemotherapies in the 1950s and 1960s, the discovery of breakthrough cancer therapies slowed for a time, before being reenergized by the introduction of new science and technologies. As we will see, the application of active immunity (i.e., vaccines) and passive immunity (mediated by antibodies derived from the laboratory rather than created in the body) foreshadowed a new and improved arsenal to be unleashed in the war against cancer.

Over time, a generation of scientists realized it might be possible not just to modify the proteins normally found in the body, such as antibodies, but also its cell-based host defense mechanisms. This realization was put into practice through the implementation of novel treatments, first performed only in the most sophisticated research hospitals in the world, but later made available to the masses through the introduction of equally impactful just-in-time technologies afforded by, among other innovative entities, Federal Express. By blending these past experiences with emerging genomic technologies, we now stand on the cusp of breakthroughs allowing even the most conservatives doctors and pragmatic patients to use the words "cancer" and "cured" in the same sentence and without a hint of irony.

As one example, we will highlight progress made in the treatment of metastatic melanoma. Only a few years ago, this diagnosis was widely and correctly presumed to be a death sentence. Equally tragic was the fact metastatic melanoma had been a focus of cancer researchers for decades. Despite all this investment, the disease had resisted virtually all attempts to cure it. As a sign of the dark humor of these challenging days, melanoma was described as the "black death of drug development," reflecting both the hallmark black skin lesions characteristic of the disease and the fate of the drugs challenging it.

Despite decades of countless failures by modern medicine to improve the prospects of patients with melanoma, the past decade abruptly witnessed a dramatic reversal. Melanoma therapies suddenly began to show promise and were approved by the FDA. Some of the outcomes can only be described as science-driven miracles. The treatment of the disease has changed radically within the past decade. A subset of patients may already have been cured of their disease and many more will happily agree to this prognosis. This brightening of their prospect can be summarized in a hyphenated word or two small letters: immuno-oncology or IO.

The advances against many tumor types have spurred many companies to entirely drop all other drug discovery activities and refocus their oncology efforts. One well-known major pharmaceutical company, Bristol-Myers Squibb, not only diverted all oncology research to this one focus but restructured the entire company to focus solely upon IO. This is a brave gamble as the entire future of some of the most storied companies in the world are now "all in," risking everything with hopes that IO will provide both health and economic opportunities for the future.

We will also discuss the potential limitations of IO, not just in terms of the business risks, but the health prospects of individual patients. While a subset of patients benefits extraordinarily from newly developed therapies, it is not yet clear if such successes can be extended to all. Consequently, it is also critical to discuss efforts to improve the breadth and depth of new IO therapies. In this light, I will highlight next-generation technologies with the potential to expand even further the impact of our understanding of the dynamic interplay between the body's immune system and cancer cells harbored within. We will also convey some risks uniquely associated with IO, including the potential, if not inevitability, that certain therapies may increase life expectancy but at the cost of acquired autoimmune disease. All medicines have side effects and IO-based therapies are no exception. Another inevitable discussion item when discussing drugs is cost and again, IO medicines are no exception. These new medicines are and will continue to be quite expensive in terms of their impact on the finite amount of fiscal resources available to insurance company. Thus, we can easily anticipate hard decisions will have to be made about who will receive such treatments and how they will get it.

With this in mind, a goal of *The End of the Beginning* is to couple the facts surrounding the history of immune oncology with the human stories of the people who have studied the disease and enabled a new generation of seemingly-miraculous medicines. The book also intends to convey the reality that the victory against cancer is not without risk—there are reflections of extraordinary sacrifices made by patients, who in many cases have contributed everything they have and are to help these technologies to succeed. I intend also to provide a forum not only to communicate past successes, but to describe how we might eliminate cancer from the repertoire of diseases we all confront. Finally, I also hope to convey the stories behind the development of astonishing new cancer treatments transforming the prognosis of individuals with diseases such as metastatic melanoma, a diagnosis which may have been a virtual death sentence a mere five years ago.

# 1

# *A Growing Concern*

We all have those moments, indelibly burned into our minds, which can be perfectly recalled and retained even years later. Beyond overtly historical moments, such as the assassination of a president or an aircraft careening into a skyscraper, there are individual flashes conveying a strong impression and shaping our lives. Yet, what may be significant to one of us is not always shared by others. I have had a handful of such experiences, and one occurred in the summer 1997, a year after beginning a career as a cancer researcher and professor at Purdue University.

I had been asked to participate in a workshop focused on the need to improve the study of prostate cancer. This first (and last) International Workshop on Animal Models of Prostate Cancer was hosted at my home institution over a two-day period during a sweltering week in mid-August 1997.[1] That time of year, known as the dog days of summer, was fitting given a focus of the workshop, which was to evaluate the strengths and limitations of our canine companions as a potential model to understand prostate cancer in people. For those squeamish souls (like myself), who are not terribly comfortable with the idea of injecting animals with carcinogens of malignant cells to cause disease, let me point out that the dog provides a great model of disease in part because it develops spontaneously, just as it does in people. The spontaneity means that the disease tends to be more diverse, unlike a chemical treatment, which provides consistent results. However, for those of us in favor of such diversity (since the disease is equally diverse in people), the dog provides a great model. This was the subject to be discussed during the conference.

My research emphasis up to this time had largely focused on breast cancer (which afflicts dogs at roughly the same rate as humans) but Purdue in general, and the veterinary school in particular, had cultivated an expertise in canine prostate cancer. A bit of trivia perhaps useful during a lull in cocktail party conversation is that the dog is the only nonhuman species that develops spontaneous (rather than chemically induced or genetically triggered) prostate cancer. The significance of that development was being cultivated at Purdue, which hosts one of the leading veterinary schools in the nation. My recruitment to Purdue was motivated in large part by the fact that prostate (and also breast) cancer in dogs shares many features with its disease counterpart in their human caregivers.

Another advantage of being a professor in a vet school was I was free to bring my own Labrador retriever, Baloo, to my office. She became widely known in our corridor as the "lab Lab" and unexpectedly became a participant when, like many orally fixated retrievers, she consumed an envelope containing a tube with a chunk of DNA (known as a *plasmid*) with the instructions to create a putative oncogene. Thankfully, she was fine, perhaps because the envelope had also contained a matched "anti-sense" plasmid, which would counteract the oncogene. I, on the other hand, had to explain to the sender why a new batch of material was being requested (and who was, thankfully, quite amused at the story and reminded me of it years later).

Baloo survived to the ripe old age of thirteen before expiring from natural causes (unrelated to the consumption of oncogenes or plastic) and her experience emphasizes the fact dogs have a shorter lifespan than most people (though the dog year conversion widely used is not quite accurate). Consequently, man's best friend develops diseases, such as breast or prostate cancer, within a comparatively short period (years rather than decades).

Dogs have also been subject to extensive inbreeding, which unintentionally has enriched the potential for certain genes betraying certain susceptibilities to disease. For example, Scottish terriers tend to develop bladder cancer and, perhaps most intriguingly, larger breeds tend to succumb to cancer (and other diseases) at a rate roughly proportional to their size (e.g., Great Danes rarely live to the age of eight whereas Malteses frequently survive twice as long). Such facts allow us to accelerate studies of cancer, both to understand the causes of disease as well as ways to treat or prevent it.

Another advantage is our canine companions either share the same diet as their masters (i.e., table scraps) or feast daily upon a highly defined diet. Either choice means the dog provides an extraordinary opportunity to control or monitor the impact of diet on the prevention or treatment of the disease. Further to what we discussed, the contrived laboratory models using transplanted cancer cells or animals subjected to intensive chemical or genetic manipulation, the disease in dogs is spontaneous and thus more natural. Lastly, many dog owners form very close bonds with their companions and are eager to participate in clinical trials while gladly sheltering their pets at home. These facts facilitate the accrual of volunteers to test new medicines and offset some of the considerable costs required for housing and monitoring the subjects.

Having arrived at Purdue only a year earlier, I was arguably as much an unknown to my intra-institutional colleagues as to the distinguished prostate cancer scientists visiting our Indiana campus from afar. Although determined to blend in and remain a wallflower during this conference, my anonymity was soon betrayed by a shock experienced during the opening presentation inaugurating the two-day workshop on that hot summer day in West Lafayette, Indiana.

Wael Sakr, a cancer pathologist and epidemiologist from Wayne State University in Detroit, was providing an overview on human prostate cancer and conveyed a summary of his life's work. Sakr had long been studying the incidence of prostate cancer using autopsy specimens from men who had had no history of prostate cancer or symptoms suggestive of the disease. Mostly, the cadavers had expired prematurely as a result of automobile accidents, violent crime, heart disease, or other reasons unrelated to cancer. Even in the youngest men in their twenties, an intensive microscopic analysis of the prostate revealed the presence of malignant and aggressive cancer cells.

This was not a rare event but quite common, being found in a quarter of all twenty-somethings. Sakr first recalled information from a paper he had published in 1993.[2] He then related the preliminary findings of an ongoing study that suggested that by the time a man reached the age of sixty, the presence of at least one outcropping of aggressive prostate cancer was a virtual certainty.

Most others in the room, who were more well-read than I in the epidemiology of prostate cancer, barely acknowledged this statement, lazily nodding their awareness, presumably sparing their energies for the long, hot day ahead of us. In striking contrast, I was subject to an entirely involuntary response, causing me to bolt from my chair, which was thankfully located in the back of the room. Undoubtedly, a component of this overreaction reflected selfish recognition that, but for an unlucky flip or two of fate's coin, I may already be afflicted with prostate cancer as a thirty-year-old scientist. I had felt invulnerable moments before, but this all quickly changed. However, most of what I felt was based on the immediate implications for defining a disease I thought I had understood an instant before.

Returning to my office after the conclusion of the day's proceedings, I made a beeline to the nearby medical library to find the details of the Detroit study (the Internet was still rather crude, and Google would not be founded for another two years). In the hours since hearing the Sakr's talk, I had convinced myself I must have misunderstood the points from the eventful early-morning seminar.

As a few years had passed since the first publication of Sakr's studies, there had been ample time for other investigators to reproduce his work, a hallmark of responsible science. These follow-on studies confirmed the overall magnitude of Sakr's autopsy study, albeit with a few caveats. As the study had been conducted in Detroit, there was a disproportionately high representation of African American men, a population known to be more susceptible to the disease.[3] Even adjusting for this, the basic facts presented by Sakr had stood the test of time and intensive scrutiny.

Looking further back in time as the evening progressed in the library, I managed to locate a scientific journal article first published in May 1934 and reprinted in 1979.[4] This study had been conducted by a Dr. Arnold Rice Rich, a urologist from Johns Hopkins University. Like the Detroit team, the Hopkins researchers had evaluated the prostates of male cadavers, though their subjects had been at least fifty years old. Despite the fact none had reported manifestations of prostate cancer, almost two-thirds of these asymptomatic men nonetheless harbored a metastatic form of the disease. A comparable study performed in the late 1970s by a team of New Orleans pathologists confirmed this study and explained why the 1934 study had been reprinted.[5] A point presciently made in a 2007 review of the subject quoted Ecclesiastes 1:9, "What has been will be again, what has been done will be done again; there is nothing new under the sun."[6] The takeaway for me remained prescient: The evidence is surprisingly old for an elderly man's disease being common in young men.

Part of the shocking personal revelation of that moment, in 1997, was a set of fundamental questions almost bordering on the philosophic: If the presence of malignant cells in an otherwise healthy person is common, might this change our view of prostate cancer? Should an indication be classified as a disease if there are no symptoms and if any morbidity or mortality might never arise, or if the symptoms do eventually arise, they will only have a clinical impact a half century later? A corollary is if most or all men have metastatic cells in their prostate (and likely cells have metastasized beyond) and yet are asymptomatic and died of other causes, should they be subjected to cancer therapy, which is often a grueling experience harkening additional problems?

From an even more fundamental perspective, what is cancer in the first place? Whereas I had awoken in the morning with extraordinary hubris I was something approaching an expert in my chosen field, I went to bed appreciating my extraordinary ignorance and yet was full of wonder. The feelings of wonder and ignorance persist to this day.

*Growth, Survival & Other Misconceptions*

The human body is a collection of something like 37 trillion cells, not counting at least as many bacterial cells that, together with human cells, comprise a "super-organism": you or me.[7] Each human cell has a distinct purpose and location. Thinking anthropomorphically, one can regard this as a cellular vocation and zip code. For example, many nerve cells remain alive for decades, carrying out the function of conveying sensory information to and from the brain and yet never move. At the opposite end of the spectrum, red blood cells (known as *erythrocytes*) may remain viable for a mere few weeks during which time they cruise all throughout the body, tens of thousands of times over again, faithfully carrying out their role of delivering oxygen to tissues. These wildly different vocations, zip codes, and life spans nonetheless all arose from instructions encoded within a single egg fertilized years before. Moreover, the extraordinary diversity represented by all the individualized vocations and locations of all 37 trillion cells must dance in tandem in an intensively complex minuet to assure that the collective (perhaps more appropriately referred to as a *cell*ective), does its part to contribute to the overall health of the organism. Quoting the late astronomer Carl Sagan (who perished from the complications of cancer), "We are, each of us, a multitude. Within us is a little universe."[8]

Given the enormous number of cells working together, it is perhaps unremarkable that from time to time some "go rogue" and cause a constellation of diseases we have imperfectly lumped into a category known as *cancer*. This catchall term is rather deceiving as cancer is an immensely multifarious disease in which not only are all cancer patients unique, but a given tumor cell can differ greatly from its benign cousins and even from other brother and sister tumor cells residing nearby. These changes reflect a hyperaccelerated form of evolution and result from extreme rates of mutation of our fundamental genetic material, DNA. A rare commonality linking virtually all cancer cells is an extreme rate of DNA mutation, both subtle (small, point changes in one gene) and catastrophic (such as the duplication or deletion of entire chromosomes containing thousands of genes). Collectively, these mutations modify the behavior of tumor cells, altering their ability to grow, survive, and move around the body.

A widely held misconception, even amongst scientists, is that cancer is a disease of accelerated cell growth. This conventional view presumes malignant cells grow faster than their normal counterparts and the resulting imbalance eventually causes the number of cells to build up and grow into a tumor, a vibrant and violent structure full of rapidly growing cells. That view further supposes a tumor continues its relentless expansion until its large size hijacks the body's nutrients, breaches the functioning of a vital organ (e.g., a lung tumor choking off the supply of oxygen), and/or sprouts metastases that travel all throughout the body, irreversibly wreaking havoc from a distance. This view is not entirely accurate.

Even fundamental words used to describe cancer are often misused. A tumor can be a generic term simply meaning an abnormal mass of cells. While we instinctively relate tumors to cancer, other physiological events can cause a large number of cells to be drawn into a specific location, where they can grow and swell into a mass generically known as a *tumor*. These particular tumors are not indicative of cancer but rather arise in response to an infection, allergens, and other comparatively minor misfiring events within the body. Consequently, the term *tumor* is used by some scientists and physicians to represent a mass *not* associated with inflammation, but others lump pretty much all lumps into the definition *tumor*. I had lazily fallen into the latter category until jolted by a personal experience.

The *tumor* nomenclature evokes a personal reminiscence from the autumn of my junior year in college at The Ohio State University. One Saturday morning, I awoke with a soreness under my armpit accompanied by a discernable lump. By late morning, the lump had swollen to the size of a grape and by early afternoon, what had begun as an oddity had evolved into a walnut-sized and painful mass that immobilized my left arm, eventually fating me to a visit to the student health center (and on a game day nonetheless). The physicians in many student health centers, even prestigious schools with large medical centers, tend toward either extreme in their career development path, usually being nearer the beginning or the end of their vocation than the middle. In this case, it was the latter and he outright declared the mass to be a *tumor*. He then handed me a sheath of papers and told me to walk across the soccer fields to the hospital emergency room. By the time of my arrival, it was a Saturday night and the ER was mostly packed with patients with high blood alcohol levels requiring rehydration and the rebalancing of their electrolytes.*

Perhaps due to the oddity of my situation (being sober), the triage nurse gave me a high priority and I soon found myself surrounded by five residents

---

* One drunken patient, who happened to be a friend from my freshman year, had lost his footing and slid from the top of Ohio Stadium to the bottom deck, which must have been a few hundred steps, sustaining severe bruising on his backside and bouncing his head off a few too many steps; he would remain in the hospital for monitoring of a possible concussion but more so because of his blood alcohol level. For those worried about his fate, he would fully recover, except for lasting damage to his reputation and dignity.

and medical students, each offering their own opinion about the mass under my arm and mostly invoking nefarious Latin-sounding terms. Rather than being flattered by all the attention, the monitoring devices revealed my blood pressure had become quite elevated. Seeing the fear in my eyes and the hypertension as reflected by my vital signs, a senior attending physician breezily walked in and, with a wave of the hand, dismissed the gaggle of junior doctors. He began his examination.

After a brief recounting of the sudden appearance of the tumor, the doctor questioned me about, of all things, my hygienic habits. He had a particular interest in my preference for deodorants, which seemed rather odd. He later returned with a large needle containing a powerful steroid. I was told the swelling should subside within twenty-four hours and was informed to regularly switch deodorants because, it turns out, the body can become sensitized to repetitive use of the same product and cause the lymph nodes near the armpit to become swollen with immune cells seeking combat with a nonexistent intruder. Relieved by a sudden reversal of my prognosis, my blood pressure returned to normal for a bit.

The relief was short-lived because the physician then told me that if the mass persisted or returned within the next week, I was to call the number on a piece of paper he handed me. In a manner meant to comfort me (but causing the opposite reaction), he assured I would be given a high priority to be diagnosed (and treated) for the potential presence of a lymphoma. Thankfully, the combination of steroids and a new deodorant was sufficient, though the week witnessed a remarkable change in the progression of time as the period until "all-clear" dragged on for what seemed like decades. Nonetheless, all's well that ends well and the experience ingrained the importance of avoiding flippancy in the use of medical terms, such as *tumor,* and the earnestness such words can impart.

Returning to cancerous tumors, it may surprise many to know most of a tumor mass is composed of dead cells and debris. Often the growth of malignant cells radiates outward and the inner cells succumb "naturally," being outcompeted for nutrients or oxygen by more vigorous, neighboring tumor cells. However, this outward growth is accompanied by a progressively more stringent Darwinian process driven by DNA mutations and the selecting of cells with the ability to thrive under increasingly harsh conditions. These events set the scene for future problems (and a reason why early diagnosis of cancer has been shown to prolong life more than virtually any other technology offered by modern medicine).

Perhaps most surprising is the fact malignant cells often grow no faster than their benign counterparts (I tend to prefer *benign* to *normal* since a proper definition of the latter is ambiguous). In some cases, the deadliest cancer cells grow more slowly.˙ The rate of growth, defined as the time required for a cell to divide into two, generally tends not to be the problem. Instead, it is more accurate to think of cancer as a disease of "inappropriate" growth. In the life of a typical cell, it faces many decisions ranging from what molecules it needs to eat (or avoid), its diligence in performing "housekeeping" chores (including repairing mutations to its DNA), and whether or not to remain a contributing member of the cellective to ensure the larger organism remains happy and healthy. These decisions entail an immensely complex series of safeguards devised to ensure each of the 37 trillion or so well-behaved citizens of the cellective are organized into a structured and well-behaving mosaic.

The myriad diseases we refer to as *cancer* might begin when any one of a trillion-plus cells forgets or ignores an instruction not to divide. The resulting division may not occur any faster than a benign cell but the instruction forbidding the cell to divide is simply ignored. This is a quite audacious action because an array of safeguards exists to prevent such whimsical decisions. For example, each cell is governed by a series of regulatory checkpoints that govern crucial life and death decisions. These checks were so-named to reflect their similarity to the checkpoint controls separating nations or protecting citizens from potential harm. In the case of the decision to grow, a gauntlet of "cell cycle checkpoints" must be overcome to assure it divides only when appropriate. These same checkpoints must retain considerable flexibility as, for example, a skin cell might suddenly need to regain the ability to divide to fill in the void created by something as minor as a papercut or severe as an amputation. Under such conditions, the body reacts by loosening or abrogating the checkpoints for a time and

---

\*     Although not a focus of this book, a subset of so-called cancer stem cells is a slow-growing fountain spawning more aggressive progeny. Due to its slow growth, these cells have proven particularly able to avoid many conventional chemotherapeutic regimens, which exploit faster-growing cancer cells.

even accelerating the process through the production of an array of substances known as *growth factors* to induce nearby cells to begin the process of wound healing. An overuse of such growth-encouraging mechanisms may explain why chronic cellular damage caused by chronic gastric reflux may increase one's susceptibility to local malignancies, such as esophageal cancers. For the most part, however, these checkpoints can prove as lethal as the famous Checkpoint Charlie in West Berlin manned by stern-faced guards toting automatic rifles. If a cell attempts to run the checkpoint and elects a decision to divide inappropriately, it is normally marked for death.

How then does a cancer cell run the checkpoint? As we have seen, the checkpoints must have some flexibility to facilitate wound repair. Random mutations acquired over the course of living one's life may arise and provide a type of pass allowing the cell to continue through the checkpoints. Sometimes, these mutations are unavoidable and arise from random chance. More often, they are triggered by intrinsic or extrinsic factors that increase the likelihood of mutation, such as chemicals, radiation, or certain genetic predispositions.

The collection of diseases known as *cancer* can also reflect choices by a cell not to perform its regular housekeeping chores, which can include tidying up mutant genetic material. By design, if genetic damage is sensed, a cell has the capacity to correct it. If the damage is sufficiently severe, then the cell is programmed to initiate a form of self-destruction. Some mutations may short-circuit these DNA repair mechanisms or self-immolation instructions and instead allow a miscreant to continue living and growing when it otherwise should not. Over time, such mutations can accumulate and impel even worse behavior, resulting in poor decision-making at an ever-higher frequency. To put this in perspective, the accumulation of these events generally takes place over years or decades before any symptom of disease is realized. However, increased exposure to environmental damage (e.g., carcinogens, certain types of radiation, or just plain old bad luck) can increase the rate of these mutations and the manifestation of disease.

Let's consider an example of how a few bad decisions can cause well-behaved cells to become a lethal menace. For this illustration, we will profile a typical keratinocyte, a major cellular component of the skin. Keratinocytes work together in a happy collective through a network of interactions with neighboring cells and the factors they all secrete, forming the thin and resilient surfaces of the skin known as the *epidermis*. Altogether, these interacting cells provide a surprisingly tight barrier (tight enough even to discourage the passage of individual protons). This helps retain the integrity of cells and higher order structures while providing protection from a harsh outside world replete with many fungi, bacteria, and viruses that would like nothing more than to gain access to the nutrient-rich interior of our bodies. To do so, keratinocytes invest much of their allotted energy and nutrients into forming a strong and tight latticework with one another and performing housekeeping functions, such as manufacturing a set of proteins known as *cytokeratins*, which help seal any holes in the barrier protecting our relatively sterile internal organs from a considerably less hygienic world outside the body. In particular, cytokeratins provide structural support to the skin cells and help organize keratinocytes to interact with one another and with other cellular components of the body to maintain harmony.

Interspersed within this cellular sheet of keratinocytes are occasional neighbors, such as fibroblasts, a distinct cell type that manufactures and exports a variety of nonliving proteins, such as collagens. Indeed, collagens (such as those that are in our fingernails) represent roughly one-fifth of all the protein in your body.[9] These collagen molecules interact with one another and with other proteins and cells to reinforce the intricate lattice outside the epidermal cells, known as an *extracellular matrix*, which provides further protection to the barrier between the inside and outside of the body. This matrix also provides a type of bumper, protecting the body from blunt-force trauma when cells crash into one another and objects during life. From the perspective of the skin cells on the hands, as one example, the simple act of clapping is an act of brutality, unleashing potentially destructive forces that could be apocalyptic were the networks of keratinocytes and fibroblasts not present nor their housekeeping functions performed with considerable rigor.

What I haven't revealed up to this point is our keratinocytes are terminally differentiated cells. The wording suggests an awful fate and to some degree, this is accurate. The skin is a surprisingly dynamic place stacked with many layers of keratinocytes (like bricks in a wall) pushed upward toward the outside world as newer cells grow beneath them. This constant replenishment is necessary given the harshness of the outside environment full of chemical and biological attacks, and a layer of dead outer skin is part of the barrier keeping the most obnoxious chemicals and organisms out. Consequently, these bricks are replenished by so-called stem cells at the basal skin surface (the lowermost layers of the skin continue to grow for the life of the organism). However, the cells pushed upward do not invest their energies into growth but instead into the production of the collagens, keratins, and other molecules comprising most of the structure of the epidermis through a process known as *terminal differentiation*. These cells remain irreversibly committed to the production of keratins for the rest of their small cellular lives, which average less than two months.

The instructions these cells receive precludes further growth (cell division) and instead, all the energies of the cell are devoted to producing protein and clinging to their neighbors as a means of keeping the outside world at bay. However, as the cells move upward toward the outside world, they encounter more environmental toxins and radioactive dangers from ultraviolet light. Occasionally, these attacks tweak the DNA and can compromise the instructions for terminal differentiation and allow a cell to regain an ability to grow inappropriately.

Beyond the constant chemical and radioactive barrage, an insidious group of microbial pathogens, known as *papillomaviruses*, can hijack our keratinocyte and rewire its control mechanisms to reinstate its ability to proliferate. From the perspective of the virus, a sudden increase in cells is beneficial because it provides more and more food and factories to produce even more virus. Eventually, this outgrowth becomes apparent through the formation of warts, which are not the result of touching frogs but rather a manifestation of a benign viral-induced tumor. These tumors rarely become more than a nuisance as they largely lack the ability to metastasize to other sites in the body and are easily removed by skin exfoliating agents, such as salicylic acid (a chemical cousin of aspirin and the active ingredient in over-the-counter medicines like Compound-W and various exfoliating washes). However, as we will see in chapter 4, papillomavirus infection of other epidermal tissues can be quite deadly.

### In the Autumn of Life

In what may come as another surprise, life is not the default setting for the cells in our body. Rather, each moment a cell remains alive is an active decision and death, or more accurately, intentional suicide, is the understood default. Stated another way: Life only persists if death is actively avoided. Such conclusions have only become clear in the past few years though the earliest foundations for this idea are almost a century old. In October 1934, the Australian pathologist John Foxton Ross Kerr published an article detailing a microscopic study of rat livers, or more accurately, the death of cells in rat livers.[10] Up to this time, life had been assumed to be the norm, and death the exception. Kerr was interested in cell death and his contemporaries had supposed that death in the microscopic world, like its macroscopic counterpart, was a dramatic event caused primarily by traumatic events. Indeed, early microscopic studies of cell death had portrayed cell death in terms of easily relatable events, such as the dramatic rupture of the cell membrane and the spewing of cell contents into the surrounding environment. This process had been widely known as *necrosis*, the Greek term for "death."

In his Autumn 1934 study, Kerr reported a very different and new type of death. Rather than the unsightly ruptures characteristic of exploding cells, he described something more akin to an implosion: The DNA-containing nucleus of dying cells would first begin to break apart and this presaged a subsequent shrinking of the cells prior to a dissolution of the cell into small pieces. Given the time of year the study was published, the name given to this process seems particularly appropriate: *apoptosis*, a Greek term meaning "falling off." Prior to its invocation by Kerr, the primary use of the term apoptosis had been reserved to describe the characteristic process by which trees shed their leaves during the autumn months.[11] Such differences between trauma-induced death by necrosis and apoptotic suicide might seem trivial to the uninitiated (after all, dead is dead), yet their implications would prove profound for our understanding of how cancer arises and how it might ultimately be defeated.

Over the half century following Kerr's discovery of apoptosis, understanding slowly accumulated about the causes and effects distinguishing apoptosis from necrosis, revealing the former to be a conscious form of suicide at the cellular level.[12] [13] Eventually, we came to understand the decision to commit suicide predominates unless prevented from doing so. It is as if each cell in the body must constantly be instructed to "stay alive, stay alive, stay alive . . ." A simple delay in this constant "stay alive" mantra may be sufficient to initiate a cascade of events culminating in intentional death. In addition, active suicide signals may be invoked under particularly noxious circumstances where elimination is good for the collective. For example, the persistence of cells infected with a virus or subjected to harsh environmental conditions might induce physical or genetic damage harmful to the larger organism.

One set of apoptosis-inducing triggers arises if a cell inappropriately circumvents the cell cycle checkpoints described above. Thus, the only way a terminally differentiated cell can grow is to override both safeguards: cell cycle checkpoints and apoptosis. The need to overcome both processes means malignant cells usually must harbor multiple and distinct mutations or invoke other tricks allowing it both to divide and to continue the "stay alive" signal. Although a tall order, experience teaches us the ability to overcome these safeguards is not foolproof. For example, the commonality of warts reflects the fact that papillomaviruses have evolved to convey machinery to promote both the "grow" and "stay alive" instructions, even in terminally differentiated cells.

Papillomavirus-associated warts are the canonical example of a benign tumor because they lack the ability to spread. The virus may spread to cause other warts, but the tumor cells themselves remain immobile and incapable of metastatic spread. A very different situation can occur with cancer-inducing transformations that facilitate movement. The migration of a cell away from the primary tumor is a complex process involving the ability to move, coupled with an ability to slice through the cells and tissues as it progresses. These feats are accomplished by reactivating the same "normal" motility behaviors that are usually reserved for use only during wound healing. For a cell to become truly metastatic, it must overcome yet another problem that is inherently not a "normal" process.

In detailing the microenvironment of the skin, we compared keratinocytes with bricks in a wall. Extending this analogy, the mortar between layers of cells is known as the *extracellular matrix*, and this material provides the chemical cues to define the aforementioned "zip code," instructing cells as to their proper location in the body. If a benign cell is suddenly uprooted and moved to a foreign site in the body, it senses a different zip code and this is generally sufficient to trigger a special type of apoptosis. This distinct form of suicide is known as *anoikis*,[14] a Greek term meaning "homelessness." This name accurately reflects the fact anoikis is triggered by the recognition that a cell has been displaced from its normal surroundings—the homelessness conveys an instruction to self-destruct.

Putting all of this together, metastatic cancer is the outcome of coordinated cellular defects. A malignant cell must be able to circumvent checkpoint controls hindering its growth and to survive the suicide signals arising when it inappropriately does so. In addition, a metastatic cell must gain the ability to move and to literally eat through the surrounding tissues in order to move to distant sites in the body. Once ensconced in its new environment, it must be able to survive and thrive within a foreign environment intent upon its destruction (via anoikis).

All these hurdles suggest a spontaneous outbreak of cancer should be exceedingly rare. The first clue this supposition is inaccurate can be found in the widespread prevalence of cancer in humans (and dogs and other species), suggesting this Houdini-like ability to migrate, invade, and survive anoikis is surprisingly routine. All this was going through my inexperienced mind with an electric shock that summer day in 1997 when I happened upon learning about the extraordinary ubiquity of metastatic prostate cancer. However, I was yet to realize the depth of my naïveté, for as we will soon see, cancer likely is not a disease arising once or perhaps twice in an unlucky few, but may literally be a daily occurrence for most if not all of us.

### A View to a Killer

Despite its prevalence, cancer remains a largely misunderstood disease. Many members of our species tend to fear what they do not understand and perhaps unsurprisingly, such views have led to a stigmatization of cancer and those afflicted with the disease. As recently as 1961, nine of ten American physicians interviewed revealed they did not inform a patient of a cancer diagnosis, in part because of the social stigma associated with the disease.[15] Although the rationale given was this might induce the patient to commit suicide, there was no evidence supporting this idea and even after such notions had been dispelled, many physicians continued to decline full disclosure, citing futility and pessimism arising from patient knowledge would negatively impact their lives or treatment. Indeed, the 1970 novel and romantic drama film, *Love Story*, was premised on such a storyline and despite being ranked by the American Film Institute as the ninth greatest tragedy ever produced, viewed by modern eyes the film seems outdated and borders on the ridiculous.

The stigma surrounding individuals with cancer is not unique to the United States and a 2007 study published by the cancer patient advocacy group LiveStrong revealed more than half of those polled in China and India agreed with the statement "people with cancer brought it on themselves."[16] Given such attitudes, it is unsurprising that proven actions, such as early screening and treatment, are not available or embraced in many parts of the world.

Thankfully, in the United States at least, such misconceptions are improving, or so many would like to believe. Nonetheless, a 2010 survey revealed 70% of Americans blamed lung cancer patients for their disease and this judgment was applied even to cancer patients who had never smoked. Indeed, the disdain felt for lung cancer patients now approaches the levels historically seen with sexually transmitted diseases and obesity.[17] Such feelings were not unique to cigarette-associated diseases as more than one third of respondents cited patient fault for the outbreak of cervical cancer (even for respondents unaware it is a sexually transmitted disease) and almost one-quarter of those polled felt patients were responsible for their bowel cancers. This compares with 9% and 15% of people who felt patients were responsible for their leukemia or breast cancers, respectively. Such findings are consistent with a psychological behavior known as the *Just World Hypothesis*, which allows some people to justify poor outcomes as a type of karma.[18]

Part of the cancer blame game may have roots in an old idea that infectious agents can cause cancers. Such knowledge has triggered a widespread perception in some communities that cancer is contagious. For example, the same LiveStrong study also reported almost a third of Mexican and Indian respondents agreed with the statement, "I worry about catching cancer from other people, who have it."[19] To get at the roots of such concerns, some of which are not founded wholly upon ignorance, it is important to provide historical context to reveal how the idea of cancer as an infectious disease entered our psyche.

*Spreading Like a Virus*

Vilhelm Ellerman was a Danish pathologist, born on December 28, 1871, in Copenhagen, where he remained for most of his life, with the exceptions of training in anatomy and pathology at the University of Heidelberg, and in Berlin and Paris.[20] Upon returning to Denmark, Ellerman served as a professor at the University of Copenhagen and took an interest in discovering new bacteria responsible for diseases in humans and animals. In the months after he married Agnes Louise Frederikke Hansen in May 1903, Ellerman published a series of reports detailing the discovery of bacteria responsible for gangrene and tuberculosis.

This notoriety gained the attention of a contemporary, Dr. Olaf Bang,* a veterinarian and professor at the Royal Agricultural and Veterinary College of Copenhagen. Bang shared Ellerman's desire to discover new bacterial causes of disease, and in 1908, the pair set out to understand the cause of a cancer in chickens with an infectious source. They focused on chicken leukosis, a form of cancer characterized by the spread of tumors throughout the liver and lymphoid tissues, usually occurring in chickens older than three or four months.

Suspecting a bacterial cause, the pair of researchers first showed they could isolate these tumors and use material obtained from biopsies of the tumor to infect otherwise healthy birds. These chickens sprouted new tumors within weeks. Convinced the culprit responsible for the outgrowths was a bacterium, Bang and Ellerman were then determined to identify the pathogen responsible for the disease and deployed a still rather new instrument to help them do so. In 1884, Charles Chamberland of the Pasteur Institute had invented a filter with pores so small they could trap and isolate even the smallest bacterial cells. Despite many attempts, Bang and Ellerman's use of the filtering technique repeatedly failed to isolate any cancer-causing bacteria. It was as if the causative agent had slipped through their net, which in fact it had.

Bang did not follow up on this finding, as his primary interest was in discovering new bacteria, so a nonbacterial cause of this disease did not satiate his interests. This would, in retrospect, be most unfortunate as it cost him a Nobel Prize. Ellerman, however, did continue to explore these findings.[21] Ellerman came to realize the pathogen responsible for causing the avian cancers was so small it had passed through the filter. Indeed, the

---

\* Not to be confused with Bang and Olufsen, a popular manufacturer of high-end sound equipment.

bacteria-free liquid filtered from their earlier experiments was sufficient to cause tumors when injected into birds. This mysterious agent was what we now know to be a virus.

Sadly, Ellerman would himself be denied the Nobel Prize for his discoveries despite the fact that he went on to discover both the virus responsible for the chicken leucosis as well as other leukemia-causing viruses. The reason for being overlooked was not (as is too often the case) a situation involving politics or personal animosities, but a requirement that a Nobel Prize recipient be alive at the time the award is announced. Despite being in the prime of his life, Ellerman could not meet this most basic criterion.

In a bizarre irony given his penchant for studying bacteria, a 53-year-old Ellerman, now a senior pathologist at Bispebjerg Hospital in Stockholm, was fastidiously attending to his personal hygiene on the morning of December 18, 1924. As he did every morning, Ellerman shaved, but nicked himself slightly, eliciting a minor blood droplet. Though seemingly trivial, the incident disrupted the integrity of the keratinocytes in his skin, providing a tempting route for some of the more obnoxious bacteria on his skin to gain access to the nutrient-dense environment they so craved below.[22] Two days later, Ellerman checked himself into his own hospital, suffering from severe inflammation on his cheek. The bacteria had not only invaded the soft flesh of his cheek but had swum upstream against the small droplet of blood flowing from a nicked capillary and used this path to gain access to his blood stream. The infection progressed and triggered a condition known as *septic shock*, in which the presence of bacteria in the bloodstream induces an overly vigorous immune response, a cytokine storm, which is often more lethal than anything caused by the bacterium itself. Ellerman's health quickly deteriorated and he died on Christmas Eve, six days after his seemingly trivial shaving accident.

Although a bit of distraction upon our focus on oncology, the anecdote nonetheless is worth expansion based on the long-forgotten controversy it triggered. Upon autopsy, it was revealed Ellerman had died from cutaneous anthrax. A subsequent follow-up revealed his shaving brush was contaminated with spores from the deadly bacterium commonly found in soil, and the occasional weapon of choice for budding terrorists.

The primary source of material used to manufacture shaving brushes prior to the First World War was badger hair. It seems the fur from the aggressive little omnivore had just the right consistency and density needed to distribute shaving lotions on the face. Most badger hairs came from central Europe (indeed the dachshund breed of dog was bred specifically to hunt badgers—the literal translation of *dachshund* from German means "badger dog"). However, the involvement of the German Empire in the Great War disrupted the lucrative trade in badger hair, even with Ellerman's homeland of Sweden, which remained neutral throughout the war and otherwise tended to side with Germany. Lower quality brushes used horsehair but again, the Great War intervened, as horses were a hot commodity during the war in Europe. Consequently, horsehair from Japan provided the source of the shaving brush used by Ellerman that fateful morning.

Although the Japanese have a reputation as fastidious germaphobes, the horsehair brushes manufactured in that country tended to be of lower quality, and some manufacturers scrimped on the procedures used to disinfect the hair prior to its use. This sterilization procedure usually entailed a combination of steam and embalming fluid but was often bypassed given the extraordinary demand for shaving brushes in Europe and North America. Usually a rare disease limited to farmers or ranchers, the anthrax-causing bacillus has a particular proclivity for horsehair.

Waves of anthrax from improperly sterilized shaving brushes exploded in cities and military installations as far afield as New York, Dublin, and, of course, Stockholm, beginning just months after the first blasts of the Guns of August in 1914.[23] The brush purchased by Ellerman in the autumn of 1924 had been manufactured from cheap horsehair riven with anthrax spores. Given its high-profile victim, this death racked the medical community all throughout Europe and North America, triggering a bit of a panic as doctors recommended to one another, their patients, and local barbers to immediately discontinue the use of shaving brushes.[24] Indeed, this incident later inspired the 1925 invention of Burma-Shave, a less dense form of shaving cream that did not require the use of a shaving brush and which remains the current mainstay of shaving hygiene.[25]

Returning to the infectious links with cancer, at the same time Bang and Ellerman were conducting their landmark study on chickens, a young Maryland medical student was graduating a year behind his classmates from Johns Hopkins University. The reason for his tardiness was not any underlying ineptitude but because of an accident reminiscent of the infection that felled Ellerman. Peyton Rous had been working on a cadaver in anatomy class during his second year at Johns Hopkins. During a lung dissection, the student cut his finger on the bone of the cadaver. Unfortunately for Rous, the cadaver had died of tuberculosis and the deadly pathogen had acquired a new victim.[26][27] The infection of the young doctor-to-be quickly evolved into axillary tuberculosis, a rare affliction in which the infection localizes to the lymph nodes of the upper arm and shoulder (similar to, but magnitudes worse than the lymph node swelling I had experienced in college). In Rous's case, the lymph node swelling likely saved his life because the localization of the disease to the lymph nodes prevented the deadly bacterium from gaining access to his lungs. Nonetheless Rous probably did not appreciate that fact as presciently as us since the next few months were filled with agonizing pain. This considerable discomfort was a symptom of an internal war between his host defense mechanisms and the bacterium, causing, among other symptoms, a massive increase in the number of lymphocytes (a type of white blood cell we will meet in chapter 2), which tended to congregate within the massively swollen lymph nodes of his arm pits and chest. Despite the agonizing and prolonged pain betraying the combat between his body's host defenses and the invading tuberculosis bacillus, Rous was not able to overcome the infection on his own. He was therefore forced to undergo an even more excruciating surgical procedure to remove a nest of infected and swollen lymph nodes. The young Rous was sent home for a year to recuperate, where he later served as a ranch hand in his mother's home state of Texas.

By autumn, Peyton Rous had recovered enough energy to return to medical school and finish his studies. He had hoped to start a research career and was particularly interested in learning more about the very same lymphocytes that had recently been the source of his great suffering. After a stint to learn more about the field of pathology, Rous took a side trip to the Friedrichstadt Municipal Hospital in Dresden, Germany, to become a specialist in autopsies (clearly bucking the cliché of "once bitten, twice shy"). Given his aptitude and experiences at such a young age, Rous was recruited to New York City in 1909 by an emerging medical researcher by the name of Simon Flexner.[28]

Though not a commonly known name today, Flexner was a superstar in the early years of the 20th century and would go on to become one of the most influential scientists of the time. Simon Flexner was born into a family of Bohemian immigrants in 1863 in Louisville, Kentucky, a neutral border state torn asunder by the Civil War. As is often the case with the children of immigrants, his family emphasized the value of an education and Flexner trained as a pharmacist and opened a practice in Louisville. All the while he was dispensing medicines, Flexner aspired to writing the prescriptions and worked toward a medical degree from Louisville Medical College.[29] After additional training at Johns Hopkins (where he overlapped with Rous, who was still an undergraduate at Johns Hopkins, though there is no record the two met), Flexner was recruited first to the University of Pennsylvania and soon thereafter to lead the Rockefeller Institute. Flexner's interests varied widely and included organ transplantation, infectious diseases, and cancer, a combination that would serve Rous well in later years.

Two years before recruiting Rous, Flexner had strongly advocated for scientists and doctors to explore the potential offered by transplanting key organs and tissues from a donor (either living or a cadaver) into a needy recipient, thus launching an entire field, which has become almost commonplace today (more than 30,000 organ transplants are conducted in the United States each year). During Flexner's time, this was an audacious proposal and required a greater understanding of autopsies (for organ procurement) and the causes of tissue rejection (in effect, giving birth to the science of immunology, which was just beginning to crystalize in the early 20th century). Although his preference was to perform the work himself, Flexner had also been appointed as the first head of the Rockefeller Institute, a newly endowed institution that would go on to become arguably the world's most prestigious research institution. An increasing administrative burden meant he needed to pull back from his own personal research and hence, Flexner hired Peyton Rous in 1909 to lead his laboratory at Rockefeller.

Rous was soon at work. On the first day of October 1909, a colleague brought a pet chicken to work. While this would hardly seem an appropriate action in most vocations, the light-colored, barred Plymouth Hen was sporting an irregular-shaped tumor projecting from her right breast.[30 31] The chicken was promptly anesthetized and the tumor removed and dissected. Sadly for avian aficionados, the operation was only a partial success and the chicken had to be euthanized on November 4. However, the sacrifice was not in vain, as Rous had determined the tumor was a sarcoma (a cancer of connective tissue cells, such as fibroblasts) and recalled the study published a year before by Bang and Ellerman. To ask whether the disease in this bird was infectious, Rous inoculated a set of healthy hens, who proceeded to develop tumors as well. What distinguished Rous from Bang and Ellerman was the successful isolation of the tumor-causing virus, a pathogen now known as *Rous sarcoma virus,* or RSV. [*][32]

Having established an incontrovertible link between viruses and cancers in chickens, Rous turned his attention to mice (the mainstay of experimental cancer research) to find out if a virus might also be linked with tumors in mammals, but these efforts proved far more challenging. Despite its potential impact, his work was also largely ignored by contemporaries and Rous gave up the whole enterprise of trying to link cancer and viruses in 1915. Thus began an almost two-decade hiatus away from oncology until in the middle years of the Great Depression, when Dr. Richard Shope, also of the Rockefeller Institute, reignited the connection between viruses and cancer. [33] That story will be profiled in chapter 4, but it suffices for now to state Shope's later studies allowed Rous to share the 1966 Nobel Prize in Physiology or Medicine, largely for his work on the chicken brought to the lab. An unintended consequence of Rous's pioneering work was it left a lingering fear in the minds of many of cancer as an infectious and contagious disease. This notion remains prevalent today, even though this is applicable only to a very small number of cancers, most of which can now be prevented with routine childhood vaccines.

## Cancer & Evolution

X-ray analyses of Egyptian mummies have revealed some of the earliest indications of cancer, suggesting the disease is at least as old as civilization. As indicated in the introduction to this book, the disease is actually far older than our species, *Homo sapiens,* which evolved from its forefathers, *Homo erectus,* a mere 200,000 years ago. Indeed, a 2016 medical imaging study

---

[*]    This cancer-causing chicken virus should not be confused with respiratory syncytial virus, also known as RSV, which causes a respiratory infection in humans and is particularly dangerous for premature infants.

of ancient hominid bones revealed evidence of an osteosarcoma (a type of bone cancer) in the toe of a 1.7 million-year-old human ancestor found in a cave near Swartkrans, South Africa.[34] As we have already seen, many animal species are susceptible to cancer, including all mammals, lizards, birds, and their progenitor species as well. Despite what you may hear on television trying to lure you into buying bogus cartilage pills in the wee hours of the morning, even sharks get cancer and those overpriced pills are a modern equivalent of snake oil.[35]

The widespread prevalence of cancer throughout the animal kingdom (and many plants) has prompted a theory that cancer may be a driver of DNA mutation and evolution (rather than the other way around). This idea was conceived and promoted in the early 1980s by an American businessman who suggested cancer has helped drive species to adapt since the earliest days of life on Earth.[36]

James Graham had a background in manufacturing and was aware every time an improvement is included in a new version of a product, the quality of manufacturing diminishes for a time (relative to an older and more familiar version of the product) before, eventually, the new manufacturing technique becomes more standardized and efficient.[37] It is widely accepted that genetic mutations (changes in DNA) are the engine driving evolution and the primary cause of cancer. Based on this understanding, Graham surmised cancer might play an active role in evolution by weeding out untenable mutations. Thus, cancer would serve as a type of quality control and remain prevalent from the oldest species to live on Earth.

The source and the theory have been contentious. Yet this idea has managed to survive through the years, though Graham's contributions have largely been forgotten.[38] [39] As a scientist, it is easy to pass off such notions as the ill-considered ramblings of an untrained amateur. However, the chauvinistic idea that a nonscientist could make a meaningful contribution to the field must be balanced against the reality that Charles Darwin, Gregor Mendel, Benjamin Franklin, and many others were amateur scientists and yet, their theories and contributions remain as relevant today as ever. While the goal of this book is neither to defend nor assail Graham's concepts, it nonetheless seems to hold true that virtually all species seem to suffer from abnormal, inappropriate growth as evidenced by tumors and/or other evidence of malignant behavior. So perhaps we ought to remember his name and provide proper credit.

Cancer might be very old indeed, as old as life itself. What is new is our ability to productively intervene against the disease and to this subject we will now briefly turn.

## Cancer Countermeasures: Past & Present

While our ancestors may have been aware of cancer, they largely lacked the means to successfully intervene against the ravages of the disease. Early writings from Hippocrates in ancient Greece reported that cancers arising in the flank of the body and lymph nodes tended to have poor outcomes even if the tumor could be removed surgically.[40] Despite the futility of doing so, surgery remained the only real option in the Western world until the advent of drug-based chemotherapy in the mid-20th century.*

Throughout most of human history, any medicines "prescribed" for cancer consisted of pastes or potions based on boiled or dried medicinal herbs. While some therapies may have had some basis for efficacy, such as the use of gnawing on bark of the yew tree for pain (which contained salicylic acid, a cousin of modern aspirin), most remedies were sham treatments meant to change the levels of the various "biles" and "humours" thought to exist in the body and whose imbalances were believed to cause disease.

A breakthrough of sorts occurred in the mid-19th century when Thomas Fowler, a physician from the West Midlands of England, concocted a mixture in 1786 that still bears his name. "Fowler's Solution" (double entendre presumably intended) was a remedy purported to heal a variety of diseases, ranging from syphilis to leukemia and skin cancers.[41] Undoubtedly, there was some truth to the advertising as we now know

---

*   The situation in Asia was marginally better since information about a variety of traditional Chinese medicines had been passed along from generation to generation over the past two to three millennia. While recent investigations have verified the efficacy of some compounds, most of these medicines have not yet proven to be terribly effective based on modern measures, suggesting that the "placebo effect" may have been responsible for beneficial outcomes.

Fowler's Solution consisted primarily of potassium arsenite, a form of arsenic. Like all heavy metals, arsenic can be toxic once it reaches high enough levels and the caking of Fowler's Solution onto skin lesions might have proven effective against the exposed tumors cells (though less so if given orally or intravenously to treat leukemia and other internal cancers). The arsenic cocktail concocted by Thomas Fowler was an early representative of a type of chemotherapy that would dominate cancer care for more than century to follow. These earliest chemotherapy drugs were known poisons, which essentially killed everything to which they were exposed.

As the 19th century gave way to the 20th, a remarkable German physician by the name of Paul Ehrlich was completing his studies of a panel of aniline dyes discovered during the heyday of the German chemical industry. Some of these dyes were looking promising in the treatment of cancers (we will meet Ehrlich again in chapter 2).[42] For example, iodoform was a powerful disinfectant directly placed on tumors to kill the tissues surrounding it.[43] Such techniques again proved useful for those tumors able to be directly contacted but were all too often also used following the surgical exposure of a tumor mass, with a prominent example being the excruciatingly painful treatment of breast cancer in a patient named Klara Hitler, which ultimately proved useless.[44] This lack of efficacy might have had implications for world history as many scholars believe her son, Adolf, who doted on his mother, was profoundly and irreversibly damaged psychologically by her death.

The modern era of cancer chemotherapy relied upon this crude kill-everything approach. As detailed in *A Prescription for Change*, cancer care entered the modern era in the latter years of the First World War with reports of anemia and even tumor regression in some soldiers exposed to mustard gas attacks in the trenches of Northwestern Europe.[45] It was not until the end of the Second World War, almost three decades later, that the chemical components of mustard gases had been isolated and analyzed for their tumor-killing capabilities. What followed in the early years of the Cold War was a veritable revolution in cancer care.

Of particular note was a paradox that the fastest-growing types of cancer tended to respond most vigorously to toxins like mustard gases (known in the medical community as nitrogen mustards). A diagnosis of leukemia not only had been accurately perceived as a death sentence, but patients were often dead within days or weeks after receiving a diagnosis. Yet these same diseases were among the first to be—and most responsive when—treated with the new chemotherapies. Why was this the case?

We now know the fastest-growing cancers tend to progress with almost a reckless abandon. Leukemia and lymphoma, cancers of immune cells, are among the fastest growing, and the speed of their growth is legendary. Indeed, this was the diagnosis most consistent with the rapid onset and progression of symptoms I had displayed during my own false alarm during my college years.

The rapid growth and need for nutrients engenders a carelessness in feeding, manifesting itself in at least two ways central to our understanding of 20th century cancer therapy. First, these cells undergo a veritable "feeding frenzy," which translates into leukemia cells stealing nutrients from the body. In doing so, these tumor cells tend to take up molecules that might otherwise escape the menu of a more selective eater. If their surroundings are rich in sickening chemicals, such as heavy metals or nitrogen mustards, then the tumor cells are more likely to acquire a particularly bad, hopefully fatal, case of indigestion.

A second feature distinguishing malignant cells from their benign counterparts requires an automotive analogy. When approaching the checkpoints discussed above, these malignant cells tend to barrel through and ram any interfering fences or walls, accumulating damage as they go. Restated in a more scientific manner, benign cells generally have the capacity to stop growing and initiate repairs once damage is detected. A hallmark of the aforementioned cell cycle is a complete halt to growth (and other activities) so the cell can expend its energy and resources to correct the damage prior to resuming normal activities. A hallmark of the inappropriate growth of cancer is malignant cells' tendency to ignore the damage and allow it to accumulate. On one hand, this is a reckless strategy and indeed, most tumor cells die (and, as we have seen, most of a tumor consists of dead cancer cells). An upside is this same recklessness favors the survival of cells able to withstand the damage and come away even stronger.

Beyond the use of heavy metals, medical scientists began to develop ways to exploit the feeding frenzy of cancer cells in a slightly more targeted manner. This second generation of cancer chemotherapeutics were designed to resemble the nutrients and metabolites preferred by somewhat pickier (i.e., slower-growing) tumor cells. These so-called "anti-metabolites" were the first anticancer drugs to be designed rather than discovered and we will now meet the innovator behind this approach.

### Like Father, Like Son

Charles Heidelberger was born in New York City on December 23, 1920, while the city was still recovering from a two-stage tragedy. On September 14, 1918, New York City health officials noted a surprising uptick in deaths from pneumonia, which was particularly surprising in the closing days of the summer. Health officers were particularly wary since, somewhat unusually, a first wave of influenza outbreaks had been experienced in late May and June, another odd time for such an outbreak in the Northern Hemisphere. Although the number of influenza patients had dissipated through the long, hot summer months, there were worrying rumors afoot of a particularly lethal variety of influenza plaguing war-ravaged France and the English colony of Sierra Leone on the west coast of Africa. Moreover, influenza was merely the opening act of a one-two punch in which influenza weakened patients' lungs to a point where pneumonia conveyed the final coup de grace.

The infant Charles's father was a young but rapidly rising chemist by the name of Michael Heidelberger. With the outbreak of war, and despite the fact that America would not become involved for another two years, Michael had volunteered for the infantry as a marksman, but given his talents, was assigned to the Sanitary Corps and stationed at the Rockefeller Institute in New York, where he focused on developing drugs to prevent or treat infectious diseases. With the outbreak of the Spanish Flu (so-named simply because Spain, a noncombatant in the Great War, was one of the few nations sufficiently transparent to admit its population was suffering from disease), the nation mobilized to combat the invisible virus as well as its partner-in-crime, the bacterium responsible for the fatal pneumonia. This particular bug, pneumococcus, became the focus of the elder Heidelberger's work when a Canadian-American bacteriologist, Oswald Avery, approached him to begin a collaboration to understand how the bacterium might be addressed. Thus began a scientific partnership allowing Michael Heidelberger to define the means by which antibodies function in the body. Antibodies had been known to play a role in defending hosts from infectious diseases, but Heidelberger went on to show how these vital proteins could recognize and bind their targets. Building upon this work, Michael Heidelberger eventually received not one but two Lasker Awards, the most prestigious American award for science and often a precursor to the Nobel Prize. However, neither Heidelberger nor his collaborator Avery, who would vault to fame for the discovery of DNA, would receive this highly coveted international award, giving them the unwanted distinction of being the most deserving scientists to never have received the Nobel Prize.

Nor would Heidelberger's son, Charles, be recognized with a Nobel Prize, despite the fact his discoveries would go on to save thousands, if not millions, of lives. Indeed, these three individuals, Charles Heidelberger, his father Michael, and Oswald Avery are considered widely to be amongst the most deserving scientists never to receive the honorific.

Like his father, Charles trained as a chemist and became a professor at the McArdle Laboratory for Cancer Research at the University of Wisconsin, where he remained for almost three decades. His early career focused on the use of radioactive isotopes of carbon, hydrogen, phosphorous, and other molecules of life, utilizing them as probes to assess the function of various enzymes (the protein-based workhorses of a cell controlling virtually all aspects of cell life and function). An interest in cancer research, matched only by a passion for sailing, was heightened by a 1962 sabbatical trip to Cambridge, England, where he learned about the emerging idea of using mouse-derived cells and tissues as tools to study the disease.

Much of Charles's career built upon the results of a 1954 study that had revealed that one of the basic components of nucleic acids (the building blocks of RNA and DNA) tended to accumulate in malignant cells. After confirming these findings, Charles conceived of an idea to make a variant of one molecule, uracil, to serve as a type of Trojan horse straight out of ancient Greek mythology. Specifically, Charles designed and synthesized a version of uracil with a fluorine molecule not present in normal uracil. Experimenting with this new chemical, he demonstrated this molecule did indeed accumulate within cancer cells and became incorporated into the DNA of tumor cells. As designed, the accumulation of the variant known as *5-fluorouracil,* or 5-FU, would then gum up the tumor cell's vital machinery in a rather clever way. The idea was the buildup of 5-FU would convince the tumor cell it had enough uracil and should shut down further uracil synthesis. Starved of this vital material, tumor cells could not make DNA, RNA, or proteins, and thus would eventually wither away (though the exact mechanism by which they die remains surprisingly unknown even to this day).

Armed with experimental evidence that the 5-FU drug might have utility, Charles tried to convince key decision-makers in the pharmaceutical industry this approach could provide a much-needed means to more selectively target cancer (as compared with toxins, such as heavy metals or mustard compounds, that essentially killed everything but cancer cells slightly more readily than benign cells). Unfortunately, his studies of 5-FU were limited by the fact it was challenging to manufacture the drug in large amounts. Consequently, a constant need for the 5-FU drug limited his ability to study its anti-cancer properties. Eventually, the water-loving Charles Heidelberger managed to find a scientific partner who mostly had his head in the clouds.

Viennese-born Robert Duschinsky spent every weekend and vacation day climbing various peaks in Europe and was an early pioneer of ski mountaineering (the idea of climbing up a mountain and skiing back down). During his less exciting weekdays, he was employed as a chemical engineer at Hoffmann-La Roche and found himself working at Hoffmann-La Roche's site in Nutley, New Jersey (lamenting the fact the Appalachian Mountains were less challenging than the Alps). Duschinsky's boss at Hoffmann-La Roche was a legend in the evolving field of drug development, Dr. Robert Schnitzer. Schnitzer had worked with Gerhard Domagk (who developed the first antibacterial medicines, known as *sulfa drugs*) while employed at the German pharmaceutical behemoth Hoechst Pharmaceuticals in the 1920s but fled Germany with the outbreak of war in 1939. Schnitzer joined Roche to lead its research and development activities in Nutley and had made a name for himself in 1948 by discovering a series of medicines to successfully treat tuberculosis, including many still used today (a particularly notable achievement given how quickly bacteria can develop drug resistance). Based on this reputation, Charles Heidelberger approached Schnitzer about his problem in synthesizing 5-FU in the mid-1950s and Schnitzer appointed the mountain-climbing Duschinsky to surmount this obstacle.

By 1957, enough 5-FU had been manufactured to allow testing in people. The early clinical trials were hosted at Heidelberger's University of Wisconsin, and the results were not only encouraging but represented a landmark toward an entirely new way to tackle the problem of cancer.[46] Over the following two decades, much work at Roche and scores of universities and pharmaceutical companies sought to identify other molecules resembling normal metabolites or substrates of key enzymes involved in the growth or survival of malignant cells. These agents became known as *anti-metabolites,* and the list of these modern-day Trojan horses includes some of the most commonly used medicines over the last few decades that will still prove their worth for years to come.

While anti-metabolites provided a means to increase the efficacy and safety of cancer treatment by targeting tumor cell enzymes, most of these same molecules were also vital for the growth or survival of many benign cells, including the fast-growing cells of the intestine, skin, and blood. Consequently, the side effects of hair loss, gastrointestinal distress, and anemia have become synonymous with chemotherapy. Although serving as miracle drugs for many fast-growing blood cancers, these medicines tended not to work as well for the many slower-growing tumors, such as diseases of the breast, colon, and prostate. Consequently, the rate of cancer deaths continued to rise throughout the latter years of the 20th century.

New thinking was needed to overcome these hurdles, and this would arrive in the latter years of the 20th century in the form of a revolution in our understanding of the science, medicine, and business of cancer. To set the stage for this revolution, it is necessary to understand the dynamic means by which cancer cells both hide and openly taunt a system of layered antitumor defenses provided by the body's immune system, a subject to which we will turn.

# 2

## *Surveillance State*

A disconcerting reality is that, despite all the body's safeguards described in the previous chapter to prevent cancer, the disease nonetheless relentlessly arises, perhaps in each of us and on a daily basis. This audacious statement is a scientific hypothesis put forward by a famous American polymath, who is perhaps better remembered for his poetry and prose (for which he was recognized with a National Book Award) than his scientific prowess (for which he was recognized with a Lasker Award, the top American scientific prize).

Lewis Thomas was born in Flushing, Queens, in 1913, at the same hospital where his parents worked. His father, Joseph Simon Thomas, was a Columbia-trained physician and his mother, Grace Emma Peck, a nurse. Despite being an average student, the affluence and connections provided by his family meant Thomas had his choice of America's top universities. He joined his father's undergraduate alma mater, Princeton University, in the autumn of 1929, just as the world's economic system was nearing calamity.[1]

The collapse of the stock market on Black Tuesday, October 29, 1929, and the resulting Great Depression overshadowed most of Thomas's time at Princeton yet did not particularly motivate him. Indeed, he later admitted lacking interest in much of anything, including his coursework, sports, or social interests.[2] In how own words, he described himself turning "into a moult of dullness and laziness, average or below in the courses requiring real work."[3] His only motivations seemed to have been invested in writing for the school newspaper, *The Princeton Tiger*, but even this exertion was minimal.

In Lewis Thomas's senior year, his passions were belatedly ignited by a Princeton biologist, Professor Wilbur Willis Swingle, who, fulfilling the stereotypic view of an Ivy League don, introduced the young Thomas both to science and popular scientific writing (as opposed to the dry manuscripts typical of professional scientific discourse). Swingle himself was quite accomplished and had developed a treatment for Addison's disease (an adrenal disorder, whose most famous sufferer was President John Fitzgerald Kennedy), but Swingle's major influences on Thomas were the teachings "science begins with the admission of ignorance" and "experiments done for the sake of curiosity often yield the most practical results."[4] Indeed, Swingle's notable scientific accomplishment arose from putting these ideas into practice in 1929, when he isolated a substance from the adrenal glands with the ability to counter the effects of Addison's disease, first in animals and then in people. With this unexpected inspiration, Thomas had suddenly been transformed into "a reasonably alert scholar," who was focused on biology and medicine (the latter career choice would also, he reasoned, assure steady employment in a nation settling into a long economic downturn). The rest of his senior year was a frenetic time in which Thomas absorbed as much information about science, medicine, and writing afforded by his limited remaining time at Princeton.

Despite unspectacular grades in his first three years, Thomas rebounded and was accepted into Harvard Medical School. His acceptance into one of the nation's finest schools, he later acknowledged, was primarily because his father and mother were close friends with Hans Zinsser, a legendary member of the Harvard faculty. Zinsser had discovered the bacterial pathogen responsible for typhus and if that were not enough, then developed an effective vaccine to eliminate the disease.[5] [6] Zinsser also shared Thomas's newly discovered passion for popular scientific writing and himself would be awarded a National Book Award weeks before his untimely death from leukemia in 1940, at the age of sixty-one.[7]

Zinsser imprinted on Thomas and further stoked the fires lit by Professor Swingle during Thomas's senior year. After graduating from Harvard Medical School, Thomas embarked upon a medical residency spent learning neurology at Columbia University. Following the surprise Japanese attack on Pearl Harbor, Lewis was drafted into the navy. As a trained physician with a predilection for science, the navy deployed Thomas into a medical research laboratory, and he endured most of the war evaluating ways to combat infectious diseases using sulfa drugs (which had only been discovered a decade before). During a posting in Guam, Thomas had been assigned a mission to study a Japanese encephalitis virus, a deadly pathogen expected to impact the troops during the invasion of the Japanese home islands, scheduled to begin in late 1945. However, the dropping of atomic weapons on Nagasaki and Hiroshima in August 1945 obviated the need for an invasion. Instead, Thomas found himself without a mission and with five months left to serve out the remainder of his enlistment and nothing much to do.

Channeling Swingle's advice from years before, Thomas's research interests while in Guam and in the years thereafter amounted to dabbling in a range of subjects from the practical (such as the creation of new ways to study infectious disease) to the esoteric (why the long ears of rabbits lost their rigidity and flopped for a few days after injection with papain, a meat tenderizer). Paradoxically, it was the latter project that inspired his greatest breakthrough.

Thomas found the meat tenderizer caused the ears of a rabbit to flop based on its ability to degrade the cartilage of the ears (the same rigid material providing structure to the nose and ears). However, the cause of the drooping was not the main source of Thomas's breakthrough. Thomas realized, given a few weeks, the ears again became rigid. This simple observation led him to realize tissues long-thought to be inert, such as cartilage, are in fact quite robust and capable of constant growth and renewal. Even decades after his tour of duty in Guam had ended, Professor Thomas (he would gain his first faculty appointment at Johns Hopkins and then move on to Yale, New York University, and his last as head of the Memorial Sloan Kettering Cancer Center) would often bring along examples of meat-tenderized-injected rabbits (before, during, and after treatment) to convey to his students and audiences the body's capacities for growth and revival were far more dynamic than had been appreciated.

During a 1959 symposium at the New York Academy of Sciences, Thomas expanded his observations on rabbit ears into a landmark talk galvanizing the creation of a field now known as *immune oncology*.[8] He hypothesized that one consequence of this vibrant new understanding that the body's cells were highly dynamic was a propensity for cancer. Thomas was among the earliest minds to appreciate cancer as a disease of excessive self-renewal and further reasoned the outgrowth of tumor cells may be ubiquitous and arise constantly in people at any time or age. This idea was perhaps more amenable to listeners in the middle third of the 20th century than today because they were familiar with the fact cancer is not a disease only of the elderly, as stories of friends and neighbors suffering from childhood cancers were far too common and rarely ended well. Indeed, a diagnosis of cancer in a young child was widely understood to be a virtual death sentence. Childhood cancers are generally fast-growing and often responsive to early cancer therapies (including mustard compounds and anti-metabolites). Consequently, cancer deaths among the young are now rare and we tend to think of cancer as a malady of the aged.

A corollary to the idea of cancer spawning at an uncomfortably high frequency raises the obvious question of why more people do not die of cancer and at a younger age. Thomas also addressed this question in his remarkable 1959 presentation in New York City.[9] He postulated while cancer cells arise spontaneously and frequently, they are subject to tight regulation by the cells and chemicals of the immune system. This was not necessarily a particularly new idea—Paul Ehrlich, a founder and leading thinker in the field of immunology, had contended in 1909 that cancer arises frequently but is kept in check by a vigorous immune response.[10] However, Thomas can rightfully be credited with rejuvenating this idea from near obscurity and helping propel it forward, ultimately leading to the creation of new medicines as revolutionary as the early treatments for childhood leukemia.

*Surveillance Mission*

Although we briefly met Paul Ehrlich in chapter 1, it is important to repeat his was arguably the greatest mind steering the course of the biological sciences in the late 19th century (and perhaps eclipsing contemporaries in others scientific fields as well, including even Albert Einstein). Ehrlich's extraordinary work in the development and advancement of the fields of microbiology and immunology have been the subjects of my two earlier works.[11] [12] Ehrlich's contributions to cancer research may ultimately be the final and greatest legacy of a man justly feted based on his contributions to the development of medicines and vaccines to combat bacterial diseases. Vaulting over his earlier work on infectious pathogens, Ehrlich found himself in his golden years celebrating the transition from the 19th into the 20th centuries as the head of the Frankfurt-based, government-supported Royal Prussian Institute of Experimental Therapy. In this role, his team was focused on the development and manufacturing of new vaccines and medicines known as *antisera*, in the struggle to overcome lethal infectious diseases. Ehrlich and his institute had provided much-needed medicines to treat or prevent childhood killers like diphtheria and tetanus.[13] While the Prussian people greatly appreciated the cures and preventative measures arising from the institute, the government was running a deficit, which provided an excuse to cut down Ehrlich. It seems Ehrlich was an outspoken advocate for liberalization of the Prussian (and then German) state and these political views did not sit well with the Kaiser or his ministers. In 1901, the Ministry of Finance demanded Ehrlich find new means of supporting this life-saving enterprise, an action perhaps also tinged by the prevailing anti-Semitism of the Prussian elite.[14]

At the same time Ehrlich was trying to determine how to save his institute, the Prussian aristocracy and people were mourning the loss of their Dowager Empress. Victoria Adelaide Mary Louisa was born on November 21, 1840, at Buckingham Palace, the first child of Queen Victoria and Prince Albert. At the age of seventeen, the young Victoria was married off to the Hohenzollern emperor-to-be Frederick of Prussia and moved to the Continent.[15] The daughter's potential for marital bliss was marred before the wedding, when the elder Victoria insisted the marriage ceremony take place in London. In part, this demand was based on the fact the English people were not happy their first princess would leave the island for the perceived backwater of Prussia. A marriage celebration in London would be one way to assuage the English masses. Queen Victoria's insistence on the location of the ceremony thus precipitated a spat with her Hohenzollern cousins, who thought, as the intended parents of future kaisers, Victoria and Frederick should be married in Berlin. The headstrong Queen Victoria of England won the day but lost popularity in Germany, particularly after voicing sentiments that the middling power represented by Prussia should be flattered even to be considered for the hand of the eldest child of the leader of the world's only superpower, the Queen of the United Kingdom of Great Britain and Ireland and the Empress of India.

This controversy likewise stoked criticism of the marriage within the Prussian aristocracy, which was further appalled to learn of the political and social views of their new princess. Despite her youth, Victoria was a vocal and faithful daughter of Prince Albert, who himself was a proud liberal and had inculcated his eldest daughter with the views of the more liberal elements of English society. Most of these opinions ran contrary to the conservative preferences of the Junkers aristocracy, which was quickly rising in the European ascendency in terms of political and military might, in part by embracing an ultra-right-wing military and political agenda. Both Albert and the elder Victoria overtly intended their daughter's betrothal, which finally took place on January 25, 1858, in St. James's Palace in London, introducing liberal reform into Prussia.

Four years after Victoria had moved from Britain to her new home in Berlin, it appeared her political views might indeed prevail within Prussia. In 1862, the liberal-leaning Prussian parliament, the Landtag, refused to grant an increase in the military budget and resisted extending the period of mandatory conscription from two years to three. Both items were essential for the Prussian emperor, Wilhelm I, who was contemplating opportunities to unite all German-speaking peoples of Europe into a single power to be overseen by Prussia. Wilhelm I dissolved parliament and, in a fit of rage, considered resignation.[16] The crisis was exacerbated by Wilhem's thin-skinned response to criticism of his hasty actions. Rumors soon began to swirl indicating Wilhelm's determination to carry through with his threat of abdication, weakening the executive at a time when strong leadership was needed to accomplish Prussia's expansionistic goals.

Channeling her own father's liberal teachings, Victoria pressed her husband to encourage his father Wilhelm I's abdication as a first step to initiate political reform.[17] Victoria's council was for naught as Frederick at the time was even more intent upon a more conservative agenda, fearing a loosening of centralized power would weaken his own prospects by the time of his coronation. Not only did this decision politically estrange him for a time from his wife, but Wilhelm and Frederick resolved the parliamentary crisis through the appointment of a new prime minister, the legendary and extremely conservative Count Otto von Bismarck. The new prime minister, despising the liberal views of the upstart princess Victoria, sought to alienate her opinons from both her husband and an adoring public. Initiating an overt and covert campaign against the princess, von Bismarck largely succeeded and, in doing so, may have fated the planet to a tragic series of hot and cold world wars to ultimately break the hold of the conservative tendencies but only after two world wars and countless millions of deaths.

Compounding her unwanted political views, Victoria was increasingly estranged from her first issue, the second in line to the throne (after her husband).[18] Since her arrival in Berlin, Princess Victoria had remained strongly prejudiced. English doctors were the finest in the world and Victoria demanded an English medical staff for herself and her family. Indeed, the delivery of her first child, the future Wilhelm II, was a challenging one as the baby presented in a breech position (bottom first). The interminable labor caused the child to suffer permanent damage, both physical (his left arm was eight inches shorter than his right) and perhaps neurological damage (the baby may have been deprived of oxygen for an extended period as his umbilical cord was pinched off and his head failed to slide through the maternal pelvis). Wilhelm survived but soon grew to resent Victoria, stating in 1889, "an English doctor crippled my arm—which is the fault of the mother, who allowed no German physicians to attend to herself or her immediate family."[19] Worse still, Victoria evinced guilt about the birth defects her son had suffered for the rest of her life. She sought to compensate by assuring her husband young Wilhelm would be able to carry out royal responsibilities, such as equestrianism. In doing so, Victoria pushed the young Wilhelm to become an accomplished rider through a brutal regimen of riding lessons.[20]

The strains between mother and son further worsened through the growing influence of von Bismarck, who continued a campaign to distance the English princess from her family, both near and abroad. Under von Bismarck's tutelage, the young prince learned to vilify both the personage and political leanings of his mother and would later eschew the liberal ideas as soon as he had become sovereign.*

In 1887, the elderly Kaiser Wilhem I was nearing death. Over the past twenty years since the marriage of Victoria and Frederick, Prussia had successfully fought off a French invasion and united most of the German-speaking principalities into a single and powerful Central European power. In this same period, Victoria's influences had taken hold of Frederick and he had become convinced to enact a series of liberal reforms upon taking power. Among his intended changes was the removal of von Bismarck and a move away from the brutal use of realpolitik, the practical use of coercion to unite German-speaking peoples and shape an aggressive, expansionist foreign policy.

By the time Wilhelm I died on March 9, 1888, Frederick himself was not a well man. A heavy smoker, Frederick had experienced excessive phlegm and mucus coating his vocal cords, causing hoarseness and occasional laryngitis. His German physicians concurred their prince (soon to be kaiser) was displaying the telltale signs of laryngeal cancer. This diagnosis was confirmed on May 17, 1887, but consistent with the practices of the day, Frederick was not told (though Victoria was). As his German doctors contemplated the complete surgical removal of the prince's larynx (an unprecedented procedure), Victoria's preferred physician, Morell Mackenzie, was brought over from England to assess the situation. A sample of the tumor was collected on May 20 and sent to the world-renowned Prussian pathologist, Rudolf Virchow, who pronounced the biopsy to be free of cancer. Mackenzie performed a second biopsy on June 9 and Virchow again deemed it to be free of any signs of cancer.

Much to the dismay of the Prussian physicians, the surgery was scrubbed, and Mackenzie instead advised Frederick and Victoria to spend the upcoming winter in the warm climes of the Italian Riviera. Frederick died there on June 15, 1888, away from their son, which further increased Wilhelm's resentment of Victoria. The German Emperor Frederick and his Empress Victoria had ruled Prussia for a mere ninety-nine days. Despite the fact a preeminent

---

\* Though Wilhelm II eventually demanded the resignation of von Bismarck, it is perhaps not coincidental given his anti-English views that Germany entered the Great War under his leadership.

Prussian pathologist had been responsible for the misdiagnosis, Frederick's son, who succeeded as Kaiser Wilhelm II, placed the entire blame squarely upon the English doctor, Mackenzie.

With his father's premature death, von Bismarck and the new Kaiser Wilhelm II quickly sprang into action. [21] [22] As a sign of contempt for his mother, Wilhelm II ordered her residences to be immediately sacked in a search for documents to incriminate the former to charges of collusion with her British relatives (though any evidence of such had been spirited away to London days before by Victoria's faithful staff). The newly widowed Empress Dowager Victoria was immediately barred from her residences and ordered into a virtual exile of solitude in the sleepy Hessian town of Kronberg im Taunus in southwest Germany. She lived another decade focused primarily on arranging the marriages of her remaining issue (Wilhelm II was the first of seven siblings) and promoting young artists. [23]

Despite suffering considerable isolation, Victoria was a sympathetic character and remained endeared, especially to the more liberal elements of Berlin society. The increasingly autocratic and insecure tendencies of its new emperor were intolerable for many citizens of the German nation, which was moving in the opposite direction, becoming more mature, confident, and, consequently, less inclined to be cowed by the new kaiser.

Victoria remained largely estranged from, and critical of, her son's autocratic policies but her ability to resist was undermined by a diagnosis of breast cancer in the closing days of 1898. [24] The former empress lingered on through mid-1901 as the disease spread to her bones and lungs. On August 5, 1901, Victoria died. In an act of rebellion against her headstrong son, her admirers decided to perpetuate the memory of her reformist ways by endowing an institution, which would actively fly in the face of the sitting kaiser.

All while the tale of Victoria was unfolding, Paul Ehrlich's mission to conquer infectious diseases had continued progressing, with the discovery of new therapies to treat diphtheria, tetanus, typhus, and tuberculosis. [25] Despite these extraordinary advances, officials from Kaiser Wilhelm II's ministry of finance informed Ehrlich in 1901 they were planning to slash the budget for his institute. [26] Ehrlich was a prominent Jewish liberal whereas Wilhelm II was a conservative anti-Semite. The Kaiser particularly disliked wealthy Jewish businessmen and Ehrlich would ultimately be personally pilloried for his entrepreneurial instincts to start a company to distribute Salvarsan, an innovative and much-needed treatment he had developed for syphilis.[27] In this context, it must have seemed logical that closure of Ehrlich's institute would mute a prominent critic from the left. The vindictive decision to undermine Ehrlich however was complicated by the extraordinary good done by his institute, which had endeared it to the German nation.

Amid these tensions, Georg Speyer, a Jewish philanthropist and co-owner of Lazard Speyer-Ellissen banking house, founded a campaign to save Ehrlich's defunded institute. Donating one hundred thousand German marks of his own money and organizing a coalition of like-minded Jewish humanitarians, Speyer's fund underwrote the costs of running Ehrlich's Frankfurt-based vaccine group.[28] The only proviso was cancer was to be included in the institute's mandate to honor the memory of the late dowager empress (which may also be interpreted as another tweak to the nose of the kaiser). Unbeknownst to Speyer, he too would soon succumb to cancer within a year. Upon his death, his widow donated an additional two million German marks to the institute in his memory.[29]

From 1901 until his death in 1915, Ehrlich devoted much of his remaining life and his institute's work to the study of cancer. Among the ideas advanced during this time was a hypothesis claiming that the body's natural defense mechanisms were capable of identifying and eliminating malignant cells. Ehrlich had coined a concept now known as a *magic bullet,* which represented the idea researchers could one day develop medicines to selectively identify and kill potentially dangerous diseases (including cancer cells, bacteria, or viruses). In doing so, Ehrlich gave birth to a concept only recently realized in modern medicine through the production of monoclonal antibodies and other targeted medicines.

These early ideas from Ehrlich were expanded upon by Frank MacFarlane Burnet, an Australian virologist who refocused his research upon the nascent field of immunology at roughly the same time Lewis Thomas was conveying his own revolutionary ideas about cancer. By this time, Burnet had already made a name for himself by introducing the concepts of clonal selection and immune tolerance, two ideas forming the backbone of our present understanding of the immune system. These contributions also paved the way to Burnet's recognition with the 1960 Nobel Prize for Medicine. Summarized succinctly, Burnet postulated that the immune system could identify and recall small variations in the molecules produced by microorganisms and deploy this immunological memory to protect against these pathogens upon future encounters. A variation to this theme was that the body similarly possessed the means to prevent potentially lethal autoimmune damage by creating a type of cellular tolerance to impair the cells of the immune system from targeting normal cells. Both ideas would later come together in an understanding of the relationship between cancer and the immune system.

Applying his disease to oncology, Burnet realized even slight modifications (e.g., those caused by mutation) could cause cancer cells to lose this tolerance. Such changes would then facilitate the directed elimination of cancer cells by the immune system. Specifically, Burnet proposed in 1957, "it is by no means inconceivable that small accumulations of tumour cells may develop and because of their possession of new antigen potentialities, provoke an effective immunological reaction with regression of the tumour and no clinical hint of its existence."[30] The multinational understanding of immune-based targeting of cancer developed by the German Ehrlich, the Anglo-Australian Burnet, and the American Thomas was further advanced by a truly remarkable scientist, who within a single individual blended many nations.

### Following A Transplant

Three years before the vindictive Kaiser Wilhelm II would be ejected from his throne, Peter Medawar was born in Rio de Janeiro, Brazil, in 1915, to a British mother and a Lebanese father. Returning to his mother's home-land for college-preparatory training, Medawar graduated with a degree in zoology from Oxford in 1935 and in 1937 and began research under no less than Howard Florey (who would go on to isolate and identify ways to mass produce penicillin). Although excited by penicillin, Medawar was assigned to a more unexciting project (in his view) to understand how certain cells of the immune system interacted with fibroblasts, a major cellular component of the skin. While Medawar performed the research under Florey neces-sary to qualify for a doctorate (Oxford is one of a few schools to award an advanced title known as a *D.Phil.,* rather than a Ph.D.), he never received the degree. This absence of a formal credential did not reflect a lack of scientific contribution but more accurately the fact Medawar had, around the time of his dissertation defense, suffered from a burst appendix, which required him to spend the money saved for the completion fee to instead pay for the surgery and rehabilitation. He later claimed it would have been overly extravagant to pay for both.[31]

As Britain entered the Second World War, the urgency to advance penicillin rose to the foreground (in recognition of an immense number of looming battlefield wounds). Given his familiarity with his mentor's work, Medawar was drafted into a project to assess the potential use of the new medicine to assist in the treatment of burn victims (a far-too-common malady in times of war). Once introduced to the grisly biology and medicine underpinning the damage caused by fire and chemical damage to the skin, Medawar advocated grafted tissues were the most effective means to treat wounds. The problem was the grafting procedure was only successful with skin isolated from other parts of the same patient's own body. There was a low likelihood skin could be obtained if the damage was extensive, which is often the case with battlefield wounds.

A logical opportunity could arise if donor skin could be used. Unless sourced from anyone other than a twin (a relative rarity), a skin graft tended not to take hold due to a process known as *rejection*. Medawar revealed the process represented a form of immunological recognition of the donated tissue as being foreign, which triggered a massive infiltration of lymphocytes into the grafted site. Conventional wisdom of the time had presumed a chemical in the blood was responsible for rejection, but Medawar's work implicated the cells of the immune system. These conclusions were soon verified by independent research conducted by other investigators (a hallmark of the research process). With enough understanding of how these defense mechanisms worked, it was presumed the responses could be controlled with drugs designed to target the immune system.

Beyond the wartime use of grafted tissues for the treatment of burns, Medawar's ideas had a larger potential to utilize grafts of entire organs to replacing failing structures, such as the heart, lungs, kidneys, or liver; a radical concept. From the perspective of a surgeon, the procedure needed to remove and replace an organ was relatively straightforward (albeit tedious). However, these organs would inevitably be rejected, and Medawar's work was the first to explain why the immune system had been triggered to mediate organ rejection. Medawar appreciated that this understanding could have clinical utility but only if this response could be prevented.

At the war's conclusion, Medawar accepted a faculty position in Birmingham, England, where he continued his studies of tissue rejection. He began using transfused blood to study the process of rejection (admittedly not an organ but a substance also susceptible to rejection due to a variety of well-known factors known as *AB* and *Rh antigens*). One of Medawar's early discoveries was that non-identical (fraternal) twins did not reject one another's blood, even when there was a clear AB/Rh mismatch.[32] [33] In contrast, non-twinned siblings did reject mismatched blood. This finding had been predicted by a theory put forward by MacFarlane Burnet that the decision to reject or tolerate tissue was determined *in utero.* In other words, the environment experienced by the fetus would define what is later considered to be "self" (and thus tolerated) versus "foreign" (and destined to be rejected). This experimental evidence in support of Burnet's hypothesis allowed both scientists to share the 1960 Nobel Prize.

Given the events causing most cancers usually arise well beyond the fetal stages of life, Medawar and Burnet again teamed up to postulate that, as a disease characterized by mutation, subtle changes in cancer cells would likewise render them subject to rejection by the body as foreign in the same way transplanted tissues were vigorously attacked by the cells of the immune system. The idea the immune system suppressed the rise of cancer was warmly embraced for a time by the scientific community of the 1960s. However, a naked rodent had become popular in the world of medical research and would derail the widespread adoption of immune surveillance for decades.

*Domestic Skills*

A surprisingly rabid debate has bred considerable contempt amongst certain scientists regarding animal domestication. Although it is generally understood that the modern canine is the first mammal domesticated by our Neolithic ancestors, a dogfight (pun intended) has occurred between scientists from different nations who are essentially marking their turf. One side maintains dogs (*Canis familliaris*) were domesticated from gray wolves (*Canis lupus*) in or around modern-day Germany over 16 millennia ago, whereas the other side claims the event occurred in Southeast Asia approximately 12 millennia ago. The dispute remains unresolved although a compromise of sorts briefly arose with the publication of a 2016 study suggesting both sides may be right, with independent domestication events giving rise to Asian (e.g., Shih Tzu) and European breeds (e.g., Golden Retrievers).[34] Although this tamed the fray for a time, the viciousness of the argument increased further a year later with genetic evidence dogs diverged from their wolf brethren closer to 40 millennia ago (without any allusion to where this event may have occurred).[35]

Far less controversial is the fact Asian societies gave rise to the domestication and breeding of what are known worldwide as "fancy mice." This practice has been popular for millennia. Although it may seem counterintuitive, a love of rodents was a hobby pursued by the elite of the Shang Dynasty around 1100 B.C.E., when small mammals, including mice, were bred for exotic variations in size, coat color, eye color, and other anatomic features. Faithful inbreeding over the ages by rodent aficionados meant the genetic background of different breeds had been culled into strains with extraordinary homogeneity. As an unanticipated consequence, scientists became interested in utilizing such mice as experimental models since genetic purity decreased variability, which often confounds the interpretation of scientific studies with animals.

The concept of laboratory mice as a mainstay of modern medical research is broadly understood, and some more mature readers may even recall a 1960s American Cancer Society fundraising campaign extolling donors to "Send a Mouse to College," starring a mortarboard-wearing gray-and-white cartoon character named Roquefort the Mouse. Roughly coincident with the launch of this philanthropic effort, a Scottish scientist made a discovery that would unknowingly revolutionize our understanding of the immune system and help foster new cures for cancer, although there were more than a few bumps in the road.

*Trouble in the Mouse House*

Norman Roy Grist was a nature-loving Scot who parlayed his interests in science to earn a medical degree from Glasgow University in 1942.[36] Surviving the Second World War despite being a participant in the Normandy landings, the disastrous airborne invasion of northern Europe (Operation Market Garden), and the crossing of the Rhine River, Grist returned to what might have seemed to others as a more mundane role in Glasgow, studying albino laboratory mice.

In the early summer of 1959, Norman and his assistant were shocked to learn their supply of white laboratory mice had been decimated by a plague of Coxsackie viruses that had invaded their animal housing facility.[37] A colony of mice had been established six years before but was now mostly wiped out. Yet, Grist noted as the infection progressed through the facility, a small number of mice seemed to flourish, even in the face of new waves of Coxsackie virus infection. He continued to breed these surviving mice with one another and ended up with a strain quite resistant to Coxsackie virus. Unlike their white-furred ancestors, this new group utterly lacked the albino-white hair of their predecessors. Instead, these mice were utterly bald, sporting wrinkled pink skin. Through repetitive rounds of breeding, Norman had established a pure genetic lineage of these bald rodents and they were forever to be known as *nude* mice.

The story might otherwise end there but these mice soon generated many questions about why they lost their hair. Sparing the reader the historical and technical minutiae behind the discovery of the changes giving rise to nude mice, it suffices to say what occurred in Grist's laboratory during the summer of 1959 was a spontaneous mutation in one particular gene, known as *FoxN1* (an abbreviation for Forkhead box protein N1).[38] This mutation altered the amount of keratin produced by certain cells in the body. Keratin, as you may recall from chapter 1, is a protein produced by keratinocytes that helps convey the durability and flexibility of skin. The particular form of keratin altered by the FoxN1 mutation is essential for the survival of a unique set of keratinocytes—ones that give rise to hair follicles. By pure chance, this mutation also disrupts a relatively small number of cells within a mysterious organ residing just atop the heart, both in mice and humans—the thymus.[39]

The thymus gained its name from the ancient Greeks based on the word for anger (*thumos*), since the thymus was presumed to be the site in the body responsible for intensely negative emotions. Although virtually nothing was known about the organ for almost all of recorded history, an early clue (in retrospect), came when the most famous medical expert of the 2nd century C.E. (and for at least the following millennia and a half), Galen of Pergamon, revealed the thymus undergoes a remarkable shrinkage as children mature. Indeed, the organ is essentially (though not quite entirely) withered by puberty.[40]

This involution of the thymus was an early indication of its function, which we now know to be a nursery for the key host defense cells in the body. The idea the thymus was involved in immune response had been first postulated during early microscopic analyses, which revealed extraordinary numbers of dead lymphocytes densely packed within the organ. Looking closer, some living lymphocytes could also be spotted and these were surrounded by a special type of tissue known as *thymic epithelia*.[41]

Based on the large number of dead lymphocytes in the organ, it was presumed the thymus was a sort of "lymphocyte graveyard or recycling plant," where dying lymphocytes went to spend their final hours.[42] Such notions were disabused in the early 1960s by a researcher born in Nice, France, in 1931 and given the name Jacques Francois Albert Pierre Meunier (later Anglicized to "Miller").[43] Jacques's father was an international banker and soon moved to Shanghai but, in the face of an impending Japanese invasion, moved his family to Australia. As the family was preparing to transition to a life down under, Miller's sister died from tuberculosis and this trauma spawned a desire by Jacques to become a medical researcher. After earning a bachelor's degree at the University of Sydney and a Ph.D. at University College in London, Miller performed postdoctoral studies in cancer pathology at the National Cancer Institute in Bethesda, Maryland. In 1966, Miller returned to Australia to lead pathology and to begin a series of studies at the Walter and Eliza Hall Institute of Medical Research in Melbourne. His work would revolutionize our understanding of the body's immune system.

Miller's pivotal study was relatively straightforward: Surgically excise the thymus from baby mice and see what happened.[44] The function of the thymus was presumed to be involved in host defense (due to large number of lymphocytes) and in the days of the 1950s following Medawar and Burnet's high-profile studies of transplantation using rodents, mice seemed a good place to start. Beyond their genetic purity, mice provided a particularly useful model as they are born without a functioning immune system. Unlike humans, which come into the world with matured host defense mechanisms, the development of the immune system in mice starts from scratch immediately after birth. Consequently, that Miller was able to demonstrate the removal of the thymus in newborn mouse pups allowed the animals to receive donor tissues without the characteristic tissue rejection (recalling Burnet's idea such outcomes are determined *in utero*). Were the thymus removed weeks or even days after birth (after the immune system had time to develop), the rejection process was as robust as if no surgery had been performed. Miller appreciated this outcome likely meant the thymus played a key role early in immune system development and helped to educate the immune system. Moreover, the fact that removal of the organ a week after birth had little or no effect on immune-based rejection meant the job of the thymus was no longer needed in mice (hence the involution of the thymus later in life).

Miller also found the mice "thymecotimized" at birth were so highly susceptible to infection they required housing within a strict germ-free environment.[45] Over the following decade, Miller and his colleagues demonstrated that their organ of interest, which had been largely neglected based on the fact it was vestigial by puberty, was the fount of the powerful immune system, both in mice and man.

To summarize, the thymus functions as the cradle, grave, and a type of military boot camp responsible for both nestling and weeding out lymphocytes during training. The training itself focused upon the ability of these lymphocytes to recognize and eliminate unwanted intruders. Miller further showed the massive death of lymphocytes within the thymus reflected the fact that most of these trainees fail and are terminated. We now know cells within the thymus fail to make the grade if they either are unable to perform the function of identifying foreign invaders or if there are potential concerns about risks for an overly exuberant attack upon host (self) tissues. In either case, these imperfect thymocytes are culled with extreme prejudice (i.e., they are given instructions to commit suicide via apoptosis [see chapter 1]), resulting in the masses of dead cells and debris observed during microscopic analyses of the organ.

In the years following his pivotal studies to assess the effects of removing the thymus, Miller advocated for the existence of two distinct populations of lymphocytes, which he broadly distinguished into T cells (for their birth in the thymus) and B cells (for their birth in the bone marrow). This idea, although proven correct, did not sit well with many of his colleagues, as evidenced by a 1968 confrontation during a seminar at Brook Lodge, Michigan, when he was challenged by Bede Morris, another Australian immunologist, who sarcastically stated B and T were the first and last letters of the word *bullshit*.[46]

A decade later, T cells gained great notoriety and acceptance, not just from the scientific community but the general public as well, largely as a consequence of the HIV/AIDS pandemic, a subject to which we will soon return. Since their discovery and characterization by Miller and countless immunologists since the 1960s, it is now understood that these T cells can essentially be viewed as the "generals of the immune system," which identify foreign invaders and command as well as participate in the attack of the body's defenses against them. Based on this overly brief introduction to the concept of T cells, we will now return to the idea of how the wrinkly and wholly unattractive nude mouse, whose baldness is attributable to a defect that selectively impairs the formation of the epithelial tissues in both hair follicles and the thymus, almost derailed the potential for curing cancer within our lifetime.

### The Naked Truth

The science of understanding how cancer arises arguably began in the 16th century with a description of a "wasting disease of miners" now generally understood to have been lung cancer.[47] With the discovery of radioactive elements by Marie and Pierre Curie in early 20th century Europe, it was presumed high exposure to radium contributed to the high prevalence of cancer in miners. Thus began an intimate connection between the emerging sciences of radiation biology and chemical carcinogenesis. The chemical side of the equation similarly came into focus following demonstrations of repetitive or prolonged exposure to certain nonradioactive chemicals that were also sufficient to induce tumors. We can now look as far back as the mid-18th century to find incontrovertible evidence coal tars, soot, and tobacco products could cause cancer. For example, surgeons in London reported a high incidence of cancers in snuff users and chimney sweeps.[48] However, scientific, ethical, and practical concerns limited the ability of scientists to do much more than epidemiological investigation of statistical risk.

These experimental limitations evaporated amid the chaos of the First World War, when two Japanese doctors were able to reproduce such findings in experimental models of cancer in animals. Yamagiwa Katsusaburō and

Koichi Ichikawa reported in 1915 repeated administration of coal tar compounds to the ears of rabbits was sufficient to cause cancerous growths.[49] The next two decades witnessed extraordinary progress in identifying chemicals able to trigger cancers in animals. Mice provided the preferred model, both because their small size translated into lower costs and because the various strains meant the inbred, virtually identical (almost clone-like) animals would minimize variability typical of animals from the wild.

Within their work, we are reintroduced to the nude mouse. Unlike thymectomized mice, the nude animals did not require a thymectomy, were far more robust, did not require germ-free conditions, and hence were more amenable to laboratory studies. Such heartiness meant nude mice could be used to address the question of whether mice lacking T cells would be more susceptible to chemically induced cancers than their hair- (and T cell) bearing forefathers. The immune surveillance theory had predicted the body's host defenses vigilantly patrol for cancers and thus the absence of an immune response in nude mice would render them more susceptible to chemical carcinogens. In a thorough set of studies published in the mid-1970s, Osias Stutman of the Memorial Sloan Kettering Cancer Center in New York City conclusively demonstrated nude mice were no more susceptible to carcinogenesis than their genetically matched cousins, who retained the ability to make T cells.[50] This seemed to settle the question, and most in the field of tumor immunology moved on to pursue other scientific questions.

A small number of scientists remained unconvinced and evidence supporting their views was hiding in plain sight: Nude mice are far too hearty to be an animal fundamentally lacking host defenses. Quite the opposite. Recall, Norman Grist had been able to isolate nude mice in 1959 because they were the sole survivors of a disastrous Coxsackie virus outbreak. These nude animals were the fighters, not the victims. Studies conducted in the early 1980s revealed that nude mice compensate for the loss of T cells by increasing the number and strength of other immune functions, including cells with functions akin to micro-sized Pac-Men (and Lady Pac-Men), which gobble up tumor cells or foreign pathogens.[51] Indeed, these changes make the mice less, not more, susceptible to cancer. Among the most pronounced compensatory changes prevailing in nude mice is an increase in a set of cells with a name reminiscent of something out of a Hollywood thriller: "natural killer cells." Their discovery, and the lives of the pioneering scientists who discovered them, were straight out of a Tinseltown script.

## Hungary for a Change

The Kingdom of Hungary was born out of the ashes of the First World War as a result of the breakup of the Austro-Hungarian Empire.[52] Naturally allied with the nearby German-speaking countries, particularly in terms of trade, the new nation aligned herself first with Austria and later with Nazi Germany as part of an effort to restore the glory of the Habsburg Empire (and to unite ethnic Hungarians within a single state). The Eastern European nation remained surprisingly autonomous for much of the war and a faithful ally to Germany, contributing troops to the Nazi invasions of Greece, Yugo-slavia, and the Soviet Union.[53] By the end of 1943, it had become apparent this partnership was no longer in the best interests of Hungary and the rapid advance of Soviet armies to the east compelled Prime Minister Miklos Kallay to begin a secretive parlay with the Allied Powers.[54] As Soviet forces neared its borders, the prime minister and his regent, Miklos Horthy, agreed upon an armistice deal with the allies. However, this was undone when word leaked out to Nazi spies before the deal could be consummated. At this time, Hitler ordered an audacious plan into action.[55] Inviting Horthy to Salzburg, ostensibly to discuss how to better relations between Germany and Hungary, Hitler enacted Operation Margarethe in March 1944, which included the capture of key Hungarian command, control, and communications centers and the kidnapping of Horthy's son as an additional bargaining chip. Under duress, Horthy was forced to discharge Kallay and rescind the armistice with the Allies. Hitler then compelled the regent to install Ferenc Szálasi, formerly the Germanophile Hungarian ambassador to Germany, as prime minister.

Thus began a crackdown in true fascist style, including a roundup of Hungarian Jews, who were forcibly relocated to Auschwitz. Alerted to the atrocities occurring within the Nazi death camps, many Hungarian Jews went into hiding, including the family of a nineteen-year-old medical student by the name of Eva Fischer. The Fischer family received forged papers from an artistic classmate, Janos Szirmai, and managed to take sanctuary within Budapest until the siege and eventual relief of the city by advancing

Soviet armies. As a result of such actions, half the 140,000 Jews in Budapest remained by war's end (which was a grim victory of sorts given the much higher proportion of Jews killed in other German-occupied regions).[56]

Amidst the rubble of postwar Budapest, Eva returned to her studies and met an enterprising and equally brilliant medical student by the name of George Klein.[57] After a brief courtship, George was offered and accepted a position at the Karolinska Institute in Stockholm. With the shadow of the Iron Curtain rapidly descending upon Hungary, George returned to Budapest for one final visit, with the goal of somehow retrieving Eva from an increasingly dictatorial state. With only one day remaining on his visa before he was required to return to Sweden, George and Eva tried to buck the extreme bureaucracy of a postwar Eastern European occupied country and managed to aggregate all the documentation needed to be married. Arriving just as the office of the magistrate was closing, the official tried to shoo them away. After a spate of prolonged and urgent pleading, the magistrate quickly looked through their documents, presumably intent upon finding a loophole to allow him to go home for the weekend. One particular certificate, a voucher indicating both applicants were free of venereal diseases, had been handwritten by one of Eva's colleagues at the Children's Hospital. This amateurish document caught the official so off guard he began laughing with sufficient gusto "tears ran down his cheeks." Apparently impressed by their chutzpa, the bemused official rewarded them with a marriage certificate, which allowed the couple to legally relocate to Sweden.

With this auspicious start, Eva and George Klein embarked on a scientific voyage that would forever change our understanding of cancer and provide the means to begin eradicating the disease. George would go on to demonstrate that a pathogen known as *Epstein-Barr virus*, which causes mononucleosis, can also trigger a distinct form of cancer, Burkitt's lymphoma.[58] His work further showed the disease is characterized by a unique alteration in the chromosomes of the malignant cells. George received many awards for his pioneering research but Eva's contributions to cancer were equally important and are the focus of our present interest.

Eva's specialty was centered upon understanding and growing cells of the immune system in the laboratory. Like George, she became interested in Burkitt's lymphoma and successfully isolated cells from patients with the disease.[59] As we will see in the next chapter, it had been well-established that the immune system of mice could be "primed" with certain vaccines to reject tumor cells, much as occurs following immunization with conventional vaccines for infectious diseases. In the course of isolating different cell populations from the spleen of these mice, Eva and her research team isolated a unique population of cells with the ability to kill tumor cells without the need for vaccine priming.[60] She termed these cells *natural killers* based on their ability to target malignant cells and the name was shortened to NK cells in the years to follow. These NK cells were quite remarkable, not only because they had an apparent "instinct" for selectively killing malignant cells, but because they were distinct from the other major types of lymphoid cells like T cells and antibody-producing B cells.[61] Further work from her group demonstrated NK cells also existed in people and possessed comparable killing activity.[62]

This work on NK cells was being performed coincident with but thousands of miles away from Osias Stutman, but would nonetheless provide direct evidence debunking Stutman's ongoing immune studies of carcinogenicity in nude mice (though it would take decades to conclusively do so).

What neither Stutman nor Eva Klein knew at the time was NK cells also function to kill virus-infected cells. We now know the compensatory changes arising years before in Norman Grist's Scottish laboratory had increased the number of NK cells and thereby allowed nude mice to survive the waves of Coxsackie virus infestations. It would require an additional two decades, from the mid-1970s until the mid-1990s, for this knowledge to come to light and longer to reveal these same changes also rendered nude mice less susceptible to carcinogenicity.[63] The scientific world might have remained utterly blinded to the potential for immune surveillance had not one of the world's greatest tragedies not occurred in the intervening period.

### Spotty Data

Among the ivory towers of academia, a former member of the Harvard faculty, Henry Kissinger, is often remembered for his quote, "The reason that university politics is so vicious is that the stakes are so small."[*] Such

---

[*]    This comment, although attributed by many to Henry Kissinger, may be more accurately credited to Paul Sayre or Woodrow Wilson.

sentiments likely reflected the feelings of the faculty in the Vienna School of Dermatology in 1880 about one of their colleagues.

Moritz Kohn was born in Kaposvar, Hungary, in 1837, but on becoming a dermatologist in Vienna, changed his last name to Kaposi (named after his hometown) because there were so many other Viennese dermatologists with the name "Kohn." The reason for the glut of specialists was Vienna hosted the founder of the field of dermatology, Ferdinand Ritter von Hebra. Von Hebra had founded and run the school responsible for the training of the world's finest skin doctors, who in turn tended to remain in the region. A reason for his colleagues' resentment was the high-achieving Kaposi had married his boss's daughter and already published a seminal book on the field with his new father-in-law. Indeed, Kaposi would rise to replace von Hebra upon his death in 1880, by which time he had already made a discovery, though relatively obscure at the time, that would cause Kaposi's name to become far more common to modern ears than those in his own day.

Back in 19th century Vienna, Kaposi was best known for his descriptions of the skin manifestations of lupus, a deadly autoimmune disease in which the body attacks its own DNA and associated proteins. However, it was a series of patients diagnosed in 1872 who were responsible for even more durable fame. In that fateful year, Kaposi was witness to skin lesions on the feet of five "elderly" men (ages forty to sixty-eight), all of whom shared a skin malady consisting of small, flat bumps (generally the size of a kernel of corn) with a brown to bluish-red hue.[64] Biopsies from these unusual lesions were examined under a simple microscope, revealing a series of sarcoma-like tumors. We now know these tumors are comprised of malignant versions of endothelial cells, which normally line the walls of blood vessels. When these cells became malignant, the integrity of the blood vessels was compromised and the resultant internal bleeding gave rise to the brown- and red-colored tumors. We now know these tumors are triggered by a virus, known as *Kaposi sarcoma-associated herpesvirus* (KSHV), which is related to the pathogen responsible for genital herpes.[65]

Kaposi sarcoma seemed destined to remain a footnote in history based on its exceeding rareness. From its initial description in 1872 until 1950, the cumulative number of cases reported in the United States and Europe did not exceed six hundred, with most cases restricted to elderly men of Mediterranean origin (where the KSHV is most prevalent). In the latter half of the 20th century, the number of cases in Africa swelled suddenly, although relatively little concern was evinced by the Western medical establishments by these distant occurrences.[66] [67] Then, something very strange started happening, first in New York City and then again three thousand miles to the west.

Whereas New York health authorities had not reported a single case of Kaposi sarcoma in the 1970s, Dr. Alvin Friedman-Kien reported in 1981 the New York University Medical Center alone had diagnosed forty-one distinct cases of Kaposi sarcoma in young men between the ages of twenty-six and fifty-one.[68] [69] Indeed, the incidence may have been much higher as most physicians, even at the NYU Medical Center, were not trained to look for these lesions, which can often be small and mistaken for typical bruises. Another unexpected finding was the patients diagnosed were all homosexual men. Kaposi sarcoma soon thereafter gained the nickname of "the gay cancer."

These early observations were among the first signs of the emergence of the HIV/AIDS pandemic, an ongoing crisis responsible for the deaths of 678,509 Americans as of 2014 and still active in the deaths of more than one million people around the world each year. As tragic as this global crisis continues to be, it nonetheless helped reignite ideas on how the immune system functions to combat cancer. This information would succor a small band of investigators, who retained faith in the idea the immune system could be co-opted to combat cancer and it is to this group we now turn.

# 3

## *That Which Doesn't Kill You . . .*

T he foundations of modern cancer therapy emerged from the ashes of two of the most traumatic plagues the world has ever experienced: yellow fever and pandemic influenza. The pathogens responsible for this pestilence unexpectedly redirected the history of medicine and would ultimately provide knowledge to help manage or even eliminate the plague of cancer.

According to recent research, a new virus is believed to have first infected humans in Central Africa approximately 2,500 years ago.[1] Although many may view the Classical period of Greek and Roman hegemony as exceedingly distant, the virus's exposure to humans for a mere two millennia makes it a relative newcomer on a biological timescale. Unfortunately, new pathogens tend to be the most devastating and this is certainly borne out by human experience with this organism.

For most of those two millennia, a virus had taken the time to first take hold and then to devastate the southern two-thirds of the African continent. This localization was perpetuated by the tendency of central Africa at the time to be more sparsely populated and weakly interactive with the rest of the world. Consequently, the virus remained largely unknown until the pernicious growth of African slave trading. By the mid-17th century, the first reports of the infection were reported in the slave-trading colonies of South, Central, and North America. The exchange of people among populations inevitably favors exposure to new diseases (e.g., the Columbian Exchange beginning in the late 15th century virtually exterminated the native populations of the Western Hemisphere). This disease was particularly insidious as it initially manifested itself with conventional symptoms, such as fever and malaise, as a presage for a later and unexpected collapse of internal organ function. The resulting jaundice (a yellowing of the skin and sclera of the eye) arising from a failing liver gave the disease the moniker it holds today: yellow fever.

Over the next 250 years, the incidence of yellow fever took a far larger toll in the New World than the Old, due largely to the fact the more temperate or tropical climes of the Western Hemisphere more closely resemble Africa than Northern Eurasia (e.g., The Tunisian capital of Tunis is further north than Charleston, SC).

Philadelphia was host to one of the deadliest outbreaks in history, which began in 1793 and killed almost one in ten residents of the new nation's capital.[2] Though an extreme case, such extremes became almost routine as yellow fever grew even more frequent and devastating over the following decades, particularly in the Caribbean islands and other warm, humid climates of North, Central, and South America.

A key breakthrough arose in the final quarter of the 19th century with an idea conceived by the Cuban physician, Carlos Finlay (although frequently misattributed to Major Walter Reed of the United States Army). In evaluating the infections arising on the island over the previous years, Finlay deduced the disease was being transmitted throughout Cuba by mosquitos. This subject was covered in greater detail in one of my earlier books but it suffices for our current story to state management of the vector (a particular type of mosquito known as *Aedes aegypti*) was sufficient to largely contain the virus.[3] Although the disease had largely (though not entirely) been managed by measures to control the mosquito population, the virus itself was not isolated until 1927 and even then, the story of this success was tragic.

Adrian Stokes was the fourth generation in a family of physicians.[4] Born in Lausanne, Switzerland, in 1888, his father, John Henry Stokes, had served in the medical corps as a civil servant in India and his grandfather, William Stokes, had gained international renown for saving countless lives during an outbreak of typhus in 1826. Foreshadowing his grandson's fate, William Stokes had contracted typhus and nearly perished. After graduating from medical school and beginning studies of pathology, the young Adrian was soon drafted into service in the Great War, where he gained a well-deserved reputation running a mobile laboratory focused on understanding and preventing the causes of infectious diseases so prevalent in the squalid conditions of the trenches. Among Adrian's specialties was the study of a series of corkscrew-shaped bacterium known as *spirochetes* that tend to be passed along to human via rat vectors. Rats were amongst the few species that actually benefitted from the filthy conditions of trench warfare.

Upon conclusion of the war, Adrian returned to a career at London University Guy's Hospital but duty would soon recall him to the battlefield.[56] This time, the enemy was yellow fever and the conflict was taking place in Lagos, Nigeria. Stokes had been recruited in the early months of 1927 to join a team of medical scientists investigating a hypothesis first proposed by Hideyo Noguchi of the Rockefeller Institute in New York City. Noguchi had been born and raised in Inawashiro, a small town in the Fukushima Prefecture of Japan. As a toddler, Noguchi had fallen into a fireplace and suffered horrific burns to his left hand. Over the following decade, he was subject to many operations, eventually recovering some use of his hand. These experiences led Noguchi down the path to dedicate his life to medicine. However, he became convinced the physical deformities to his left hand would preclude a medical career in Japan. Consequently, Noguchi moved to the United States in 1900 to perform research with Simon Flexner (whom we met in chapter 1). During his time at the Rockefeller Institute, Noguchi identified the bacterial pathogen Treponema pallidum, a spirochete bacterium, in the brains of patients with syphilitic brain disease, a manifestation of the sexually transmitted disease responsible for dementia and paralysis. Although this achievement would be remembered as a notable advance in the war against infectious diseases, scrutiny of his methods revealed suspect rationale and interpretation of much of his work.

From an ethical standpoint, Noguchi's discoveries with syphilis had been facilitated by experimentation on orphan children. The studies overseen by Noguchi had included highly invasive research through intentional exposure of many orphans to syphilis. In part, Noguchi deflected criticism by stating he had not performed any research on the orphans he had not already conducted upon himself. Indeed, by 1913, Noguchi had infected himself with syphilis so many times his own chronic infection would cause neurological pathology and Noguchi would soon begin displaying increasingly erratic behavior, a telltale sign of the brain damage so often associated with syphilis.

Noguchi was charged in 1911 with a felony based on his controversial studies with syphilis and was the subject of high-profile exposés in *Life Magazine* and other publications. Despite these taints, Noguchi was eventually acquitted of the charges, though the stigma remained. Nominated nine times for a Nobel Prize between 1913 and 1927, persistent allegations about the reproducibility of his findings and a broken ethical compass precluded the honor. Worse still, Noguchi's reputation was about to face another body blow, which would preclude any possibility of more Nobel Prize nominations.

Based on his experience with syphilis, Noguchi postulated yellow fever was caused by a new spirochete he had discovered. This work, he claimed, was based upon materials collected during yellow fever outbreaks in Central America. By this time, Noguchi, to be generous, was viewed as diffident and at least one colleague referred to his actions as "erratic" and "paranoid," possibly outcomes from his progressing syphilis. These traits worsened as one study after another failed to reproduce Noguchi's findings with yellow fever, including even internal investigations by fellow Rockefeller scientists using material provided by Noguchi (on the rare occasions he would assent to do so). Facing embarrassment, the Rockefeller Institute sought to resolve a rapidly escalating and openly public dispute among its internal staff and joined by scientists around the world.

In 1927, Rockefeller commissioned a study in Lagos, Nigeria, a region of endemic yellow fever, to try and isolate this bacterium from monkeys displaying the symptoms of yellow fever. Adrian Stokes, who had been working in Guy's Hospital in London, accepted an opportunity to participate in the Rockefeller project and moved to Lagos.[7] Problems arose almost immediately when the Lagos team was unable to identify a spirochete from these monkeys or from human patients with yellow fever. Likewise, the team failed to isolate spirochete-specific antibodies, a telltale sign of an immune response in these animals or patients. Instead, Stokes and his Lagos team found that the agent responsible for the disease could be filtered away from spirochetes and all other bacteria: a definition consistent with what we now know to be a virus. Further work showed this virus could infect mosquitos and thereby transmit yellow fever.

In a particularly awful irony, the conclusive proof this new virus was indeed responsible for causing the disease was revealed to and by Stokes himself, who was bitten by the mosquitos with which he was working. Although Stokes's grandfather had been infected by typhus while at work, he had survived. Stokes himself was not so fortunate and succumbed to yellow fever just as he was verifying the viral identity of his murderer. Following his funeral and burial in Lagos, his colleagues at the Rockefeller compound in Lagos completed the last of Stokes's unfinished experiments and began the process to publish his final paper just as his obituary was being read in newspapers throughout the world.[89]

As a postscript, Noguchi seemed more troubled by the apparent refutation of his identification of a spirochete responsible for yellow fever than by the death of Stokes. He endeavored to travel to Africa and harangued his friend, mentor, and boss, Simon Flexner, to allow him to go.[10] Conceding to the pleas, Flexner relented and by the end of 1927, Noguchi was in Lagos, performing research and traveling back-and-forth to Accra, capital of modern-day Ghana in West Africa and another hot spot of yellow fever. Over the following weeks, Noguchi was frustrated in his efforts to reproduce his own findings linking yellow fever with a spirochete. Heartbroken, Noguchi was traveling from Lagos back to Accra by sea when he began to experience chills and soon thereafter developed a debilitating fever. Within a week, the symptoms had progressed to jaundice followed by the prodigious vomiting of blood, foretelling Noguchi's own death to yellow fever days later.

Although Stokes's manuscript, published in 1928 after his death, was received by the medical and scientific communities with considerable acclaim, buried within this seminal work was an inexplicable finding. The team had actually discovered not one, but two different forms of the yellow fever virus. One variant tended to seek out the tissues of the nervous system, which placed it in a category defined as a neurotropic virus. Infection with the neurotropic form of the virus triggered a terrible but short-lasting fever. As awful as an infection of the brain and spinal cord can be, an even more dangerous form of the yellow fever arose from a viscerotropic (later to be known as a *pantropic*) form of the yellow fever virus, which invaded not just the nervous system but spread to multiple organ systems throughout the body. As such, the pantropic form of the virus was far deadlier, as evidenced by the fact this form of the virus was responsible for the deaths of Adrian Stokes and Hideyo Noguchi.

As the Lagos team was evaluating the different forms of the virus, they noted (but did not emphasize) a puzzling finding[11]: Infection of a monkey with a neurotropic virus tended to protect the animal from infection with the far deadlier pantropic killer. This outcome did not reflect conventional immunity as was known at the time because these protective effects could be seen within hours rather than the days or weeks required to recognize a foreign attacker. The puzzling finding was soon verified by other teams but otherwise remained virtually unexplored for a decade.[12][13]

The discovery of the exotic yellow fever virus was noted with extreme interest by a young Canadian medical student. Born in 1909 into an academic family (his father was an ophthalmologist and his mother the niece of the founder of McMaster University), Frederick Ogden MacCallum immersed himself into the rapidly maturing field of virology.[14] An eighteen-year-old Frederick closely followed the tragic but uplifting story of Adrian Stokes and jumped at a chance to move to London to study virology shortly after graduation. While serving as a researcher at the Medical Research Council of Great Britain, MacCallum almost suffered the same fate as his hero when he contracted psittacosis (an exotic bacterial pathogen able to causes deadly fevers in a wide variety of birds). MacCallum verified the pathogen could cause disease in humans by suffering from its effects himself. Thankfully, MacCallum survived but his close call with psittacosis thereafter convinced him to execute a particularly high degree of cautiousness to protect his personal safety as well as the research teams he would lead.

In 1937, a 28-year-old MacCallum made a discovery, which would unknowingly change the research of viruses and cancer forever. In a series of studies with monkeys and hedgehogs (two species susceptible to infection with yellow fever virus), MacCallum verified the old observation that infection with the neurotropic variant of yellow fever quickly protected these animals from infection by the deadlier form of pantropic virus. The truly unexpected part and major breakthrough was in demonstrating the neurotropic form of yellow fever also prevented these animals from being killed by Rift Valley fever virus as well. Whereas yellow fever is caused by a pathogen from a family now known as *flaviviruses*, Rift Valley fever is caused by a different virus wholly unrelated to yellow fever. This protective effect lasted but a few days and quickly diminished thereafter. These findings eliminated the possibility that exposure to the neurotropic virus might have elicited some sort of immunity. Specifically, the development of protective antibodies or cells would have taken days or weeks to unfold and would have mediated long-term protection thereafter. Exactly the opposite had been observed by MacCallum: a form of protection developed almost immediately but expired within days. Such an outcome was truly unexpected and MacCallum labeled this strange behavior as "viral interference" in which infection with one virus prevents infection by an unrelated virus in the days thereafter.[15]

The timing of this breakthrough was unfortunate as the clouds of war obscured an efficient follow-up. As a rising star in the infectious disease arena and a citizen of one of its primary combatants, MacCallum was given vital roles in developing vaccines against yellow fever and other pathogens likely to be encountered in the many exotic climates that hosted key campaigns of the Second World War. Among his contributions were the identification and separation of two viruses, which he named hepatitis A and hepatitis B viruses (a subject to which we will return in chapter 4). After the war, MacCallum would later develop a vaccine against both of these deadly infectious diseases of the liver. Although a hero for his work on yellow fever vaccines and hepatitis, MacCallum narrowly avoided infamy.

In the months following the attack on Pearl Harbor, the Allied forces were struggling with prioritization of their wartime efforts. Much of the Soviet Union was occupied by Nazi forces and Joseph Stalin and his foreign minister, Vyacheslav Molotov, were clamoring for a second front in Europe. The Americans, still reeling from the loss of their Pacific fleet, were unprepared for such a venture while the British were being pushed halfway across North Africa by Erwin Rommel, the Desert Fox. As a show of appeasement and to foster Allied unity, Churchill elected to visit Stalin in Moscow to explain how these predicaments had necessarily forced a delay of the much-anticipated second front. An adamant Churchill believed delivering the message in person would prevent a widening of the rift between the Soviet Union and its Western allies.

As is often the case in times of war, the public health infrastructure in the Soviet Union was crumbling. Infectious diseases were rampant throughout the Soviet Union and hepatitis pandemics were particularly common all throughout the remaining Soviet-held territories. Churchill's doctors strongly recommended he seek protection via immunization with one of MacCallum's yellow fever vaccines. Churchill, always in a hurry, was troubled to learn the immunization would take weeks to become effective and despite his advisors' pleas, declined to delay the trip and thus refused immunization.[16] In retrospect, this was a little-known, historically crucial decision, as the vial of vaccine MacCallum had intended to administer to his prime minister himself had been inadequately prepared. The same vial would instead be administered to an otherwise healthy Royal Air Force officer, who became deathly ill.[17] Given yellow fever is particularly deadly to individuals with stressed liver function, Churchill's notorious drinking habits (more on that later) help suggest MacCallum would likely have killed the 67-year old prime minister and at a key point just before the Battles of Midway and the First El Alamein, and thereby could have shattered Allied morale and unity, irrevocably altering the tides of history.

*Interfering with Influenza*

Building upon MacCallum's work, we now turn to the second infection-based trauma of the early 1900s, which unexpectedly underpinned radical advances in oncology a century later.

The Spanish Influenza outbreak began in 1917, continued through 1920, and left permanent scars on the psyche of the world's population. The pandemic that might have felled as many as 100 million people world-wide (roughly one in twenty-five of all humans alive at the time) was in fact two different infections working together.[18] First, a particularly nasty variant of influenza virus would either directly kill its victims or weaken them, thereby increasing their susceptibility to a follow-on infection with a bacterium known as *Streptococcus pneumoniae,* which would deliver the coup de grace. In my earlier book, *A Prescription for Change*, I reported how the pandemic drove studies of the obnoxious bacterium and unexpectedly gave rise to a scientific revolution in biotechnology, beginning in the early

1970s.[19] For now, we will focus our attention on how the headliner in this terrible pandemic unexpectedly drove advancements toward a potential cure for cancer.

Beyond horrific pandemic forms of influenza, which naturally arise every few decades (as typified by the Spanish Influenza outbreak), thirty thousand or so Americans perish each year from seasonal influenza virus infection, qualifying it as one of the most persistent and deadly serial killers in the developed world. Such realities have propelled much research into understanding how we might combat the disease. One line of investigation was advanced by a team led by Alick Isaacs and Jean Lindenmann at the National Institute for Medical Research in London.

Alick Isaacs was born in 1921 into a family of Jewish Lithuanian immigrants.[20] His paternal grandfather had entered Britain as a refugee from the pogroms and eventually settled in Scotland, where Isaacs's father was, like most immigrants, determined to make a better life for himself and his family. Isaacs's entry into the world under such tutelage helped encourage an interest in science and medicine. He earned a medical degree with honors from Glasgow University in 1954. During his subsequent studies, he received many honors, including a Rockefeller Travelling Fellowship, which underwrote a voyage to Australia, where Isaacs would be mentored by none other than MacFarlane Burnet (who we met in chapter 2), thereby triggering a lifelong interest in influenza virus.

While studying under Burnet, Isaacs learned the basics of how to study influenza, including the use of chicken eggs as a preferred medium to propagate the virus (indeed, most modern influenza vaccines continue to grow the virus in eggs before they are inactivated). During this time, Isaacs became acquainted with MacCallum's idea of viral interference and was immediately and irreversibly enraptured by the concept. After returning to London, Isaacs continued his research and verified the same behavior applied to influenza virus as well.[21] [22] Moreover, his work demonstrated not only could an active form of influenza virus prevent a cell from becoming infected by another virus, but prior exposure of a cell to an inactive (killed) batch of influenza virus could likewise prevent infection by an otherwise viable influenza virus. This suggested to many researchers at the time that perhaps the dead virus might have somehow engaged with the cells of the body to prevent a subsequent living virus to infect the cells. In this way, one could think of the dead virus as a means to physically block its living brethren.

Two years after receiving his medical degree, Isaacs was joined in London by a young Swiss researcher, Jean Lindenmann, who had traveled to work in London supported by a fellowship from the recently established World Health Organization.[23] The pair began growing viruses in the laboratory not using eggs, but instead deploying the new technique of "tissue culture" in which chicken egg cells were seeded into large bottles and incubated within a large, heated drum. This system provided a more efficient means than eggs to generate massive amounts of influenza virus. This technique was used to collect enough material to allow the investigators to isolate the agent, presumed to be the carcass of a dead virus, which was responsible for the interference phenomenon.

To the surprise of the two scientists, they observed that the exposure of these tissue cultures to dead virus triggered far more interference than might have been expected from the simple competition by dead virus particles. Scratching their heads, Isaacs and Lindenmann were the first to appreciate the carcasses of dead viruses were not the source of the viral interference. Instead, they postulated the chicken cells themselves had produced something able to block influenza virus infection. They named this material "interferon." At first, Isaacs and Lindenmann suspected interferon had an antibody-like function to selectively block influenza. However, follow-on studies revealed the interferon produced in response to influenza could protect against myriad unrelated viruses, thus eliminating the idea this protection had been mediated by antibodies.[24] [25] [26] Within two years, Isaacs's team had purified interferon from virus-infected chicken embryos (the process used to make influenza vaccines).[27] Their work would soon link interferon with cancer.

### Interferons, Evolution & Cancer

Over the next two decades, it was revealed there wasn't one interferon, but multiple and sometimes overlapping systems of different interferons. Some of these interferons were produced by virus-infected cells while others were actively synthesized by the cells of the body's immune system as part of host defense against other pathogens. Yet, all shared the ability to interfere with viruses. In humans alone, there are more than twenty different interferon genes. These different genes have evolved over time to protect us from a constant onslaught of viral pathogens, which were always changing in parallel. In a situation reminiscent of the arms race between American and Soviet superpowers during the second half of the 20th century, the creation of a new interferon put Darwinian pressures on a virus to evolve a means to escape the interferon. As some viruses were successful in doing so, other interferons would evolve in people to address this new threat and so the competition persisted over the millennia.

Along the way, some of these interferons had gained the ability to block the growth of tumor cells. It is unclear whether this arose by mere chance, but it seems likely similar evolutionary pressures propelled the selection for interferon molecules with antitumor properties. Isaacs and Lindenmann's early studies had utilized interferon from virus-infected chicken eggs, but this material produced was relatively crude and expensive to manufacture. Nonetheless, these early studies were promising, particularly when interferon was found to block the growth of tumor cells in mice.[28] Despite the extreme costs needed to treat the average person (who is slightly larger than the average mouse and thus requires a proportional scaling of medicine), a precious reserve of limited interferon, arduously collected through hundreds of hours of toil, was first tested in people within a few years of Isaacs and Lindenmann's first report of its isolation.

Unsurprisingly, the initial focus of early clinical trials emphasized viral infections, which did show some promise. All the while, the potential for utilizing interferon to treat cancer loomed large in the background. Simply put, the high cost and low quality of material collected from the techniques of the day (such as harvesting material from virus-infected eggs) was insufficient for sustainable investigation. Moreover, this lack of reagents threatened to scupper the study of interferon entirely as the subject slowly faded into the background in light of other exciting, contemporaneous subjects. However, interferon would regain its footing and again move to the forefront with support from a remarkable advocate.

Mathilde Galland was born in 1926 near the shores of Lake Como to a Swiss Protestant father and an Italian Catholic mother. Raised in Geneva, she always felt the outsider: a German- and Italian-speaking Protestant in a predominantly French-speaking Catholic environment.[29] As such, she developed a fierce independent streak and had a soft spot for other ostracized populations. As she was matriculating into the University of Geneva, the world was just coming to grips with the realities of the Holocaust. Galland's sympathies, rooted in her own background as an outsider, were captured by the plights of the Jewish people, particularly in light of the international strife associated with the dream of creating an Israeli state. Galland surrounded herself with many Jewish friends in Geneva and became impassioned about Zionist causes in the restive days before the United Nations adopted the controversial Resolution 181, which portioned the British Palestinian mandate into autonomous Jewish and Palestinian territories. These strong sentiments propelled Galland to convert to Judaism and marry a Bulgarian Jewish medical student, David Danon. Danon also happened to be a member of the outlawed Zionist paramilitary group, Irgun. The rebellious but clean-cut former Protestant, Galland soon found herself transporting guns and ammunition back and forth across the Franco-Swiss border on the back of her bicycle as part of a larger effort to smuggle weapons destined for the new state of Israel, which was subject to a weapons embargo by most established world powers. While these dramas were unfolding, Galland was working first toward a bachelor's degree and later a Ph.D. in the field of genetics, which she completed in 1953.

When Danon accepted a job in the nascent Israeli Air Force, Galland took a position at the Weizmann Institute of Science in Rehovot. Despite her relocation to the Middle East and the birth of a daughter, the marriage didn't last, but she remained in Israel and at the Weizmann Institute. As part of her duties, Galland provided tours of the facility to wealthy potential donors. In 1957, a tour of the institute given to a Jewish American attorney would forever change her life.

Arthur Krim was born in New York City, the son of a Russian immigrant who ran a fruit and vegetable stand on the Lower East Side. Krim was a voracious student and graduated from Columbia University in 1930 and stayed on to earn a law degree.[30] These outcomes are particularly impressive given his humble beginnings and the prominent anti-Semitism of Columbia in this era.[31] By the time of his visit to Israel, Krim had risen through the ranks of Hollywood to take the helm of Eagle Lion Films and then to manage the successful turnaround of United Artists, a struggling firm founded by Charlie Chaplin, Douglas Fairbanks, Mary Pickford, and

D.W. Griffith three decades before. Krim helped engineer the production of *The African Queen* and *High Noon* within the first year of his leadership, and the studio quickly became profitable and would dominate Hollywood for years to come.[32]

During a 1957 visit to Israel, Krim became infatuated with the young scientist Galland, who served as his tour guide. They continued a long-distance relationship until 1959, when Galland agreed to move to New York and marry Krim. All the while, she had been performing research in the field of human cancer viruses and had been particularly intrigued by the work of Alick Isaacs and Jean Lindenmann on interferon. Galland sacrificed her research career by moving to America, but the newlywed began a lifelong quest to advocate for medical research in her new position among the fashionable, wealthy, and powerful pillars of New York and Hollywood. Over the two decades following her arrival in America, Mathilde Krim took a strong role advocating for cancer research and was recruited by the Memorial Sloan Kettering Cancer Center to help lead fundraising and increase the visibility of the research conducted there. The power couple held numerous cocktail parties with Manhattan society to raise funding for Sloan Kettering and advance Mathilde's pet projects. These soirees allowed her to raise the funding and prestige for interferon research, culminating in a highly publicized 1975 conference focused on the promises for treating cancer with interferons.

The potential of interferon in cancer was showcased at this Manhattan event and boosted by Mathilde Krim in the months and years thereafter. Receiving the title of the "Interferon Queen," Mathilde's advocacy was at first highly respected but eventually was regarded with growing disdain as critics leveled charges that the promise of interferon she advocated did not match the results of clinical studies. Accusations began resonating that Mathilde had lost her objectivity in a blind advocacy of the potential cancer-fighting properties of interferon.[33][34] Mathilde shrugged off such criticism as bureaucratic politics but her passion began to cross over the invisible line between advocacy and hype. As we will soon see, the drug did not live up to the very high expectations confidently and loudly broadcast by Mathilde and, eventually, even her own powerful advocacy began to wane.

Over time, Mathilde would largely put aside her interests in interferon and would fill this vacuum by embracing a cancer-related subject about which she had become even more impassioned. In the early 1980s, Mathilde began hearing whispers about a strange type of cancer concentrated in Manhattan, afflicting friends, who happened to be homosexuals. This disease, which soon became known as *gay cancer* (Kaposi sarcoma), had been exceedingly rare but cases were suddenly being reported all over New York City. The cancer was one manifestation of a disease we now know to be HIV/AIDS. Although concentrated in New York City even before its more famous spread to San Francisco, the administration of Mayor Ed Koch was still recovering from the depths of the economic crises and deficits New York had suffered in the 1970s and the city largely ignored the quickly escalating health crisis. To fill this void, Mathilde mobilized her energies and resources to help raise awareness and funding to combat the new epidemic and, in doing so, became even more well-known for her advocacy of HIV/AIDS than for interferon.[35][36] However, it is to the story of the latter which we will now return.

Part of the reason why Mathilde Krim's advocacy of interferon was so invaluable was that for two decades after its initial description in the late 1950s, the production of interferons (there were quite a few from which to choose) had remained prohibitively expensive. Exceedingly deep pockets were needed to underwrite the expenses required for their isolation and purification from virus-infected cells. Moreover, the purification techniques were not only inefficient, but the material was often contaminated with other substances, which is particularly problematic given this interferon had originated from virus-infected cells. Indeed, Krim and other interferon advocates routinely invoked contaminants when a particular clinical trial failed to meet expectations.[37] All this changed with the advent of the biotechnology revolution, which sparked in the early 1970s and quickly gained momentum. The cloning of the various interferon genes meant highly pure, recombinant interferon could be manufactured faithfully in batch after batch. These new interferons were relatively inexpensive, at least compared with how it had been purified previously, and the gene could be manipulated to modify both its production and to improve biological activity.

Given the expectations surrounding interferons, many researchers were impatient to investigate their clinical potential. In the interregnum between the discovery of interferon activity and the availability of recombinant material, scientists took an unusual approach to try and trick the bodies of cancer patients to produce interferons. This was accomplished by injecting cancer patients with killed viruses, which could convey a false impression to the immune system that the body was under attack. This approach proved quite laborious to procure, concentrate, and isolate the virus particulars. Consequently, dead viruses were soon replaced by various chemicals, such as polyinosinic:polycytidylic acid, which could trigger the production of natural interferon in the body in a means that largely showed (though not entirely mimicked) the response following viral infection. These treatments came with their own risks, particularly if the inactivation of the viruses was incomplete, as even a few surviving viral particles could become lethal in cancer patients with weakened immune systems. Unsurprisingly, the approach of tricking the body into thinking it is under attack by a virus proved to be particularly toxic, as an exaggerated immune response would cause spikes in prolonged fever, muscle aches, cramping, and general malaise.

Of particular disappointment for the many patients who suffered through these significant side effects, interferon treatment generally did not ultimately prove widely effective. A small number of patients did see their disease go into remission, but this was all too few and all too brief, often conveying just a few days or weeks of additional survival and at the expense of rather substantial side effects. There were, however, promising exceptions. Particular efficacy was observed for hairy cell leukemia, a rare B cell cancer, where virtually all patients demonstrated a shrinkage of their tumors.[38] Less spectacularly, interferon-based drugs showed promise against other blood cell malignances, such as chronic myeloid leukemia (CML). Indeed, interferon-based medicines were included for a time in the standard treatment regimen, though these would soon be displaced by newer medicines, which were both more effective and less toxic. As importantly, these early patient pioneers in interferon therapy contributed to a rapidly growing understanding about the immune system and cancer, which would eventually translate into breakthrough therapies to benefit future generations.

As compared with the impact of interferons on lymphoid cancers, most results with solid tumors tended to disappoint. This differential responsiveness likely reflects the fact immune-based cells had evolved to be particularly responsive to interferon stimulation. However, there were some exceptions to the general rule of interferons' limited efficacy against solid cancers. For example, certain cancers of the kidney, known as *renal cell carcinoma*, tended to respond quite well and shrink in about one of six interferon-treated patients. While the duration of the effect lasted only an average of four to six months, these outcomes were superior for a disease for which physicians and patients were desperate for any therapy improvements. In the end, a handful of interferon-based medicines were approved by the FDA and continue to be used for diseases, such as renal cell carcinoma, today.[39]

Although interferons themselves did not convey the much-hoped-for panacea for malignant diseases, our understanding of these molecules did provide the foundations for a new science describing how the immune system interfaces with cancer cells. This would ultimately prove essential for facilitating the discovery of truly curative treatments for cancer but before conveying this story, it is necessary to describe another key milestone surrounding a molecule that would overshadow interferon for a time as "the next great thing": interleukin-2.

### Don't Read This If You Like Raspberry-Flavored Foods . . .

In a direct sense, the concepts propelling present-day attempts to manipulate the immune system to target cancer have their foundations in a commercially valuable, nocturnal mammal. The beaver is one of the more highly recognizable mammals in North America, not just because of its cute appearance, but because trade in the creature helped drive early colonization of the more northern regions of the Western Hemisphere, particularly among the French colonies in Ontario and Quebec. Whereas most typical American history books and lectures will convey the beaver pelt as the sole reason for this prodigious trade, this oversimplification neglects a rather uncomfortable fact: Beyond their fur, traders harvested the perineal glands (midway between the anus and the sex organs) to collect an oil-filled sac, and then sold them for a neat profit. Indeed, the government of the Canadian province of Ontario still today includes this greasy product, known as *castoreum*, in their annual auctions of products gathered from native wild animals.[40]

The beaver coat has come into and out of fashion but arguably had its heyday in the Roaring Twenties of the 20th century due to its frequent association with Ivy League grandees. However, most of the same elites who were kept warm by their fur coats during the Harvard-Yale football games were probably unaware the genitourinary fluid seeping from the species adorning their backs were also playing a part in a time-honored tradition that directly appealed to other senses of the rich and powerful.

The castoreum from the Eurasian beaver (Latin name *Castor fiber*) had for millennia conveyed a source of scents and flavorings. In particular, the oily, brown exudate from the anal sac beavers use to mark their territory was a staple for luxuries. Having no direct experience smelling the behinds of beavers myself, I can only pass along the word of others: raw castoreum is extraordinary foul-smelling. This is unsurprising given its role is to help animals mark their territory and most wild creatures generally do not intend to convey a pleasant experience for interlopers but rather a rude warning to stay far away. However, if left to dry for at least two years, the smell becomes less offensive and, to some, quite attractive. When prepared properly, castoreum allows perfumers to create novel fragrances and food flavorings, conveying a "leathery" impression.[41] Indeed, beaver-based castoreum is still routinely used in high-end perfumes, including Chanel Antaeus and Jacques Guerlain's wildly popular fragrance, Shalimar.

In another sense, a distant ancestor brave enough to have decided to taste the aged secretions of a long-dead mammal would have found aged castoreum conveys hints of raspberry and vanilla. Indeed, many high-end foods and drinks today still use beaver castoreum and the FDA certifies this material as safe. Arguably, the most fitting name for a castoreum-based product is a type of vanilla-flavored Swedish schnapps known as *Bäverhojt*, which translates into English as "beaver shout" (presumably since Bäverslem, or "Beaver slime," might not inspire quite the same marketing appeal).

The medicinal properties of beaver castoreum were also quite well known back in the heyday of European beaver trapping, much to the chagrin of the originators of the product. The product had been in the European *materia medica* since Roman times based on its ability to alleviate headaches, seizures, and fever. The Romans also believed the foul smell resulting from the burning of fresh castoreum could induce abortions and address painful menstrual cramps and hysteria (a word based on the Greek term *hysterika*, which means "uterus"). Whereas many traditional natural cures are based more in folklore than research, there may actually be some science behind the use of castoreum. It seems willow tree bark was a mainstay of the diet for a European beaver. It is well-known willow tree bark contains a chemical known as *salicylic acid* (the caustic ingredient of wart medicines, such as Compound-W). Once ingested, metabolic conversion of salicylic acid can create a more popularly known chemical, acetylsalicylic acid. In doing so, high levels of salicylic acid and/or its cousin, aspirin, may explain the medicinal properties widely attributed to beaver castoreum.

Based on the popularity of beaver pelts and castoreum, European beavers were hunted to near extinction and the population has never recovered. As is known to virtually every Midwestern American school child, the French took an interest in the Western Hemisphere in large part because of the beaver trade. At its peak in the first half of the 18th century, a single trading station located at York Factory, near Hudson Bay, processed nearly sixty thousand beaver pelts in 1731 alone.[42] Given this was just one trading center and the English colonies were less known for beaver trapping than their French competitors, one can see how things did not look good for North American beaver by the late 18th century.

As overhunting of the North American beaver (*Castor canadensis*) appeared to fate it to the same outcome as its European cousins, perfumers and chefs were forced to seek alternative sources of scents and oils. Before progressing to telling the story of how this alternative helped ignite the modern-day revolution in immune oncology, we will provide a brief epilogue to assure the reader that a wicked combination of the American Revolution and the brutal displacement of Native Americans (who did the bulk of beaver trapping) from the woodlands of the United States allowed the North American beaver population to rebound. Although the number of animals in the wild still suffer from habitat loss and occasional swings in the popularity of beaver fur (though thankfully not because of castoreum), the animal is now protected in most of its remaining native American habitats. Though once a prominent member on the endangered species list, its prospects for a full recovery look damn good.

A suitable replacement for castoreum was found in the seeds of the *Ricinus communis* plant. Indeed, the more commonly used name of the plant, castor, reflects the connection with beavers. Although castor oil largely lacks salicylic acid, its oil can impart many of the same perfume and medicinal properties. Consequently, approximately 300,000 tons of castor oil are produced each year.[43] Perhaps the most well-known of its medicinal properties is the treatment of constipation. In a far darker time, castor oil was deployed in the 1920s by Benito Mussolini's black shirt fascists to humiliate (and occasionally kill) their enemies, prompting an early slogan of the Italian fascists that their power was backed by "the bludgeon and castor oil."[44]

Beyond the oil, the castor bean also has a comparably shadowy past as the source of ricin, a powerful toxin used by real-life James Bond-like assassination plots by Russian and other irresponsible state actors and terrorists as detailed in *Between Hope and Fear*.[45] Ricin was first described in 1888, arising from the doctoral research of Peter Hermann Stillmark while at the University of Tartu (now known as *Dorpat*) in modern-day Estonia.[46] Stillmark had identified ricin as one of a family of proteins known as *lectins*, which share the ability to bind quite strongly to sugar molecules.

Although meat is not known for its sweet taste, the outer surface of most animal cells are coated in sugars and sugar-coated proteins. These sugars play essential roles governing key decisions by the cell (e.g., whether to grow or die). A key breakthrough for cancer research and our story was the discovery that certain lectins have the ability to bind the sugars on these cells and, in doing so, alter such decision-making. In part, this knowledge helped explain the toxicity of ricin (when the signals cause death) whereas other lectins were beneficial. Key for our understanding of the interplay between cancer and the immune system, a small number of lectins allowed scientists to discover an underappreciated molecule and, in doing so, gave rise to a revolution that first swept immunology and now offers opportunities to cure cancers.

### Going Nuclear

Nineteen sixty was an *annus mirabilis* for a young immunologist at the University of Pennsylvania. A Philadelphia native, Peter Nowell spent most of his life in his hometown, departing only to attend college at Wesleyan University in Connecticut and later for a two-year stint as a young doctor at the Naval Radiological Defense Laboratory (NRDL) in San Francisco.[47] Otherwise, his entire career was spent at his medical school alma mater, the University of Pennsylvania. This Bay-area excursion is worth noting not just because it drew him away from the City of Brotherly Love for a time but because the NRDL had been tasked with analyzing the effects of ionizing radiation on the body. In particular, NRDL was interested in determining the effects of such radiation in causing damage to the DNA found in the nucleus of our cells.[48] As the owner of the laboratory for these studies, the military had intentionally created a unique resource in the form of heavily irradiated warships.

You may recall from hazy films in history class the early days of nuclear testing featured above-ground explosions, often conducted in exotic South Pacific paradises (rendered utterly inhospitable by the fallout). If you look closely at some of the vintage films, you will note the United States Navy had intentionally arrayed obsolete ships at different distances from ground zero to assess both the direct damage from the explosion as well as the effects of radiological contamination arising from the nuclear fallout. What you can't see (even if you squint) is evidence that the navy had placed various laboratory animals on the ships either at the time of the explosion and/or various times after the ships had become irradiated. The purpose of these experiments was to assess the extent of biological damage from the radiation. In particular, investigators harvested the DNA from these animals (from both living and otherwise unwilling volunteers) and measured gross evidence DNA damage.

Given these tests occurred in the 1950s (more than a half century before DNA sequencing technologies could be affordably deployed), the precision of these tests was relatively crude and largely relied on a technique known as *karyotyping*. This technique takes advantage of the fact that the long, wiry strands of DNA (which end-to-end, extend up to one yard long in a single human cell) tend to condense into distinct, densely packed chromosomes just before a cell divides. The average human has twenty-two pairs of chromosomes plus a pair of sex chromosomes (XY for male and XX for female), and the shapes of these condensed chromosomes have been highly studied and thus provide a means to identify gross damage caused by, for example, the ionizing radiation arising from a nuclear blast.

During his time at the NRDL, Peter Nowell had mastered the art of karyotyping. He was eager to apply this laborious technique to painstakingly compare irradiated or diseased cells with "normal" specimens. The idea to be tested was that the condensed chromosomes in irradiated cells (or cells from irradiated animals) would betray gross changes in shape as compared to the chromosomes in non-exposed control animals. Unfortunately, only a small fraction of cells in any given sample are actively dividing and so a karyotyping analysis would entail the assessment of thousands of even millions of cells per sample just to find enough dividing cells to reach any conclusions. Consequently, this technique required hours of backbreaking visual analysis while hunched over a microscope in a completely dark room. Having spent the early part of my career performing similar work, I can confirm one can easily disrupt their circadian rhythm, ensuring a sleepless night complemented with an added bonus of considerable neck and back strain, requiring ample consumption of aspirin (or castoreum, if you happen to have some lying around).

Upon his return to the University of Pennsylvania, Nowell deployed karyotyping to study DNA in cancer cells. One of his major breakthroughs in 1960 was a demonstration of a distinct subset of patients (fewer than one in twenty of individuals with the disease) with chronic myeloid leukemia (CML) displayed a shrunken form of chromosome number 22.[49] This defect was present only in their tumor cells but not surrounding benign cells, suggesting the altered chromosome might be responsible for the disease. Given his passion for his hometown, it is quite appropriate Nowell would name this aberration to commemorate his city. This first identification of the "Philadelphia chromosome" would greatly aid the documentation of those patients with this particular form of CML.[50] [51] Later studies would reveal this gross change triggered an unnatural form of a cancer-causing molecule. Thankfully both for our story and for the many patients diagnosed with CML each year, the discovery of the Philadelphia chromosome would ultimately result in a highly specific and effective cure (a subject to which we will return).[52]

While Nowell would rightfully be celebrated for the rest of his life for this 1960 discovery of the Philadelphia chromosome, a less recognized study conducted in the same year would prove to have an even more lasting impact on cancer. All the while Peter Nowell was working on CML and defining the Philadelphia chromosome, he was also studying a phenomenon associated with lectins.[53] Like contemporary aficionados of karyotyping, Nowell was aware lectins were essentially "sticky" molecules used to agglomerate cells together. This may sound trivial but is an essential tool for those individuals who spend hours, weeks, and years analyzing cells under a microscope. When the technique is perfected, one can get just enough cells within a single field to affect a substantial time savings if you don't have to go searching around the microscope slide to find more cells. It may sound trivial, but requiring seconds, rather than minutes, is much valued, particularly since a typical study often entails the study of thousands of samples. Consequently, the use of lectins greatly improved efficiency (and back health).

One of the lectins used for this purpose is known as *phytohemagglutinin* (PHA), a molecule obtained from castor oil. In a fortuitous accident in 1960, Nowell left a sample of lymphocytes exposed to PHA over the weekend. He was studying lymphocytes because they were easily obtained from the blood and, unlike the more numerous red blood cells, the lymphocytes have DNA and chromosomes whereas the red blood cells do not. Rather than throwing the sample away (which would be the instinct of most investigators), Nowell instead viewed the sample under the microscope and was shocked to see far more lymphocytes than were expected. Although the red blood cells were present at the expected number, the lymphocyte population had expanded rather dramatically. Looking further, Nowell noted a large fraction of these lymphocytes were dividing. He immediately realized this to be a useful technique because, as you may recall, karyotyping is only useful to analyze cells that are preparing to undergo division. The fact PHA could drive a larger fraction of cells to divide meant a large fraction of a sample would be the useful lymphocytes and these cells would be properly "posing" in the right way for his analyses, increasing the efficiency of karyotyping studies.

This observation might have remained a mere footnote and of use only to the tiny subset of squinty-eyed microscopists who earn their keep by studying chromosome shapes. However, Nowell and his colleagues realized the ability to drive the proliferation of lymphocytes could have important scientific and medical applications. Prior to Nowell's discovery, it had been assumed lymphocytes, which comprise only a small proportion (roughly one out of a thousand) of the cells in the blood, were static creatures performing some unknown yet presumably mundane function. Whereas we now understand lymphocytes to be dominant regulators and mediators of the body's defense network, the pioneering scientist, Steven A. Rosenberg, has noted the word "lymphocyte" is nowhere to be found in the index of the 1958 edition of the flagship journal of the American Association of Immunologists, *The Journal of Immunology*.[54]

Nowell's revelations with PHA revealed lymphocytes were capable of dynamic growth, and also allowed scientists to grow enough lymphocytes to beginning studying what they did in the body. This timing arose none too soon as a killer was soon to plague the planet. The murderous villain was HIV, a virus with the ability to infect and kill a subset of lymphocytes known as *CD4 T cells*. Unbeknownst to Nowell or anyone else in the 1960s, HIV was already well on its way to exploiting its own intimate knowledge of lymphocytes as part of a modus operandi to inactivate the body's defenses. This ability to identify and eliminate CD4 T cells increased the ability of HIV to spread within and between people (and becoming the focus of Mathilde Krim's next major advocacy project after interferon, not to mention the final link connecting a weakened immune system to the rise of cancer).

It is quite unsettling to consider the potential consequences for our species had the HIV pandemic begun just a few years prior to when it did. Indeed, it has already been established the disease had jumped from primates to humans coincident with the onset of the First World War. However, the disease essentially sat dormant for a few decades, largely due to the fact transportation in that place and time limited the spread.[5] Had the virus gained hold in a more densely populated area or nearer a major site of international travel, our species might have suffered a very different fate than the relative fortune we experience today.

Over the two decades after Nowell's 1960 study with PHA, progress in understanding how this castor oil–derived compound could promote the growth of white blood cells was frustratingly slow, largely because the scientific understanding of the immune system itself was just beginning. Although medical breakthroughs, such as the smallpox vaccine and various antisera, had been in use for decades prior to the studies of PHA-treated lymphocytes, virtually the entire emerging field of immunology was focused upon antibodies as the primary means by which the body protected itself from foreign pathogens. T cells were considered passé and not worthy of much interest. Indeed, Nowell's contemporaries, many of whom were focused heavily upon antibody research, might have been surprised to know these remarkable assemblages of protein had been produced by one population of lymphocytes, known as *B cells*. However, Nowell's finding with PHA would allow these same investigators not only to stimulate the growth of B cells, but to study T cells, which proved to be as interesting, if not more so, as their B cell brethren.

Among the first studies forming the foundation of this emerging field of immunology, investigators in the months after the discovery of PHA's remarkable activity study soon learned they could elicit a similar induction of lymphocyte growth simply by co-incubating lymphocytes from two unrelated donors. Whereas lymphocytes had seemed to many investigators to be relative quiescent cells, the demonstration that chemicals, such as PHA or mixing lymphocytes from different donors, could elicit such vibrant activity triggered a dramatic awakening. The field of immunology had unknowingly begun a period of frenzied growth to enlighten the world as to the power of the immune system. With this in mind, we now return to a subject, initially broached earlier in our story, about the desire to transplant tissues and organs from one person to another.

The raging growth of lymphocytes first observed in the 1960s was soon linked to the body's decision whether to reject (or tolerate) donor transplants. In the course of dissecting the causes of tissue rejection and coincident lymphocyte growth, investigators discovered the cells responsible for the rejection process (we now know these to be T cells). The T cells had become activated by the presence of perceived foreign interlopers and, as one of their first responses, had secreted a factor into the cell culture media with the ability to alert the lymphocytes around it to prepare for battle.[56][57] In other words, an activated lymphocyte could elaborate a factor to stimulate its own growth as well as the growth of other lymphocytes throughout the body. This same factor could be triggered by treatment with PHA or by mixing lymphocytes from unrelated donors, suggesting that this was a key regulator of the immune response. The identity of this molecule would remain elusive for years but would eventually be revealed by a young expert emerging from the world of interferon research.

### Would You Prefer Red or White?

A year after the description of this soluble lymphocyte growth factor produced following PHA stimulation, a young Kendall A. Smith graduated from Denison University and matriculated just up the road as a medical student at The Ohio State University in Columbus. While crossing the campus's main quadrangle (called The Oval) in 1967 as a third-year medical student, Smith struck up a conversation with another colleague nearing graduation. Rather than being excited to start their careers, both men fretted leaving the relative protection provided by the campus. The Vietnam War was near its peak and Ohio State was a hotbed of anti-war sentiment (indeed, the campus would

erupt into violence in the days following the May 1970 Kent State mas-
sacre, causing the National Guard to quarantine the campus and triggering
the paving of all streets to prevent the underlying bricks from being pried
up and used as projectiles). In the course of this spring 1967 conversation,
Smith learned selected medical students could perform a research internship
sponsored by the National Institutes of Health (NIH) at various research
institutions across the nation. This service to the nation could substitute for
military service and thereby allow them to avoid military duty in Southeast
Asia. As similar concerns about fighting in Vietnam had hardened the resolve
of many of his contemporaries, Smith quickly appreciated the competition
for these few research slots would be particularly fierce.

Though he was at the top of his class, Smith seized upon his friend's
advice and sought to gain much-needed experience in research, which might
distinguish his NIH research internship application from those of others. He
found a sponsor in Dr. Charles Mengel, the director of hematology at the
Ohio State Hospital. Mengel had been a bit of a wanderer, being recruited
to Ohio State from Duke University just a few years before, and would
leave the Buckeye State at the same time as Smith to chair the department
of medicine at the University of Missouri.

Unlike the research institutions of contemporary times, the fraction of
medical school faculty performing research in the late 1960s was quite small.
Mengel was an exception and had a vibrant laboratory studying hemolysis
(the science behind understanding the causes and effects of red blood cell
destruction). Although his initial motivation to explore medical research
may have been a bit suspect, Smith's early experiences working with Mengel
turned him into a complete research convert. In his final year, Smith performed enough research to publish a scientific manuscript coauthored with
Mengel.[58] In return, Mengel recommended Smith for a two-year, NIH-
funded research internship at Yale University followed by a two-year stint
at the National Cancer Institute (NCI) in Baltimore, Maryland.[59]

During his research internships, Smith was introduced to the interplay
between viruses and lymphocytes, which inevitably entailed exploring
the role of interferons. These experiences led to a later fellowship in Paris,
where he continued his studies of lymphocytes and began a collaboration with another American ex-patriot, Torgny Frederickson, who was on
sabbatical from the University of Connecticut.[60] The two researchers had

shared experiences in Connecticut and in red blood cell biology and these common interests favored a collaboration focused on identifying soluble growth factors responsible for the promotion of erythrocyte production. The collaborative studies would culminate in the discovery of erythropoietin, a natural protein that selectively promotes the manufacture of red blood cells (without affecting white blood cells). This protein (better known for its shortened name, Epo), would later be approved to treat the anemia, a lack of oxygen-carrying red blood cells, which frequently plagues cancer patients undergoing chemotherapy (and would gain far more notoriety as the preferred doping agent abused by Lance Armstrong and as heartily endorsed by the Russian Olympic team).

Following the discovery of Epo and its effects on red blood cells, Smith would also deploy the experiences gathered during studies of red blood cell growth to identify the protein responsible for the proliferation of white blood cells. He returned from Paris to a faculty position at Dartmouth and, as is often the custom in academia, would later invite a more senior colleague to give a talk on their work. The speaker was Robert Gallo, a NCI scientist, who would go on to discover retroviruses and garner considerable controversy in the 1980s as a codiscoverer of the virus responsible for AIDS.[61] [62] At the time Smith invited Gallo to speak at Dartmouth, the nation was celebrating its bicentennial and Gallo was publishing work on the isolation of a crucial growth factor that promoted the growth of T cells.[63] [64] Smith and Gallo exchanged ideas on the best way to identify and characterize this molecule, ultimately leading to an invitation by Gallo for Smith to come to NCI and conduct some experiments with Gallo's NCI team. The productivity of this visit was almost destroyed when Smith learned upon his arrival from Gallo that the key cells responsible for the production of the magical growth factor had been killed as a result of a freezer malfunction. However, the visit was saved because this unfortunate mishap allowed Smith to meet Frank Ruscetti, a scientist who also was working with Gallo.

Together, Ruscetti and Smith initiated a series of experiments meant to recapitulate the biological activity propelling the growth of T cells. This activity had first been identified by the Gallo team but was soon lost following the freezer failure.[65] Gallo, who has a reputation as a fierce competitor, had tried to block a partnership he may have regarded as not in his own best interest, and urged Ruscetti to work with another NCI researcher,

Ronald Herberman. However, the collaboration between Ruscetti and Smith persisted over the protests of their more senior colleague and resulted in the identification of this vital factor.

This new protein could allow investigators to grow T cell lines in the laboratory. Although Ruscetti and Smith had described the biological effects of this T cell growth factor, its identity remained elusive and would remain so for years since there were vanishingly few T cells from which the molecule could be purified. Nonetheless, they persisted and pooled as many sources of T cells as they could find and seized upon the emerging technology of monoclonal antibodies (the subject of chapter 6) to help them purify the growth-stimulatory factor from these T cells. The identity of the magical substance was finally revealed in the early 1980s.[66] [67] Although it was the first T cell growth factor identified, this substance would forever be known as *interleukin-2* (IL-2). This downgrading of its name reflected the fact another lymphoid factor had been found to be able to induce IL-2 production (i.e., IL-1 leads to IL-2, etc.).

Despite the years of agonizing work required to generate enough material to analyze, IL-2 soon became plentiful within months after its first formal description. The sudden availability can be credited to a combination of science, free market incentives, and luck. On the side of science and luck, the coincident advent of recombinant DNA technologies meant, once the gene had been cloned, recombinant IL-2 could be generated in bacteria and other systems en masse. The economic incentives logically followed upon the hype and hope accompanying the discovery of IL-2, a substance able to induce the body's immune system to effectively combat cancer. These emotions carried the day starting in the 1980s but did not go entirely according to plan and, indeed, almost derailed the looming benefits of immune-based cancer therapies altogether.

We will now turn to the antagonist in this story, one of the world's oldest and most deadly villains, and see how this culprit nearly claimed immune oncology as one of its many victims.

*Burrowing into Moles*

A discussion of body piercing seems rather a severe tangent in a work focused on cancer but the connections are surprisingly intimate. Beauty marks are not just a recent fad but have remained in vogue for centuries, being first referred to by Alexander Pope in his 1712 poem, *The Rape of the Lock*, and modern equivalents have positively influenced the celebrity of supermodels, such as Cindy Crawford, and actresses including Marilyn Monroe.[68] Indeed, these signature looks have inspired the sincerest forms of flattery, which range from simple make-up fixes (using eyeliner) to more invasive body piercings with circular or shaped gold studs.

The presence and patterns of moles has a rich history even beyond the aesthetic as, for example, the pattern of moles on the torso of a two-year-old boy, Lhamo Thondup, convinced a team of pilgrims in 1933 they had at last identified the modern incarnation of a religious leader, the man who today still represents Tibet to many as the fourteenth Dalai Lama.[69] Similarly, disparate cultures in the Eastern and Western world have long used the presence and patterns of moles on the body as sources for divination.[70] [71]

What these imitations seek as a source of divine inspiration are in fact a potential killer. The medical term for a mole is a melanocytic nevus. This particular moniker likely causes pause to most readers since it embeds the term *melanoma*, one of the deadliest forms of cancer. The cancer known as melanoma has been documented as far back as Hippocrates's description during the Classical period of ancient Greece.[72] Although reports of this deadly disease have blackened medicine throughout history, it remained a rare disease until relatively recently. In the past half century, however, the incidences of melanoma have skyrocketed, particularly in fair-skinned Americans and northern Europeans, presumably due to an ironic desire to achieve a "healthy tan."[73]

High-profile patients, such as Senator John McCain, have waged high-profile battles with the disease, though the victims of melanoma are not limited to Caucasians or indeed to lesions on the head or upper torso due to a failure to wear proper covering. For example, an otherwise healthy, 32-year-old Jamaican singer noticed a mole growing under his toenail one day in 1977. Ignoring advice from his doctor to have the toe removed, the singer was basking in the attention received for his landmark album, *Exodus*, and preparing for a world tour. Instead, he elected for minimal intervention and within four years, the world had lost the Rastafarian legend Robert Nesta "Bob" Marley.[74]

Part of the reason why melanoma is so dangerous is its ability to metastasize throughout the body. As such, elimination of the original tumor (e.g., Bob Marley's toe) may be insufficient if the disease has already spread from this primary site. Historically, a diagnosis of melanoma has been a virtual and irreversible death sentence. Despite innumerable attempts, few if any medicines had ever shown promise in stopping the disease and even the few that had only increased average life expectancy by mere days or perhaps a few weeks.

What was needed to fight such a disease is a body-wide mobilization of cancer-fighting potential. This was the conclusion of a New York-born physician by the name of Steven Rosenberg at the NCI, who realized broad stimulation of the immune system provided such an opportunity. Rosenberg was responsible for an audacious series of clinical trials. Though suffering from initial setbacks, this work would later be realized as a foundation for a new field allowing some physicians to cautiously contemplate and even at times whisper the "c-word" for melanoma: cure.

As he related in a book cowritten with John M. Barry, Rosenberg was born in the Bronx into a Polish immigrant family, which eked out a living running a group of luncheonettes.[75] His working-class roots translated into a strong work ethic and served the Rosenberg family as both he and a brother endured the training needed to start a career in medicine. Following an intensive six-year program encompassing both undergraduate and medical training at Johns Hopkins, Rosenberg moved to Boston, where he performed both his clinical residency and received a Ph.D. in biophysics. In search of a career in which he could blend his love of medicine and research, Rosenberg accepted a position at the NCI in 1970. Despite high-profile offers to be the chief of surgery at the prestigious Dana-Farber Cancer Institute, Rosenberg remained at NCI for the rest of his career (becoming chief of surgery there in 1974 at the still-tender age of thirty-four).

Along the way, Rosenberg became thoroughly engrossed by the body's natural ability to cope with cancer. Inspired by a 1968 case in which a patient had survived for decades despite the presence of metastases all throughout the liver, he realized the immune system must have risen to the challenge and eliminated the cancer (a surgery Rosenberg conducted twelve years later revealed no trace of the disease and the procedure performed was only needed to remove an inflamed gallbladder).[76] [77] His passion for understanding why this patient had so thoroughly recovered from what should have been a fatal disease almost led Rosenberg to call off his engagement to his future wife as he feared family obligations might distract him from his passion to perform cancer research. As is usually the case, diligence itself is insufficient to ensure scientific and medical breakthroughs and often requires the added assistance of patience and good fortune. A prominent example of this can be seen with his experiences with IL-2.

In the days immediately following the identification and cloning of the magical substance with the ability to induce lymphocyte growth, Rosenberg partnered with Cetus Corporation (a start-up company considered by many to be the first biotechnology company) to explore its potential new medicine. For almost half a decade, Rosenberg tested IL-2 in patient after patient, sixty-six in total, without achieving any meaningful impact on their diseases. Actually, the results were arguably far worse, as the IL-2 itself was toxic and some patients were succumbing to the extreme side effects of treatment. All this would change and in dramatic fashion at a time when most of the nation's attention was focused upon the presumed reelection of President Ronald Reagan.

Around the time of Reagan's first election in 1980, a 29-year-old naval officer, Linda Taylor, was in training at the Defense Intelligence College and reported to the infirmary after noting a dark, irregularly shaped mole on her back.[78] The diagnosis was melanoma and after surgical removal, the young officer was informed there was a one-in-two chance it could return.

Return it did. In the summer of 1984, Taylor was serving in Guam, when dark shapes again appeared, this time not one, but three—tumors indicating a violent return of the disease. She was evacuated stateside to family outside Pensacola, and was hoping to receive treatment at an Air Force hospital in nearby Biloxi. However, this hope was countermanded when a superior officer sent her to the Bethesda Naval Center, in Maryland. Another federal organization, the NIH, was immediately across the street, and Linda would have been treated exclusively by naval doctors had luck not intervened. To her good fortune, an NIH-based doctor was present and informed her of an NIH team assessing the effects of interferon on melanoma in clinical trials being conducted just up the road in Frederick, Maryland. Unfortunately, the interferon was ineffective, and she was given only months to live. Her medical file was stamped, "Death Imminent" as additional melanoma lumps proliferated across her body.[79]

Back in Bethesda, Rosenberg had been dealing with one failure after another with his IL-2 therapy but remain undeterred. Although Taylor was steeling herself for the inevitable, she met with Rosenberg and agreed to participate in his IL-2 study. Not responding to the conventional dosing levels Rosenberg had relied upon up to this time, he dramatically increased the dose of IL-2 Linda would receive. This was a particularly bold decision as, you may recall, the drug itself was likely responsible for hastening the deaths of some trial participants.

Linda Taylor, as a robust naval officer, withstood the tortuous treatment, whose side effects were comparable to the worst case of influenza one could imagine and included extreme fever, chills, and swelling all throughout her tissues. By mid-December, she was allowed to return to her family in Pensacola, but the unmistakable black and swollen tumors still covered her body. As she recovered, one noticeable improvement was no new tumors had formed. Moreover, upon a return visit to Bethesda, a biopsy revealed the blackened masses of melanoma nodules no longer had any living cells—the malignant cells within had been killed by an IL-2-induced lymphocyte frenzy. Another few weeks were required for the body to absorb and clear the debris from these dead masses, and the tumors soon began to fade away. Further testing revealed the cancer remained in remission (the word "cure" was and is still a hard word for most of us in the cancer profession to contemplate), and has remained so for the three decades since her IL-2 therapy began.

Taylor's response to IL-2 therapy was truly remarkable but sadly a rare oasis in a desert of melanoma treatment failures. Over time, the extraordinary optimism born from Taylor's experience began to fade and IL-2 as a stand-alone therapy was largely abandoned, even by stalwarts like Rosenberg himself, based upon insufficient responses. Nonetheless, IL-2 was incorporated into therapeutic regimens along with other more conventional chemotherapeutic medicines. Rare cases like Taylor's convinced Rosenberg and other cancer researchers of the potential for immune-based therapy if only the immune system could be induced to kill the cancer in a more safe and effective manner. This would require later breakthroughs, but at last, an opportunity to cure cancer seemed within sight.

# 4

## *Deadly Sins*

As promised in the introduction, this chapter begins with drinking and, as is often the case, ends in sex.

For the story to move forward to fulfill the early promise arising from studies of IL-2, it must again move backward a bit. When we last left off with Frederick Ogden MacCallum (F.O. to his friends), the scientist who had discovered viral interference, he had barely avoided infamy when Churchill refused to be immunized with MacCallum's yellow fever vaccine. You may recall the particular batch with which MacCallum was planning to inject Churchill had a propensity to cause an inflammatory disease of the liver, widely known as *hepatitis*. This would likely have been fatal for a notoriously heavy drinker like Churchill.

Reportedly, a typical Churchillian day began with an early morning "mouthwash" of whiskey and soda followed by a pint-sized bottle of champagne at lunch and a glass of cognac.[1] Perhaps unsurprisingly, he would then nap and awake to a tumbler always filled (again) with whiskey and soda and work until an aperitif of sherry before dinner, which of course included a second pint of champagne. His after-dinner work schedule included a glass of port or brandy. As an aside, despite all of this work, Churchill remains one of the most accomplished politicians and prolific writers in history. As unique and exceptional as Churchill's accomplishments have remained, far more impressive is the story of his liver, which endured and overcame hardships that would and indeed usually does kill the vast, vast majority of people who have shared his habits. Whereas many famous people have had their brains preserved for future analysis, in the case of Churchill, one might have pickled his liver for future study as well (especially as the liver was quite accustomed to being pickled). However, it is safe to say, with all the damage alcohol imprints upon the liver, an acute case of hepatitis would undoubtedly have felled the great man.

The liver is an extraordinarily complex organ, whose functions include the clearance of toxins in the body. Many of these toxins are a natural outcome of life, being the waste products of metabolism by the trillions upon trillions of cells in the body. One example, well known to many, is the consumption of ethanol. If left unchecked by the liver, the presence of alcohol would swell the cellular membranes in the body (including those in the brain, causing the sensations associated with intoxication).[2] When the membrane swelling reaches a literal breaking point, the cells rupture. For those prone to consume excess alcohol over a relatively short term (from days to a few years), the liver can respond to repeated insults by manufacturing more of the enzyme tasked with neutralizing ethanol (alcohol dehydrogenase), precipitating the well-known phenomenon of alcohol tolerance. However, the need to focus on one activity necessarily means the liver has fewer resources to devote to other detoxifying activities (such as poisons in the environment or radical-containing metabolism by-products), thereby sensitizing the body to damage from other natural and environmental toxins.

Even the extraordinary capacity of the liver to adapt to this constant assault can become overwhelmed. First the organ and then the body begin to flail as a consequence of the death throes of an increasing number of cells. The liver itself becomes and early victim as instead of detoxifying these toxins, the cells of the organ succumb to the damage.

Analogous to the damage caused by a cut or puncture of the skin, the death of a large numbers of liver cells causes scars to form and these remnants of prior damage increasingly disrupt the architecture of the liver and, in doing so, cut the tissue off from its sources of oxygen and nutrients. Yet the liver continues to fight back, and one response is for the organ to simply to grow as rapidly as possible in an attempt to replace these lost regions. Unfortunately, the new tissues are far less efficient and the growth continues. As the rate of damage is likely to persist (unless the drinker accepts complete abstinence), the organ can swell to many times its original size and yet never achieve the efficiency of its younger self. One example of this is the propensity of alcoholics to suffer from cirrhosis of the liver, which can be characterized by a swollen abdomen caused in large part by an outsized liver. Eventually, the liver will be unable to cope, and its failure is shown first by the classical symptoms of jaundice (a yellowing of the skin and eyes).

The situation can become far worse when these same liver cells come under assault from outside predators, and this is where F.O. MacCallum rejoins our story. As the frequency of tainted yellow fever vaccine increased, MacCallum became increasingly uneasy about the implications of the trend. For example, the United States Army suffered one of its largest setbacks in the early days of the Second World War, when more than fifty thousand soldiers were infected by a batch of contaminated yellow fever vaccine and began to show signs of jaundice, a sure sign of hepatitis. This outbreak occurred just as the nation was trying to recover from the psychological and military consequences of the bombing of Pearl Harbor (not to mention the loss of the Philippines and fears of an impending invasion of the West Coast). The outbreak of hepatitis threatened to become an existential crisis as thousands of troops were bedridden at a time when invasion fears gripped the West Coast of the United States and the northern coast of Australia. Consequently, the hepatitis outbreak sidelined a large number of troops, which could not be deployed to war zones. MacCallum's concern about such events mixed with confusion because the contamination caused a type of jaundice seemingly unlike anything seen before (ironic given the vaccine was intended to prevent a different form of jaundice caused by yellow fever).

A diagnosis of hepatitis itself was not a particularly new idea and references to an indication known widely as *catarrhal jaundice* had been cited as far back as Classical Greece and Rome.[3] In these cases, however, the manner by which hepatitis was transmitted had implicated contaminated foodstuffs. The disease witnessed (and indeed caused) by MacCallum was quite different.[4] This contamination was associated with the human blood products used to generate the yellow fever vaccine. In hindsight, we now know reports of an indication referred to as an "icterus epidemic" had been published as early as 1885.[5] In that case, the jaundice was linked to a serum-derived smallpox vaccine responsible for sickening hundreds of German dockworkers in Bremen. Intrigued by the dichotomy differentiating between a food-borne versus a serum-borne form of hepatitis, MacCallum began studies to further distinguish the diseases and their causes. He was quickly able to eliminate a bacterial cause of either disease, as serum (or contaminated foods) remained contaminated even when passed through the most sophisticated filters of his day (and which removed virtually all bacterial pathogens). Such a finding meant the mysterious biological entity must be among the mysterious substances known at the time as "viruses."

In these early days, the term *virus* was a bit of a catchall, reflecting nonbacterial pathogens that shared the property of being so small they could not be seen with conventional microscopes. Although scientists knew viruses were not intact bacteria, that demarked the extent of their knowledge, and many conceded these perplexing pathogens might not exist at all. For example, they could not distinguish whether these viruses reflected a non-filterable toxin released by a bacterial pathogen or a new form of submicroscopic life. For a time, the term *viruses* remained the default response to the question of the causes for infections in which a bacterial pathogen could be eliminated.*

Given this assumption of a "viral" cause, in 1945 MacCallum began referring to the different causes as infective hepatitis viruses or serum hepatitis viruses.[6] As these terms themselves created confusion as both described seemingly different causes for otherwise similar infectious diseases of the liver, he later changed the designation to "hepatitis A" and "hepatitis B" viruses, respectively, monikers still used to this day.[7]

Although first described in 1945, decades were needed for the maturation of the scientific and technological prowess necessary to isolate and

---

* Beyond viruses, certain infectious proteins, known as *prions*, could also have played a role in disease transmission. As luck would have it, these even more exotic pathogens were neither known at the time nor were responsible for the hepatitis observed by MacCallum.

characterize the hepatitis viruses. For example, the hepatitis A virus was seen for the first time using an electron microscope in 1973, revealing an elaborate icosahedral-shaped protein containing RNA (not DNA) as its genetic material.[8] In this same time period, the city of Philadelphia again enters our story as the setting for a most unusual way in which the hepatitis B virus came to be identified.

## Invisible Needles

The discovery and eradication of the hepatitis B virus was made possible by a scientist who emerged from a working-class neighborhood in the Flatbush section of Brooklyn. This locality was a collection of ethnic enclaves and is arguably best known now for the fact its accent gave inspiration to Mel Blanc for his distinctive voicing of the cartoon character, Bugs Bunny.[9] A young, third-generation Jewish immigrant, Baruch Samuel Blumberg was the son of an attorney and became interested in mathematics and science following immersion within exceptional public high schools in Brooklyn (James Madison High School boasts among its alumni senators Bernie Sanders and Charles Schumer as well as Justice Ruth Bader Ginsberg and the entertainers Carole King and Chris Rock) and Queens (Far Rockaway High School alumni include physicist Richard Feynman and financiers Carl Icahn and Bernard Madoff).[10]

Although originally drawn toward math, Blumberg became impassioned by the science and application of medicine upon matriculation to Union College, receiving his medical credentials from Columbia University in 1951. His particular interest was in understanding the differences among people and how this impacted their susceptibility to disease. Such understanding was evolving in the 1950s with the recognition of minor genetic differences that could distinguish amongst individuals as well as differences amongst different populations based on geography or ancestry. This seemingly esoteric science would enthrall Blumberg as it was becoming clear these minor genetic differences were not simply mistakes in DNA but had evolved for some unknown purpose. An examination of these subtle differences suggested they might provide an advantage only in a particular geographical context or under uncommon circumstances that perhaps had long since been extirpated by modern society or diluted by long-distance travel. Consequently, assigning a function, if any, to such genetic variation was not (and still is not) easy work. Despite and perhaps because of these challenges, Blumberg persisted in his endeavors and this dedication would ultimately save or improve the lives of countless millions worldwide.

According to the venerable Oxford English Dictionary, the term *polymorphism* was first recorded in 1839 as a means to describe something arising in several different forms. The word was hijacked by Charles Darwin to describe the array of subtle differences between individuals, which cumulatively drive evolution.[11] A full century later, the term was further co-opted by the British evolutionary biologist Julian Sorell Huxley (who also founded the World Wildlife Fund) to indicate differences in the composition of a particular gene, able to distinguish one individual within a species from another.[12] It was this version of the word that so intrigued Blumberg, largely as the result of a service trip he undertook with Harold Brown, a Columbia professor, between his third and fourth years of medical training.

During the summer of 1950, just as Communist forces were crossing the 38th parallel in a surprise attack on their southern neighbors in the Republic of Korea, Blumberg was immersed in the South American country of Suriname. Dominated by dense tropical forests, the country had for many years been a blend of indigenous populations and colonists from northern and western Europe. The climate favored an economy based upon sugarcane farming, a labor-intensive crop dependent upon the forced labor of slaves. Following the abolition of slavery by Dutch overlords in 1863, the nation began importing indentured laborers from other Dutch colonies in modern-day Indonesia (and later from India when a British presence became dominant). By the time of Blumberg's arrival, Suriname had also recruited laborers from China and a variety of Middle Eastern nations.

Given this mishmash of peoples from across the planet, Suriname provided an ideal location to evaluate the similarities and differences in how people responded to disease. Though Blumberg, as a medical trainee, was still learning the basics of his intended profession, he and his professor noted certain ethnic populations tended to differ in terms of their susceptibility to infectious agents. For example, certain individuals or nationalities tended to be more prone to lymphatic elephantiasis (a disfiguring condition caused by mosquito-borne worms, *Wuchereria bancrofti,* which cause dramatic swelling to the lymph nodes and surrounding tissues). These genetic differences intrigued Blumberg as he completed his medical training and decided upon the next steps to devote his budding career to such studies.

The next few years for Blumberg were divided between serving as a physician at New York's Bellevue and Columbia Presbyterian Hospitals. All the while, his intrigue about the emerging science behind genetic variations and disease susceptibility progressively expanded. In 1955, he left the United States to begin doctoral studies in biochemistry at Oxford University, where he evaluated polymorphisms in both animals and people. During this time, Blumberg traveled the globe in search of blood specimens from individuals separated by thousands of miles. His intention was to inquire whether there were differences able to predict susceptibility to particular ailments.

By definition, a polymorphism is a subtle change in DNA that may (or may not) relate to a noticeable change in biology. The DNA from a single human cell can be stretched to a length greater than a yardstick and at the time, DNA sequencing technologies were nonexistent. Consequently, Blumberg faced the challenge of trying to identify tiny differences akin to the proverbial needle in a group of one hundred haystacks, which may be further compounded by seeking an invisible needle. Rather than sampling enormous numbers of people at random from around the world, Blumberg soon developed an innovative approach meant to maximize the likelihood of identifying polymorphisms. His idea was to take advantage of the fact the immune system had evolved to recognize and eliminate such subtle differences between people by producing antibodies. These antibodies were known to play a role in the rejection of tissues grafted from one individual to another (along with T cells, which we now know to be the primary mediators of rejection). Blumberg therefore reasoned if a person's immune system has been exposed to the polymorphisms from another individual, then the person would generate antibodies against this foreign substance. In thinking about how one person might be exposed to the differences in another, he considered the still rather new medical procedures of blood transfusions. Although most people go through life without ever receiving blood from another person, some do and at a high frequency. A key question was to identify a group of people whose blood had been frequently exposed to the blood of others. Blumberg reasoned these people would likely have made antibodies against the features of others, which differed from themselves.

## *A Bloody Mess*

In the years following the decline of the Western Roman Empire, an era commonly referred to as the Dark Ages, the practice of medicine virtually collapsed throughout most of Europe. We can all recall vivid, albeit implanted, mental images of dank, muddy villagers or even high nobility being treated with leeches or literally bled to death. A stark exception arose in the lands conquered by Arab invaders, who spread the new religion of Islam starting in the 7th century C.E. Whereas the cumulative knowledge developed by the Greeks and Romans and passed down in the form of texts and manuscripts (most of which had been largely lost in the Christian world), these texts had been studied and translated into Arabic during the Islamic Golden Age (from the 8th to the 13th centuries) in some places, such as the House of Wisdom in Baghdad.[13] Rather than continue its steady erosion as experienced in the West, the scientific basis of medicine continued to make great strides in the Islamic world. A prominent example is exemplified by an Andalusian physician by the name of Abu al-Qasim Khalaf ibn al-Abbas al Zahrawi (or Al-Zahrawi for short).[14] Although this 10th-century physician from the Iberian Peninsula is best known as the modern "father of surgery," he enters our story based on his observations that a propensity for excessive, and sometimes lethal, bleeding disorders tended to cluster within certain families and to be passed along to new generations.

Al Zahrawi's observations were an early rational evaluation of a disease commonly known today as *hemophilia*. Hemophilia is arguably best known for its prominence in the royal courts of Europe, as passed along by Queen Victoria to her many offspring, who would eventually rule the courts of Britain, Germany, Russia, and Spain and pass the genetic susceptibility to the disease along to each.[15] Indeed, the rise of the fascinating but troubling figure of Grigori Rasputin, who catalyzed the demise of the Romanovs, was attributed to his apparent (though inaccurate) ability to manage the hemophilia of the only male royal heir of the Russian line, Alexei Nikolaevich.[16]

The primary cause of hemophilia is the transmission of a polymorphism impairing the function of one of the twelve factors in the blood responsible for clotting. Setting aside Rasputin's mystical approach to treating hemophilia (which did not actually work), the diagnosis of hemophilia was essentially a death sentence as even the most incidental mishap could cause disproportionate bleeding, both externally and within the body.

A breakthrough therapy for the disease arose with the supplementation of a hemophilic patient's blood with blood or blood products obtained from healthy donors. The English physician William Harvey had attempted the first blood transfusion at St. Bartholomew's Hospital in London in the mid-17th century and more than two centuries later, another London physician, Samuel Armstrong Lane, used the technique to treat hemophilia. However, transfusions were exceedingly risky due to the risk of rejection, much as we have seen with organ transplants.

The ability to transfuse blood from person to person without rejection had been enabled for widespread use by Dr. Karl Landsteiner's discovery in 1900 of the ABO blood group system, another set of human polymorphism. The ABO system reflects a subtle change in how carbohydrate chains are added to certain red blood cell proteins and critically controls whether donated blood will be compatible in a recipient.[17] The ability to recognize compatibility arising from this set of polymorphisms, eventually facilitating the widespread adoption of blood transfusions. As Blumberg realized, a hemophiliac would therefore be exposed to blood from many different donors. As the body's immune system had evolved to distinguish self from non-self, Blumberg appreciated hemophilic patients would likely generate antibodies distinguishing between their own genetics and polymorphisms found in the blood of their donors. Blumberg's goal was therefore to isolate and characterize these antibodies.

Blumberg isolated antibodies from sufferers of hemophilia and anemia who had received transfused blood components. He then began to ask if any of these antibodies could distinguish amongst different people. Stated another way, the question was whether exposure of the patient to the blood of another person had triggered the production of antibodies able to identify subtle differences between the blood donor and recipient. This work began in earnest after Blumberg's return to the United States to accept a position at the NIH in Bethesda, Maryland, and continued after Blumberg moved to the Institute for Cancer Research in Philadelphia. As part of his study to evaluate genetic differences among people, he requested and soon received samples of blood from around the planet, with emphasis upon maximizing racial and geographic diversity.

In 1963, a vial of blood arrived at Blumberg's office from a hemophilia patient in the United States. After testing the sample against a collection of known blood donors from around the world, Blumberg was surprised to find a sample from one particular hemophiliac who had produced antibodies with a robust ability to recognize a protein found in a vial of blood obtained from a foreign donor. Looking through his files, Blumberg realized the matching sample had been sent by a physician from the west coast of Australia, who in turn had collected the blood from an Aboriginal donor. This unknown molecule was therefore termed the *Australian antigen* (or *Au* for short).

Follow-up investigation revealed Au antigen was relatively rare, being found in roughly one in a thousand samples. Consistent with its name, the Au antigen was present in the blood of approximately one of sixteen indigenous Australians and even higher in some Asian populations. Indeed, the highest levels reported to date include prevalence in 15% of people found on certain islands in the South Pacific.[18]

Although this distribution of the Au signature at first seemed to be consistent with the idea the gene for Au was focused in Australasia, this neat hypothesis was shattered by a series of unexpected findings. For example, the Au antigen was also sporadically found in the blood of people all throughout the world independent of their geography or race. Even more odd was the finding Au was also prominent in patients with certain types of leukemia, again regardless of their geographic location, ancestry, or race.

Thinking they might have stumbled upon an underlying genetic marker predisposing these people to cancer, Blumberg and his team focused on identifying Au and soon discovered a far more surprising and disconcerting result. In 1966, Blumberg had initiated a study to ask if the presence of the Au antigen might render children susceptible to Down's syndrome. In the course of this work, a Down's syndrome child by the name of James Bair had been tested and found not to express the Au antigen. A later test revealed the opposite finding—he now had Au antigen. After eliminating the possibility the earlier test had been wrong (a false negative), wonderment turned to shock when the investigators learned James had just been diagnosed with icterus (a.k.a. serum) hepatitis, also known as *hepatitis B.*

Blumberg soon realized they had accidentally linked the Au antigen to the cause of hepatitis B.

Blumberg's team mobilized into action, requesting serum samples from any and all patients diagnosed with any form of hepatitis. Whereas those patients with food-borne disease (hepatitis A) did not express the Au antigen, those with icterus (or viral) hepatitis were consistently positive. This suggested the source of the Au antigen caused viral hepatitis. As you may recall, the designation of "viral" hepatitis was presumed to be a virus but it had never been conclusively proven nor the virus isolated. Within a year, Blumberg's team had confirmed this hypothesis but in a most unfortunate manner. In early April 1967, a technician in Blumberg's Philadelphia laboratory who was tasked with working with patient samples, suddenly felt unwell. Thinking fast, she tested her serum for the Au antigen and, whereas she had been reliably negative weeks before, the results were now positive. Sure enough, she was then admitted to the hospital and was treated for viral hepatitis and thankfully recovered within a few weeks. Nonetheless, this experience provided firm evidence, not only linking the Australian antigen related to hepatitis, but indicating the virus harboring Au was infectious.

The implications from the fact the Au antigen had identified the cause of viral hepatitis (soon to be known as the hepatitis B virus) were far-reaching. First, the outcome provided an opportunity to identify infected individuals and carriers of the virus. If they express the Au antigen, then they harbor the potential for disease. Within months, Blumberg's own hospital excluded donors who tested positive for Au antigen from donating blood and this precaution was soon adopted nationwide and globally.

Second, antibodies able to recognize the Au antigen could be used to capture the virus. In brief, these antibodies could be attached to the surface of a solid support (like a Petri dish) and then be used to enrich and purify the virus for study. This was accomplished in 1968, and by 1970 enough experience had been gained in isolating the viruses to facilitate analysis using a high-powered electron microscope.[19] A series of studies by the English pathologist David Maurice Surrey Dane revealed the virus as a particle with a size of 42 nanometers (roughly one thousandth the width of a human hair). Much to the chagrin of Dane, this structure soon gained the moniker of a "Dane particle" and his colleagues incessantly teased him for the rest of his life, frequently inspiring anger by mentioning the name of the particle or even referring to it as "DP."[20] Subsequent studies revealed the virus genetic material to be based on double-stranded DNA, which although similar to humans and most other living organisms, is relatively exotic for a virus (which often use RNA or single-stranded DNA as their genetic material). This new virus was named the hepatitis B virus (HBV).

Blumberg quickly deduced that his findings supported the feasibility of an HBV vaccine. Indeed, his identification of the Au antigen was only possible because a patient in Philadelphia had made antibodies able to target the virus. Blumberg therefore reasoned they could develop a technique to isolate the Au antigen (which was later renamed the hepatitis B surface antigen or HBsAg) from the serum of infected individuals and use this material as a vaccine to make antibodies that could block the virus.

This was an audacious plan as all vaccines until then had arisen from killed or weakened infectious agents. In contrast, Blumberg was proposing to develop a vaccine from material isolated from known carriers of the disease.[21] He filed a patent in 1969 for this technique and Blumberg's idea was circulated among pharmaceutical companies around the world. However, this idea did not generate much interest.[22] After two years of searching, the HBV vaccine found its champion eighteen miles away in the truly legendary figure of Maurice Hilleman. As profiled previously, Hilleman championed vaccine research at Merck Pharmaceuticals and is credited with the discovery and deployment of far more vaccines than any other person in history.[23] [24] Hilleman's list of achievements includes the vaccines to prevent mumps (which he isolated from his sickened daughter), as well as for Japanese encephalitis, measles, Rubella, chicken pox, meningitis, multiple types of pneumonia, and hepatitis A. Six days before the United States celebrated its bicentennial, Hilleman published a seminal paper reporting the success of an HBV vaccine in animals and the intention to begin human clinical testing.[25] Five years later, Merck received an approval for Hepatavax-B from the FDA. Unexpectedly, this milestone launched a new era in cancer research as, for the first time, the public was able to prevent not just an infection but as we will soon see, eliminate an entire class of cancer.

My earlier book on the history of vaccines revealed controversy virtually always accompanies the introduction of a new vaccine.[26] The HBV vaccine was no exception. As envisioned by Blumberg and put into practice by Hilleman, the Hepatavax-B entailed the purification of HBsAg from infected individuals, which would then be injected into healthy patients as a vaccine. Given this serum was highly infectious, Merck had invested considerable resources into the development of a purification schema to separate the relatively small HBsAg protein from the much larger HBV viral particles. As part of the manufacturing process, the material was treated with formaldehyde and other virus-killing agents to kill any viruses that might have survived the purification process, thereby increasing the safety of the vaccine.

Based on epidemiological evidence, gay men and intravenous drug users tended to have the highest frequency of chronic HBV infection. Consequently, this population served as key serum donors for the new vaccine. Infected donors were paid, starting in the late 1970s, to provide serum for the manufacture of the new HBV vaccine. This timing was particularly unfortunate given a small number of gay men and addicts began experiencing rare infections and an equally uncommon skin malady quickly dubbed "gay cancer" (Kaposi sarcoma). These unusual maladies were the early warning signs of a pandemic and medical crisis eventually responsible for killing more people in the developed world than any postindustrial infectious disease outbreak (other than Spanish influenza).

With the recognition of the emerging HIV/AIDS pandemic, Merck confronted two problems. As the world came to appreciate the magnitude of the rising pandemic, rumors began swirling linking it to the HBV vaccine. Such irresponsible rumors became fodder for a fringe element of hate-mongers. Prominent among these false prophets was Leonard Horowitz, a self-described author, filmmaker, whistle-blower, music industry evolutionary, and natural medicine pioneer who touted himself as an "internationally-recognized genius."[27] Overlooking this subtle absence of humility, Horowitz added the HBV vaccine to a list of manmade threats intentionally foisted upon a naïve American public by government officials and "big-pharma" executives perpetrating "political genocide" via AIDS and Ebola. Along the way, Horowitz enriched himself through the publication of books targeting a gullible general public. All these claims would, of course, be proven false, but not before the false prophet had endangered the lives of many.

All the while, the pool of potential donors was literally dying away in the 1980s as the HIV/AIDS pandemic raged through their donor pools. A cold calculation revealed the loss of donors could threaten a steady supply of HBV vaccine. This outcome was avoided by an early victory emanating from the emerging biotechnology revolution. In 1986, a small company in the Bay Area of California by the name of Chiron had gained an FDA approval for a hepatitis B vaccine based on HBsAg produced in a genetically modified, benign bacterium. This new approach precluded the need for continual sources of HBV-infected plasma and utterly undercut the concerns expressed by a fringe group of anti-vaccinators, who had invoked their extreme theories to justify the shunning of a vital vaccine. Unbeknownst to many at the time was the fact that FDA approval would soon prove to be an opportunity to eradicate one of the world's deadliest forms of cancer.

### Help Me, Obi-Wan Kenobi

One morning in early August 2000, an elderly Merula Silvia Salaman was diagnosed with a rare type of hepatocellular carcinoma, a liver cancer afflicting roughly 6 of 100,000 people in the developed world.[28] Her symptoms included pain in the abdomen, nausea, and fatigue. At the time, the patient was preoccupied with caring for her ailing husband of sixty-two years, who had previously been diagnosed with prostate cancer and was bedridden. As the doctor shared the diagnosis with the couple's only son, he elaborated how the symptoms led to the diagnosis. The son then responded his father had been suffering from the exact same symptoms. After a brief house call, the doctor pronounced to the son the same diagnosis for his father he had made earlier in the day for his mother. Within days, the father had passed away and he was joined by his wife a mere seventy-two days later.

The remarkable fact that two people would be diagnosed with the same exceedingly rare disease is all the more so given the personages involved. The husband was best known to one generation as Lt. Nicholson from *The Bridge on the River Kwai* and to another as Obi-Wan Kenobi from *Star Wars*. His wife, Merula, had been born into a wealthy family and became an actress. Repressed by a domineering husband, Merula abandoned the craft to become a stay-at-home mom.[29] As Alec Guiness's career blossomed, the couple did not participate in the glamorous Hollywood lifestyle. While Alec himself was known to imbibe, he did so less than most of his contemporaries and this made the diagnosis of liver cancer all the more perplexing.

How, then, was it two people from the same household had expired from a notoriously rare disease? As we have seen, their lifestyles did not at first glance seem to play a key factor nor did geography or demographics. For example, the highest rates of liver cancer prevail in relatively poor regions of Southeast Asia and Melanesia, where, according to statistics compiled by the World Health Organization, it is five to ten times more prevalent than in the sleepy, upscale market town of Midhurst, England, which housed the Guinness family.

While geography, demographics, and intimate relationships play key roles in solving this mystery, the culprit is hepatitis B virus. As you may recall, HBV was originally discovered through the detection of the "Australia antigen," a marker found in the serum of an Aborigine from down under. This moniker accurately reflects the fact HBV is endemic within large regions of Southeast Asia, including among the native tribes of the Australian outback. Moreover, HBV infection is transmitted sexually (as well as via contaminated tainted blood) and is most prevalent among the homosexual community. Sir Alec had struggled with his sexual identity for most of his adult life and while he mostly remained monogamous to his wife, he participated in occasional dalliances. Indeed, it seems likely one of these indiscretions served to infect the legendary screen and stage actor and, in turn, he had unintentionally communicated the disease to his wife.

The insidious part of this story is the fact that it has only become recognized comparatively recently that HBV causes hepatocellular carcinoma, which explains the tragedy encountered by the Guinness family. The means by which an infection can cause cancer may reside within a single gene with the mysterious name of the hepatitis B "X gene" or HBx. The function of the "X gene" lives up to its mysterious name as it has many functions in the promotion of hepatitis B virus infection (although we have only unlocked a few of these mysteries). What we do know is the protein helps to promote the expression of many genes in the host cells that prevent the host cell from dying. Consequently, the virus-infected cells remain alive long enough to manufacture more virus. Indeed, many infected cells actively proliferate, all the while slowly shedding new viruses.[30] This slow but persistent reproduction contrasts dramatically with, for example, its distant cousin the Ebola virus, which burns through its food sources within a few days and thus constantly must seek out new victims.

Although it may not be intuitive at first, the approach utilized by HBV is quite a brilliant strategy from the perspective of the virus. While keeping its quarry alive and reproducing itself slowly necessarily restricts the number of viruses able to be produced within a given host cell, it does prolong the duration of infection. This strategy is rather dazzling because it allows the virus not only to shelter from the immediate consequences following infection (not the least of which is the immune attack triggered by infection), but by keeping its host (i.e., its foodstuffs) alive for days, months, and decades, and slowly shedding new progeny, the virus can assure its continued propagation for years to come.

One consequence for the host experiencing this enhanced emphasis upon cell growth is a propensity for a less well-regulated form of cellular proliferation typical of the early stages of cancer. Thinking in an anthropomorphic way about this outcome, it is important to recall the virus does not necessarily "want" the host to die of cancer but likewise is not terribly troubled if the host expires a bit earlier than would have otherwise, as, by this time, its progeny have likely hopped into new hosts.

HBV is also rather unique as it is one of the few viruses able to integrate its genetic material into the host. This strategy is not entirely unprecedented as we know the viruses responsible for HIV and a few types of leukemia share this property, but these are all in the family of pathogens known as *retroviruses* (a family of RNA-based viruses, which synthesize a novel protein allowing their RNA to incorporate into the chromosomal DNA of its hosts). HBV is not a retrovirus, but in the interest of not having to jump constantly into new hosts, it has evolved a strategy to integrate itself into the host and remain along for the ride for years or even decades.

Like HIV, HBV infection is chronic and the damage caused by HBx accumulates as the virus sneaks its way into more and more liver cells, promoting their growth and survival as it does. Given liver cells play vital roles in detoxifying the poisons associated with everyday life, this might even be a convenient relationship. Inevitably, one or more of these cells crosses a key threshold where the growth is no longer controllable, and the cell acquires a malignant character, gaining the ability to move away from the liver and to vulnerable sites, such as the lungs and bone marrow, where it disrupts the functions of these organs and eventually becomes fatal.[31]

In this context, it is important to review the extraordinary contributions of Baruch Blumberg and Maurice Hilleman. In their development of an HBV vaccine, these two scientists were responsible for the potential to thoroughly eliminate a type of cancer from the face of the planet. Long a scourge in Asia and beyond, HBV immunization will forever block the cause of hepatocellular carcinoma. Such an achievement requires the public health community emphasize the availability and benefits of vaccination, a challenge confounded by the continued growth of a fringe anti-vaccine movement (a key member of which is the forty-fifth president of the United States).[32]

Within the United States, the adoption of the vaccine has already had already reduced the incidence of acute hepatitis B infection by 75% from 1990 to 2004 and should proportionally reduce the hepatocellular carcinoma to almost zero, assuming of course the anti-vaccinator fringe does not undermine these efforts. Such achievements were possible because health care providers targeted certain groups as having the greatest risk of HBV infection. Even so, only one-third of Americans have received the vaccine. As is the case with more familiar vaccines, such as the measles-mumps-rubella jab or the diphtheria, pertussis, and tetanus vaccine, many in the public remain skeptical of vaccination.

Despite the extraordinary good arising from the ability to eliminate a preventable form of cancer, irrational reactions against these preventative measures proved even more fierce when health care providers had to fight against the Bible-thumping moral outrage that arose with the introduction of "the promiscuity vaccine," a subject to which we will now turn our attention.

### All Ears

The moral outrage over "the promiscuity vaccine" is rather fascinating given its indirect connections to religion. In the year 612, a child was born into a prominent Jewish family in the Arabian village of Yathrib (known now as Medina). The child lost his father as a toddler and in her grief, his mother, Umm Sulaym bint Mihan, embraced a new religion with its genesis just months before. The new creed was founded when the prophet Mohammed became enlightened by the archangel Gabriel in the Cave of Hira outside Mecca, a rival town to Medina.[33] Although only one of a handful of adherents to this new faith, Umm Sulaym bint Mihan was resolute. Known widely as a local beauty and the scion of a prominent family, the new widow was soon pursued by potential suitors, but she required her new husband convert to Islam and raise their child in the new religion.

The child, Anas ibn Maalik, was immersed in Islam from the beginning and, from the age of ten, began recording Mohammed's sermons in person, eventually being granted the nickname *"yaa dhal udhnain"* (o' you with two ears) by the Prophet himself. Anas ibn Maalik, like his mother, remained an adherent to Islam through its many tribulations and narrated hundreds of hadiths during his lifetime.

As his mother was a companion to the Prophet, Anas ibn Maalik remained a prominent figure in Islam and, following Mohammed's death, migrated to Basra to help spread word of the burgeoning religion. His family gained prominence as scholars for generations to come. Centuries later, a grandson of Anas ibn Maalik with the name Zakariya ibn Mohammed al-Qazwini continued his Persian family's tradition of authoring works on religion, expanding his portfolio to include science, and may have been the first person to popularize the science fiction genre.

Instead of his fictional stories, we will focus upon the most famous non-fiction work from Zakariya ibn Mohammed al-Qazwini: *Marvels of Things Created and Miraculous Aspects of Things Existing.*[34] As the title indicates, the book catalogued both the common and the most unusual aspects of nature, including artwork of the creatures and places described therein. Due to the fantastic nature of the subjects and images, the work was a huge success and was transcribed by hand and later printed by machine all throughout the Muslim world for more than five hundred years after its initial publication in 1283. Within the opus are images and discussions of cosmography, geography, and anatomical wonders of the world, both human and animal. While some hybrid images reminiscent of centaurs and griffins are clearly fanciful to modern eyes, al-Qazwini sincerely intended the work to convey his belief in real-world events and creatures. Indeed, even some of the most ridiculous images stand the test of time and one particular image has retained a mythology in the 21st century and yet has also been verified using modern scientific experimentation.

Buried within this volume of almost one hundred pages is an image of a horned rabbit. This depiction is an early rendering of a creature sighted on many continents. In Germany, the beast is known as a *Wolpertinger* and has a Swedish cousin with the title of a *skvader*. Its Western Hemisphere manifestation, as recognized by both Native Americans and later European immigrant, was first documented in 1829 when a veteran trapper by the name of Roy Ball strolled into the frontier town of Douglas, Wyoming, to report a rabbit with prominent horns protruding from its head. Old Roy might not have been the first man in Wyoming to witness such an event because one member of the famed Lewis and Clark expedition, John Colter, reportedly confided to friends about such a creature during his time in Wyoming during the 1804–06 Corps of Discovery mission.[35]

In America, the sightings of these horned beasts have been fairly common from the mountainous regions encompassing Wyoming, Colorado, and to the flatlands of Nebraska and Iowa. The animal has been commemorated with songs and children's books and portrayed in countless websites. The beast was even the subject of a 2014 Wyoming legislative bill to become the official state mythical creature.[36] However, this creature is not mythological but is quite real.

This odd creature has been named a "jackelope," a playful combination of jackrabbit and antelope, and has spawned its own mythology as to its origins. Faked versions of jackelopes can be purchased in some taxidermy shops (by placing deer horns on a rabbit head) and a "Jackelope Award" is presented annually at the annual Electronic Photojournalism Workshop to bestow a dubious award for the most digitally manipulated picture of the year."[37] Unlike counterfeit creatures, such as Sasquatch or the Loch Ness monster, the authenticity of the jackelope has been proven by scientific researchers and can be readily reproduced in the laboratory. Importantly for our story, the verification of the very real nature of the jackelope facilitated the potential to forever eliminate some of the deadliest forms of cancer.

The idea of a real mythological creature seems about as much of an oxymoron as a naval captain from Iowa. Nonetheless, these two analogies are intimately linked. Richard Shope was born on Christmas Day, 1901, in Des Moines, Iowa. His childhood was spent hunting and wandering in nature and he enrolled at Iowa State University with the intention of majoring in forestry. In a fateful but fortuitous happenstance, the registrar's office for the Forestry Department had just closed so Shope went across the hallway and instead registered to become a premedicine major. His college matriculation occurred just as the Spanish influenza plague was gaining speed and this disease would forever shape Shope's career.

Shope became obsessed with viruses and would go on to help identify the virus responsible for Spanish flu, receiving the 1957 Lasker Prize. In

1931, while working at the Princeton branch of the Rockefeller Institute, Shope successfully identified a virus from pigs and determined it was able to infect humans and also that the pig was the likely reservoir responsible for Spanish flu (the world's deadliest outbreak is now believed by many to have originated in swine farms in Haskell County, Kansas).[38] This work would be confirmed two years later by a team led by the British virologist, Sir Patrick Playfair Laidlaw, by which time Shope was already onto other discoveries to cement his fame as an expert virus hunter.[39]

During the Second World War, Shope was drafted into the navy to continue his studies of viruses. The United States Navy has always been particularly interested in exotic viruses because its sailors and marines often find themselves in tropical climates. Of high priority during the Second World War was understanding the causes of rinderpest, a disease of cattle and other two-toed ungulates (e.g., buffalo and deer). Amid the conflict among humans, the Nazis were known to have displayed interest in weaponizing the highly infectious disease and releasing it in enemy territories as a means to eliminate a primary source of protein. For example, the German veterinarian Erich Traub was an expert in rinderpest and reported directly to Henrich Himmler, leading a Schutzstaffel (SS) biowarfare laboratory located on the island of Riems off the Baltic coast. This program was so sensitive that Traub was kidnapped by the British special services after the Allies learned he was in the Soviet zone of occupation and were fearful the former Nazi scientist might be conscripted into the burgeoning Soviet bioweapons enterprise.

By the time Traub had been secured, the Iowa-born Captain Shope of the United States Navy was finalizing his work on a vaccine to protect cattle against rinderpest and, with his release from military obligations, returned to civilian life to renew his studies of other viruses. Before, during, and after the Second World War, Shope pioneered the study of animal viruses in rabbits. These models would not only be of use for discovering new viral pathogens but also for developing and testing vaccines to prevent viral diseases. The unexpected fact would be these same models would provide the foundations for one of the most impressive victories in the war against cancer.

As we have already seen, a connection between viruses and cancer had been suspected since the first months of the 20th century with landmark reports from Peyton Rous of a virus responsible for cancer in chickens.

Beyond this exotic finding in poultry, the field had remained largely stagnant in large part because of a need for models to test the relationship between viruses and cancer. All this changed with Shope's 1932 isolation of one particular rabbit virus that could cause an unusual series of growths on the paws of cottontail rabbits.[40] Upon autopsy, the growths were revealed to be benign, largely containing mucous with a texture comparable to Jell-O. Consequently, the virus causing these tumors was appropriately named a "myxovirus," derived from the Greek term *myxo*, for "slime."

The myxovirus-caused tumors were not overtly stunning since the growths had remained benign, lacking the malignant and dangerous characteristics of a fully developed cancer. However, this finding reenergized the largely dormant concept viruses might contribute to cancer. Shope's discovery of the myxoma virus might have been relegated to the dust bins of medical history had it not been for two events. First, a modified myxoma virus would be deployed by the Australian government six decades later as a bioweapon to help reign in an out-of-control proliferation of rabbits on the continent. More importantly for our story, this work primed Shope to make a far more dramatic discovery a few months after concluding his myxoma work.

### Mythbusting

The town of Cherokee, Iowa, tucked into the northwest corner of the state, is a six-square-mile hamlet of approximately five thousand people. Its primary claim to fame today is its listing on the National Register of Historic Places for the Cherokee Sewer Site, where prehistoric native Americans processed buffalo carcasses. Nearby is the Phipps Site, a midden betraying the fact the Late Prehistoric Mill Creek native Americans had populated the site for centuries.

Cherokee enters our story as the home of a Mr. Thomas Archibald McKichan, who had an unusual encounter with wildlife in 1932. The 66-year-old native Cherokee resident spotted a rare and much rumored sight: a wild cottontail rabbit with horns. Word spread until it reached Shope, who was still at the Rockefeller Institute in Princeton, New Jersey. Although a thousand miles away, Shop had retained many interactions with friends and colleagues back home in his native Iowa.

Following up on his work evaluating the gelatinous outgrowths on the paws of rabbits infected with myxoma virus, Shope became interested in this more dramatic manifestation and made it known he would love to see a specimen. Within weeks, Shope was excited to take possession of a live jackelope, which had been trapped by another Cherokee resident, Mr. Clifford Peck. Three additional horned rabbits soon arrived from a Mr. Earl Johnson of Rago, Kansas. The sudden abundance of these animals provided conclusive evidence the jackelope of yore was quite real.

While studying the animals, Shope realized they were in good health (other than sprouting horns and warts all over their bodies).[41] Upon analysis, these warts and horn materials were quite distinct from the outgrowths detected on the paws from his myxoma-virus-infected rabbits. For one thing, the tumors were solid and had gained the ability to spread throughout the body, key hallmarks of cancer. Critically, Shope demonstrated ground up material from the horns could be rubbed onto the skin of other rabbits and cause them to undergo a similar transformation within two to three weeks. He had just created the first manmade jackelope.

In subsequent studies, Shope began studying the pathogen responsible for this disease and demonstrated it was far smaller than a bacterium, thus placing it in the mysterious bin known as a *virus*. In subsequent years, Shope isolated the virus responsible for this transformation, labeling it a papillomavirus (named so for the Greek word for "wart"). This was a prescient nomenclature, as a closely related virus of the same family would later be shown to cause the benign warts adorning the hands and feet of many sufferers (and the noses of an occasional wicked witch). However, most of these warts tend to be as benign as the gelatinous myxovirus tumors Shope had earlier discovered. Moreover, these warts tend to disappear when trated with skin debridement therapies, such as salicylic acid or freezing with liquid nitrogen. Lacking a direct connection to the more dangerous malignant diseases, the study of papillomaviruses soon declined to a few specialists and would largely remain a backwater of research for decades to come.

### The Truth About HPV, Warts and All

Warts have coexisted with humans for thousands of years, as evidenced by analysis of Egyptian mummies, who bore such blemishes. Arguably, one of the most famous wart sufferers was Oliver Cromwell. Following his overthrow of King Charles I during the English Civil War, the new Lord Protector of England, Scotland, and Ireland commissioned a portrait. The artist, Peter Lely, was instructed by the recently elevated Puritan to convey a painting not intended to flatter but rather to be as accurate as possible. The result was an image inspiring a saying still used today that the work was to depict Cromwell, "warts and all."[42]

The causation of warts has its own mythology, which includes anecdotes well-known by most schoolchildren to include direct contact with toads, particularly during a full moon. While most of this lore is inaccurate, one truism is warts are indeed infectious. Modern science has implicated a special family of viruses, first discovered by Shope, and has shown these are responsible for these disfigurements of the epidermis. There are at least 170 different types of papillomaviruses that target humans (and perhaps twice as many to be discovered), as well as the countless variants able to infect other species (including, of course, toads).[43]

Most direct encounters with human papillomavirus (HPV) cause minor, benign outgrowths like warts. Upon rare occasions, some of the more malicious versions of the virus cause a more severe disease. An extreme version is the human equivalent of the jackelope. A disease by the name of epidermodysplasia verruciformis is exceedingly rare yet equally sensational.[44] Also known as *treeman syndrome,* uncommon strains of HPV combine with inherent genetic susceptibilities in its victims to cause massive outgrowths on the hands and feet.[45] The growth of tissue causes the digits to coalesce into masses resembling gnarled tree trunks. No effective treatment exists and periodic surgical removal, which can entail more than a dozen pounds of tissue during each procedure, tends to be temporary, as the consequences of infection inevitably recur.

As disfiguring as "treeman syndrome" can become, the tumors tend to remain benign. Consequently, the field of papillomavirus research continued to remain stagnant. This all changed with an understanding that some papillomavirus-infected individuals are not so fortunate and develop a deadly cancer. The genesis of this understanding began in the 1970s following a series of remarkable contributions to scientific thought from a German professor who received his scientific training in yet another Philadelphia laboratory. Harald zur Hausen was born in 1936 and grew up in an industrial part of North Rhine-Westphalia. As the local specialties included coal production and oil refining, zur Hausen's hometown was subjected to repeated bombing from Allied aircraft during the Second World War, and damage to the local schools impaired his ability to receive a formal education for much of the first ten years of his life. A powerful curiosity about nature and biology overcame these setbacks and zur Hausen was able to finish high school and enroll in the University of Bonn. Following graduation, he obtained a medical degree in Dusseldorf but struggled for a time with the question of whether to dedicate his life to treating patients or to medical research.

Zur Hausen soon realized his passions lay in research, but his opportunities for scientific training were limited in Germany. Consequently, he began seeking opportunities in the United States and landed an offer from the Philadelphia laboratories of a German émigré couple, Gertrude and Werner Henle. This couple, who were pioneers in the field of virology, had contributed to a wide variety of breakthroughs, including a diagnostic test for mumps and contributions toward the influenza virus vaccine. At the time zur Hausen started his work in Philadelphia, the Henle laboratory was focused upon a virus newly discovered by a trio at Middlesex Hospital in London.

### A Hot Discovery

One morning in 1957, an evangelical, Ulster-born surgeon by the name of Denis Parson Burkitt noted a child in his adopted hometown of Kampala, Uganda, whose swollen jaw betrayed the presence of a lymphoid tumor. The child had "bizarre lesions involving both sides of his upper and lower jaws."[46] The more he looked around his community, the greater his realization this cancer and unique disfigurement was uncomfortably common, and the unique swelling of the lower face was observed in roughly one of every twenty thousand boys in Uganda. This might sound obscure but would translate into roughly 1.5 million diseased individuals were the same disease to arise at that frequency in the American population. Thereafter, Burkitt began a meticulous study to assess the abnormally high frequency of this rare cancer in children across the region and ultimately expanded this study to include much of the African continent. Uganda has a notoriously warm climate and a remarkable outcome of Burkitt's study was a determination the unique cancer did not occur in areas where the temperatures fell below 15 ºC (60 ºF).[47] For example, the incidence of Burkitt's lymphoma in Holland is exceedingly low and is likewise absent in South Africa. Even Algiers, which will never be considered as a host city for the Winter Olympics, does not experience Burkitt's lymphoma as the temperatures there occasionally dip below the threshold in the winter months.

Beyond temperature, another intriguing finding from Burkitt's studies was the occurrence of the disease was likewise restricted to areas receiving an annual rainfall of at least 20 inches (which also helps explain the lack of the disease in Algiers and other Saharan regions of the African continent).

This strange climactic dependence remained a mystery for a time. Diseases borne by mosquitoes, a bane of Africa, were an obvious suspect but this was quickly eliminated. Likewise, a constellation of infectious agents associated with malaria could be excluded as the cause. Eventually, it was deduced the cancer arose in individuals with a depressed immune system, but this alone did not explain why the tumor had begun in the first place. For the final piece in this puzzle, we return back to a fateful seminar at the Royal College of Surgery in London on May 24, 1961. On this date, Denis Burkitt reported his findings about the unique lymphoma. In the audience was a young physician by the name of Michael A. Epstein. Epstein was so deeply impacted by Burkitt's seminar he saved a copy of the flyer announcing the talk, which remained in his files for more than two years while he attempted to identify what he was convinced was causing the disease: a virus.

To isolate this virus, Epstein requested specimens from lymphoma biopsies (by this time, it was known as *Burkitt's lymphoma*—the name that persists today). Epstein required one sample each Thursday, promptly delivered by air on a night flight from Kampala to London. Epstein had developed a strict routine in preparing the samples and despite much work and considerable frustration, all attempts to isolate the virus were fruitless.[48] [49] On December 5, 1963, Epstein was awaiting yet another specimen but the weather in London was particularly cold and for reasons lost to history, the flight was diverted to Manchester.[50] Consequently, the sample of virus arrived a day late. Worse still, when Epstein looked at the specimen, he found the fluid around the sample to be cloudy, usually an indication of bacterial contamination. The presence of bacteria in the specimen would have been compounded by the long time the package sat rotting in airports. Being a Friday night and during the holiday season, Epstein considered trashing the sample altogether. To be sure about this decision, he took a drop of the fluid to analyze under the microscope to confirm his suspicions, expecting to see flocculent bacteria swarming about the fluid.

What Epstein instead witnessed was quite shocking. The cloudiness in the sample had not in fact been an indication of bacterial contamination. Instead, the tumor cells had detached from the mass and had begun to grow in the fluid. Furthermore, the cells continued to grow, even though it was rare for cells from a clinical specimen to retain the ability to grow in the laboratory.

Epstein's night was clearly ruined as he began efforts to evaluate these tumor cells. After removing the tumor cells and any other bacteria in these growing specimens, Epstein then asked if there might be any viruses in the sample. Much to his delight, analysis of the fluid using a high-powered electron microscope revealed copious amounts of an unknown virus. The shape of the virus was unlike anything Epstein or indeed anyone else had ever seen. Working with his colleagues, Yvonne Barr and Bert Achong, the team identified and catalogued the virus as a novel virus distantly related to the pathogen responsible for herpes. The virus would eventually be named Epstein-Barr virus (EBV; Bert Achong, the expert in electron microscopy, was for some reason snubbed in the naming of the pathogen). Although best known as the infectious agent responsible for mononucleosis, "the kissing disease," the virus is far deadlier and has demonstrated an ability to survive outside the climatological constraints first described by Denis Burkitt. Among the first actions taken following the isolation of the virus, Epstein sent a sample of the virus across the Atlantic to the laboratory of some old colleagues, Gertrude and Werner Henle. Shortly after his December 1965 arrival in Philadelphia, the study of this new virus would be assigned to the Henles' newest trainee, Harald zur Hausen.

The young zur Hausen's first major contribution to cancer research was a demonstration that EBV infection of normal B lymphocytes was sufficient to trigger malignant cell behaviors.[51] This finding was the first direct demonstration a purified virus could confer malignant character upon human cells. This finding was groundbreaking, providing enough fame for the young German to return to his homeland and receive an appointment as the chair of the Institute of Clinical Virology in Erlangen-Nurnberg.

As his career unfolded, zur Hausen focused upon strengthening the virus-cancer connection. Beyond Burkitt's lymphoma, EBV would eventually be linked to almost half of the cases of another B cell cancer, Hodgkin's lymphoma. In another remarkable geographic twist, it was found that EBV contributes to a variety of cancers, particularly among the populations of Japan, China, and Southeast Asia, including stomach cancer and nasopharyngeal carcinoma. Whereas these indications are exceeding rare in the Western Hemisphere and Europe, both the virus and the diseases associated with it are endemic in many parts of Asia. As such, the development of a safe and effective EBV vaccine is a high priority for medical researchers and public health professionals. A candidate developed by investigators at the NIH has not yet been approved, but has garnered considerable interest in recent years.[52]

Beyond the ability of EBV to cause the malignant transformation of human B cells, zur Hausen began a quest to identify other human cancers with a viral genesis. Based on epidemiological and sociological behaviors of the disease and its sufferers, it had long been suspected cervical cancer was in fact an infectious disease spread by intercourse. Zur Hausen suspected the disease might be caused by the same virus responsible for genital herpes (HSV-2) but this idea was eventually refuted.[53] He then considered the potential that papillomavirus might be involved, in part based on the findings of Shope and diseases, such as "treeman syndrome."

In the period around 1980, it was becoming clear there was not one papillomavirus but rather hundreds, and perhaps even thousands, of different forms of the pathogen. This realization was coupled with an increased ability to isolate, identify, and clone new viruses and compare their genes. These techniques allowed zur Hausen to identify two variants of papillomavirus associated with cervical cancer. These variants, eventually designated HPV-16 and HPV-18, were found at a high frequency in women suffering from cervical cancer. In particular, these viruses were present in the cells donated in 1951 by a young African American woman from Baltimore, Henrietta Lacks, whose life, disease, and cells were the subject of Rebecca Skloot's outstanding 2010 book, *The Immortal Life of Henrietta Lacks*.[54]

The breakthrough studies by zur Hausen demonstrated the appearance of these viruses was not simply correlative, but the infection was sufficient to trigger a complex process driving normal cervical cells to become malignant. As the scientific understanding linking cervical cancer with papillomavirus matured, it became clear virtually all cervical cancer was initiated by HPV. Indeed, the two variants discovered by zur Hausen alone were responsible for more than two-thirds of cervical cancer cases (with a handful of other variants responsible for the remaining). These findings earned the investigator a 2008 Nobel Prize in Medicine for demonstrating the culpability of a sexually transmitted disease in cancer.

### Greeks & Romanians

In science, it is remarkable how often the same (or a very similar) breakthroughs have arisen at roughly the same time by people on opposite ends of the world. This was certainly the case in 1927 when two physicians, working thousands of miles apart, stumbled upon the same finding within weeks of one another. The first researcher was a Romanian investigator by the name of Aurel Babes. Born into a family of intellectuals in Bucharest, Babes's father was a professor of chemistry and his paternal uncle, Victor, was an internationally recognized microbiologist who is credited with the discovery of the bacteria for which he was memorialized: babesiosis.[55] After winning awards for his aptitude all throughout his academic training, the young Babes remained in Bucharest and became a pathologist, specializing in the diagnosis of gynecological diseases.

On January 23, 1927, Babes was invited to present an overview of his research at a meeting of the Romanian Society of Gynecology.[56] During a groundbreaking presentation, Babes revealed a new procedure in which smears from gynecological lesions were obtained using a platinum instrument and spread onto glass microscope slides.[57] After these were air-dried and stained with a chemical dye, the slides could reveal the presence of cancer. An update on the work was presented again to the same society in Bucharest on April 5, 1927, and was published in the international medical literature via a report in *La Press Medicale* in April 1928.[58]

Three months before Babes's article appeared in the international medical literature, an American pathologist by the name of Georgios Papanikolaou published his own study. A former army physician who served in the Greek army during the First Balkan War of 1912 (a predecessor of events presaging a trigger for the First World War), Papanikolaou emigrated to the United States with his wife and served as a rug salesman and then a part-time violin player in a restaurant before landing a pathology position at New York University in 1914.[59] His academic activities evolved as he first began studying the female reproductive system of guinea pigs and later applied his learnings to people. Specifically, he found swabs of material from the cervix onto glass slides could allow one to detect the presence of uterine or cervical cancer.[60] The technique was published in January 1928 and included in a landmark book published in 1941.[61][62] The latter publication created a standard for an assay named after Papanikolaou. Well, sort of. Given the length and complex spelling of the discoverer's last name, the name of the procedure would soon be known simply as a Pap smear (rather than a more cumbersome "Papanikolaou smear").

This technique, which is still in practice today and was independently discovered in Hungary and America, is credited with saving the lives of at least 6 million women worldwide. Although Papanikolaou was nominated five times for a Nobel Prize, he never received it. As it turns out, though a gifted researcher, Papanikolaou did not keep up with the medical literature as closely as he should have. Consequently, he was not aware of the work by Babes (even up to the time of his death in early 1962) and thus was viewed by many on the Nobel committee as snubbing the Romanian doctor's independent contributions. Though one can argue the techniques developed by the American and Romanian doctors were substantially different, the principle was the same, and so history has not been as kind to Papanikolaou while the contributions by Babes have been all but forgotten, except in Romania, where the procedure is referred to as the *Methode Babes-Papanicolaou*.

Having established how the disease is diagnosed, it is important to provide information on the disease it reveals. Worldwide, cervical cancer is the fourth most common cancer and the fourth leading cause of cancer death in women.[63] Absent an early diagnosis of the disease with the assistance of a Pap smear, the primary symptoms include vaginal pain and bleeding, as well as pelvic pain, particularly during intercourse. Unfortunately, these symptoms tend to betray advanced forms of cancer, which likely has undergone metastatic and spread throughout the body. For women with advanced disease, a mere 20% of those with stage IV cervical cancer are expected to survive two years. Treatments are generally considered minimally effective at this advanced stage and those who opt for chemotherapy generally suffer from a decreased quality of life with little benefit in terms of increased survival. Despite these grim statistics, the recent approval of a new vaccine offers a much-needed opportunity to prevent and thereby eliminate this horrific disease altogether.

*Shell Games*

The investigation, which ultimately provided an opportunity to utterly eradicate cervical cancer, was an extraordinary partnership between two gifted researchers with its own share of tragedy. Ian Hector Frazer was born in Glasgow, Scotland, in 1953, and moved to Edinburgh two years later.[64] The child of two medical researchers, his father led a diagnostic pathology laboratory while his mother studied diabetic nerve damage, obtaining her Ph.D. while Frazer was in high school. Growing up in such an environment and being inherently curious, it is perhaps unsurprising Frazer embraced science at a young age and, like virtually all children of the Space Age-dominated 1960s, wanted to be an astronaut. Instead, he left home to attend a private high school in Aberdeen, where he became interested in biology and later medicine. After a successful college experience at the prestigious University of Edinburgh, Frazer focused upon kidney diseases.

According to a 2008 interview conducted by Robyn Williams on behalf of the Australian Academy of Science, Frazer chose to focus upon renal diseases based in large part on exciting new discoveries arising throughout the 1960s in the nascent field of immunology.[65] The fields of cancer immunology and transplant immunology have historically been closely linked (since roughly the same cells and systems provide key players for both fields). Many of the same investigators contributing to cancer immunology were in parallel contributing to the emergence of organ transplantation. As one example, Peter Medawar, who had teamed up with MacFarlane Burnet to conjecture mutations betrayed cancer cells to a vigilant immune system, also developed the tissue-typing system used to predict donor compatibility.[66] Indeed, many of the same drugs developed for the treatment of leukemia and lymphoma were also used to suppress the immune systems of organ recipients.

The kidney is a particularly useful organ for studies of transplantation, as most healthy individuals have two kidneys, one more than is needed for a continued healthy life. Consequently, the spare organ can be donated to others if an adequately matched recipient is identified. Whereas most other transplanted organs originate from cadavers, the time needed for transport, not to mention the trauma the body undergoes during death, contrasts with a kidney transplant, where the donor and recipient might be located in the same or adjacent surgical suites.

The early-to-mid-1970s, when Ian Frazer became intrigued by renal diseases, was the beginning of a golden era in kidney transplantation. In the course of his training in immunology, Frazer consistently noted that groundbreaking research was taking place in the Walter and Eliza Hall Institute of Medical Research (WEHI) at the University of Melbourne. When offered an opportunity to train with Professor Ian Mackay, the head of the immunology clinical research team at WEHI, Frazer did not second guess his opportunity and was soon headed for the land down under. Early in his clinical research training, Frazer met MacFarlane Burnet, who had been at WEHI since 1923, and, like this idol, Frazer remained in Australia for the rest of his career.

Over the years, Frazer's interests slowly expanded to include liver diseases. This was a logical choice because liver transplantation was beginning to thrive clinically and because many forms of hepatitis are considered to be autoimmune disorders. As his work in studying the liver progressed, Frazer unexpectedly found himself amid a swirl of activity bringing his immunological expertise to the forefront. Starting in the early 1980s, Frazer was one of the first researchers to appreciate gay men with chronic hepatitis B virus infection also tended to have a severely suppressed immune system. His work would critically contribute to the solidifying evidence of what we now know to be the HIV/AIDS pandemic, which was gaining momentum all throughout the world. In this same period, Frazer also was in the right place and time to recognize another fact that would help eliminate cervical cancer. During the frenzy of medical science surrounding the HIV/AIDS pandemic, Frazer realized the same gay, immunosuppressed men (who would later be diagnosed as infected with HIV) had a prevalence of genital warts. Genital warts, in turn, were known to be caused by papillomavirus, the same infectious agent responsible for cervical cancer.

In summary (and for those trying to track the twists and turns), Frazer's fascination with kidney transplantation led to an understanding of liver diseases, which contributed to the discovery of HBV. Increased understanding of HBV in turn coincided with the outbreak of HIV/AIDS and, finally, HIV/AIDS renders its victims susceptible to HPV-mediated genital warts, which are also a cause of cervical cancer. This complex but logical progression of interests would prove critical for setting the stage for Frazer's most important contribution to science.

In 1985, Frazer moved to the University of Queensland in Brisbane and continued to treat and research HIV/AIDS patients while remaining one of only a handful of investigators interested in papillomavirus (despite the fact this was a half century after Shope's description of papillomavirus-mediated tumors in rabbits). The need to identify potential collaborators and to share reagents led Frazer to perform a sabbatical in 1989 half a world away in the English countryside laboratory of Martin Evans in Cambridge. Evans was an early pioneer in the field of embryonic stem cells and Frazer reasoned these cells might provide a means to produce much-needed papillomavirus. In effect, his goal was to infect these stem cells with HPV and have them produce large amounts of infectious virus. The problem was the HPV virus was too toxic and tended to kill the stem cells before new progeny could be collected.

While in Cambridge, Frazer met married traveling scientists, Jian Zhou and his wife, Xiao-Yi Sun, a pair of clinical researchers who were likewise visiting the University of Cambridge from China. With the clock ticking until he had to return to Australia, Zhou and Frazer struck up a valuable partnership. Zhou's expertise was in molecular biology, the isolation and expression of genes. The two had shared interests in determining how to use molecular biology to modify HPV to favor its propagation in stem cells but Frazer was almost out of time. As Frazer was packing his bags for a return to Australia at the end of his year-long sabbatical, he convinced Zhou and Sun to relocate to Brisbane and arranged for visas (which was no easy task, as immigration to Australia was still dominated by xenophobic laws intended to exclude non-European migrants).

Thus began a productive partnership with a challenging beginning and tragic end. Their early scientific frustration centered on the fact that while

Frazer and Zhou were among a few, who had learned how to culture stem cells while in Evans's laboratory, the papillomavirus remained far too toxic. They tried cutting back on how much virus was used for infection and on other environmental conditions, but regardless of what each attempt, the virus proved too destructive. Rather than serving as a factor for further viral production, infection simply killed the cells before the amount of virus had grown appreciably. The pair quickly realized they needed an alternative means to grow papillomavirus for further study.

This inability to use the native form of virus led to a decision by Frazer to employ Zhou's molecular biology skills to eliminate the means by which HPV had killed the cells. Specifically, Zhou began to deconstruct the virus gene by gene, with the goal of finding the minimal number of genes necessary to propagate virus growth without killing the host cells. After years of painstaking work, the team of Frazer and Zhou had exceeded their original goal. Eventually, they had mutated enough components of HPV to propagate the virus before it killed the host cells.

This ability to isolate papillomavirus allowed Frazer, Zhou, and, indeed, the rest of the scientific community to study the virus. Among the work performed was the realization the viral particle was the shape of a 55 nm icosahedron (resembling a sixty-sided symmetric sphere far more complex than a soccer ball) that surrounded the virus's DNA genetic material and a smattering of enzymes, which controlled the ability of HPV to reproduce and infect other cells. Critical for our story is this complex structure was comprised of unique arrangement of a protein known as *L1*.[67] Important for our story is the fact L1 is faithfully conserved amongst the multiplicity of HPV variants, which would ultimately have massive clinical implications.

In the goal to create an HPV-like structure utterly lacking pathogenicity, Zhou ultimately created a viral variant consisting of only the L1 protein. The key breakthrough was to identify conditions to allow L1 to spontaneously self-assemble into icosahedrons. One trick, for example, was to modify the genetic code so the virus would optimally express even more of the modified L1 protein.[68] When properly done in just the right way, the resulting structure looked remarkably like the virus as it existed in the wild.[69] However, the resulting particles lacked genetic material and other proteins needed to cause disease, essentially serving as empty shells. These protein shells of L1 were not viruses but instead gained the moniker of virus-like particles

(VLPs). With this advance, Zhou and Frazer realized not only could they study HPV, but they also had created the potential for a vaccine with the ability to confer immunity against HPV.[70] Zhou and Frazer worked first to create a VLP for HPV-16 and reported this in 1991. Within a year, a team at the NCI had demonstrated these VLPs could trigger HPV-specific immunity in animals and this finding launched a race for human testing.

In the years since the 1991 discovery of VLPs, two key players emerged in the race to develop an HPV vaccine. A small Gaithersburg, Maryland, company by the name of MedImmune utilized VLP technology to develop a vaccine to include the major forms of HPV linked with causing genital herpes (HPV-6) and cervical cancer (HPV-11, -16, and -18).[71] The company developed the vaccine and demonstrated remarkable protection in both animals and through phase II clinical trials to establish the safety and efficacy of the disease. Confronted with a large-scale trial to obtain licensure from the FDA, the company realized it did not have the resources to conduct a phase III clinical study and instead partnered with a large pharmaceutical company, GlaxoSmithKline, to carry the product over the finish line.

Their competition was led by the Australian company CSL, which had taken a license to the patent submitted by Zhou and Frazer, but they too soon realized an overwhelming amount of resources would be needed to advance a vaccine to licensure and elected to partner with Merck. The two competitors battled both in the clinics and courtroom, each accusing the other of intellectual property violations while advancing their work in clinical trials. In the end, a compromise was reached whereby the Merck product, known as Gardasil®, would be marketed in the United States while the GlaxoSmithKline product, Cervarix, would be marketed in the rest of the world.[72] Gardasil gained an FDA approval in 2006 and began to be marketed in the United States.

Jian Zhou and Ian Frazer continued to study HPV. Although the two colleagues continued to collaborate, each had his own research laboratory and they saw each other less and less frequently. In January 1999, Zhou and Frazer met in South Carolina and the former looked and felt tired. Zhou decided to take some time off to return to his home in China and rest. Three days later, Frazer received a phone call indicating his friend and colleague had been hospitalized and within a day, Zhou was dead. Although the word is frequently over-used, this death was not only tragic but truly ironic as Zhou had died from complications associated with hepatitis B virus infection, a disease preventable by the only other vaccine to prevent cancer (other than the one for HPV).[73]

## The Promiscuity Fallacy

Before moving on to discuss some of the extremist reactions to the HPV vaccine, it is important to clarify some widely held misconceptions about HPV. Unlike other sexually transmitted diseases, HPV cannot be prevented by abstaining from sex or by using female or male condoms. This is because HPV tends to reside all throughout the groin region, from the midthigh to the lower waist. Consequently, heavy petting or other direct contact of the upper thighs, even while partially clothed, can allow the virus to be transmitted from one person to another. Another misconception is an HPV vaccine is only useful to protect against cervical cancer. This again is inaccurate because the virus contributes to other malignancies, including anal cancer (which claimed the life of Farrah Fawcett at the age of sixty-two) and throat cancer (which killed Erin Moran of *Happy Days* fame and afflicted the actor Michael Douglas).

Although Gardasil/Cervarix provided an extraordinary opportunity to eliminate a deadly disease and sailed the through clinical trials necessary for licensure by the FDA, it faced an unexpected hurdle. As word of the vaccine spread, public awareness increased of the fact cervical cancer was a sexually transmitted disease. This recognition caused more radical elements of the religious right to preach the HPV vaccine was a "promiscuity vaccine."[74] Their reasoning suggested teens would be encouraged by the vaccine to have sex knowing they would be protected from cervical cancer decades later.[75]

A spokesperson for the conservative Family Research Council, led by the television preacher James Dobson, was quoted as stating, "Giving the HPV vaccine to young women could be potentially harmful because they may see it as a license to engage in premarital sex."[76] Prominent Republicans, such as Texas governor Rick Perry, who had advocated for the HPV vaccine, reversed course to kowtow to the right wing of his party in preparation for a failed 2012 run for his party's nomination to be president of the United States.[77] The rhetoric became even more aggressive and irrational in 2009 following the publication by an FDA panel recommending boys aged nine to twenty-six also be immunized.

The expansion of the vaccines to males served to amplify the outrage expressed by the religious right. These passions ignored both the facs these boys would be protecting their future partners from disease and may even protect themselves from other HPV-linked cancers (e.g., anal, penile, and esophageal carcinoma). Indeed, recent studies suggest HPV may play a role in even more diseases, including breast and prostate cancers.[78][79] Consequently, Gardasil and Cervarix may convey far greater protection than is widely appreciated and further study will be necessary to delineate the full benefits of the recipients for these vaccines.

There is no reason to believe the examples conveyed in this chapter—hepatitis B, EBV and human papillomavirus—are the only viruses contributing to cancer. We are in the early days of defining and understanding the *human virome*, a term used to describe the constellation of viruses we live with on a day-to-day basis, both beneficial and harmful. The complexity of these viruses is likely to be at least as daunting as the microbiome of bacteria with which we cohabit and may be even more so given the recognition viruses infect and alter the functions of both bacterial and human cells. Thus, it is reasonable to expect the number of cancers able to be eliminated through the use of future vaccines will blossom in the coming years, hopefully leaving dreaded diseases, such as liver and cervical cancer, to be vaguely recalled as past scourges of our ancestors.

# 5

# *An Old Story*

The Rockefeller Institute has featured prominently throughout our story, being the source of many medical breakthroughs as evidenced by its employment of Simon Flexner, Michael Heidelberger, Hideyo Noguchi, Alick Isaacs, and Richard Shope, to name but a few. Although most people are aware funding for the institute (and later university) originated in the form of one of the wealthiest men the world has ever known, John D. Rockefeller, less is known of the motivations for the philanthropic deeds leading to the establishment of an institution serving as arguably the most well-known legacy of the great man (other than, perhaps, the center in midtown Manhattan bearing his name). This is worth a moment of reflection, particularly since it defines the direction of our story of immune oncology.

John Davison Rockefeller was born on July 8, 1839, in the town of Richford in upstate New York. Rockefeller was the eldest son of a lowlife huckster, William "Bill" Rockefeller, who earned the nickname of "Devil Bill."[1] Bill was a miscreant in every sense, even justifying stealing money from his young sons with the statement, "I cheat my boys every chance I get. I want to make 'em sharp." When John was ten, his father was accused of pulling a gun on their housekeeper and then raping her. Bill's father-in-law posted bail but the scoundrel upped sticks and moved the family farther upstate to Oswego, causing the father-in-law to file a lawsuit in a failed attempt to recover his money. By the time court officers had arrived at the new Rockefeller home to serve the papers, Rockefeller's mother Lucy, (and the daughter of the plaintiff), informed the officers Bill had skipped town and left his wife and children stranded in Oswego. Bill changed his name to "Doctor Bill Levingston, Celebrated Cancer Specialist" and moved throughout the Midwest and Canada as a literal snake oil salesmen, hocking the fake substance (which wasn't even snake oil but rather a concoction of petroleum) for a few dollars as a cure for cancer.[2] As most Americans know, his son John made just a bit more money from selling petroleum than his father had.

The fatherless Rockefeller family wandered a bit, eventually settling just west of Oswego in the Cleveland, Ohio, suburb of Strongsville. John became a bookkeeper and entered into a small business of oil drilling in the months before the outbreak of the Civil War. As the war was winding to an end, Rockefeller's younger brother, William Avery Rockefeller, entered the oil business as well, emphasizing refining rather than drilling. The two brothers merged their mutual interests in 1870 to form Rockefeller, Andrews, and Flagler, which quickly became the largest oil refiner on the planet. The company, whose name was later changed to Standard Oil, became such a behemoth it captured more than 90% of the world's refining capacity and was eventually declared a monopoly and broken up by the United States Supreme Court in 1911.[3]

By this time, Rockefeller had sired four girls and a boy. His youngest, John Davison Rockefeller Jr. was born in Cleveland but moved with his family to New York City. The young John D. Rockefeller was quite shy and self-conscious, which challenged his ability to make lasting friendships. Nonetheless, he found a soul mate with a schoolmate's sister. Her name was Elisabeth "Bessie" Dashiell and John Junior often introduced her to others as his "adopted sister."[4] The two were inseparable and whereas John Junior remained reserved and guarded, Bessie was quite adventurous. In 1890, at the age of seventeen, Bessie began a summer vacation involving a train journey from coast to coast and then up to Alaska. This might not seem tremendously daring by today's standards but keep in mind the first transcontinental railroad had only been completed twenty years before. The West was still quite restive and this journey began months before the murder of the famous Lakota chief, Sitting Bull (who had defeated Custer at Little Bighorn a few years earlier).

Bessie and John Junior kept up a frequent correspondence all throughout the trip and the latter was troubled to read Bessie had pinched her hand when it became stuck between two seats of the Pullman car. Although this event left a bruise, it was otherwise not noteworthy except the pain continued to worsen and the hand became quite swollen. This malady continued even after her return to the East Coast and as the month of September passed, the pain and swelling increased further, preventing young Bessie from getting any sleep. Although her local doctor in Lakewood, New Jersey, had tried to immobilize the arm and otherwise convince Bessie and her parents the hand would heal, they became sufficiently alarmed and took a trip into New York City to see a surgeon.

The surgeon to whom they were referred in the summer of 1890 was a recent graduate of the Harvard Medical School. Although young, William Coley had already developed a reputation as a top-notch surgeon who specialized in diseases of the bone.[5] He would examine Bessie's hand and note a bump "about the size of half an olive" and tender when touched. Suspecting an infection, Coley sliced into the hand, expecting to trigger an outpouring of foul-smelling pus but instead essentially nothing happened. The tissues seemed normal and the young surgeon consulted his boss, William Bull, arguably the most famous surgeon of the era. Bull advised Coley to practice what we now refer to as "watchful waiting," which essentially meant to observe over time under an expectation the situation would resolve itself.

As summer gave way to autumn and Halloween approached, Bessie was once again in his office, complaining of even greater pain and swelling.[6] This time, Coley enlarged the cut and noted "grayish granulations" on the bone beneath the swelling but again, no trace of infection Coley also scraped these granulations off the bone, which provided some relief to Bessie's pain. But the respite lasted but a few hours. As even greater waves of pain eventually spread, Bessie began to lose feeling in her fingers. Coley remained perplexed at the lack of any signs of infection and considered the possibility of cancer. He ordered a biopsy of tissue cut from the hand, which confirmed his fear. Bessie was diagnosed with bone cancer, a cruel disease often afflicting children and young adults. Worse still, the pathologist report indicated the most aggressive form of the disease, round cell sarcoma. In the days before chemotherapy, this was a death sentence and Bessie's only hope was to remove her right arm below the elbow. The family then again entered a period of a "watchful waiting" while praying the disease had not already metastasized throughout the body.

Around the Thanksgiving holiday (which was still a relatively new event in America, having started a few decades earlier in 1863), Bessie complained of abdominal pain and days later, multiple tumors began to be found all throughout her body. Some tumors might arise within the course of a single day or new ones found after a night's rest. As the tumors grew (Coley estimated her abdominal tumor had grown to the size of a "child's head" and multiple lesions on her body to the size of "a goose's egg"), Bessie's body began to give way under the onslaught. She died on January 23, 1891, and was buried in Woodlawn Cemetery in Lakewood, New Jersey, less than six months after returning from her train journey. Coley attended her bedside until the end and signed the death certificate.

All the while, Bessie had John Rockefeller Jr. as a constant companion. John Junior had been preparing to move up the road to matriculate at Yale University in nearby New Haven but was so overwrought by Bessie's declining health and rapid death that his grief precluded his departure. These dark days were lightened only a bit by the fact the painfully shy John Junior had made a new friend in the form of William Coley. The two had spent much time together caring for Bessie in her final days. This friendship would continue throughout their lives amidst many twists and turns.

Needing a change in scenery, John Junior spent time at the family estate in Cleveland but still could not bring himself to start college at Yale. During this time in the Buckeye State, the young Rockefeller had a pivotal conversation with another native Ohioan and family friend, William Rainey Harper.[7] Harper was a renowned professor of religion, a loyal member of the Baptist church and was working with John Junior's father following a generous endowment to launch the modern-day University of Chicago as a school of higher education closely aligned with the Baptist Church. Harper encouraged John Junior not to enroll at Yale, which was affiliated with the Episcopal church, but at Brown University, which held a Baptist affiliation. Brown has earned a long-term reputation for educating upper-class Americans. John Junior enrolled and coming out of his shell a bit, even taught a class in Bible studies, graduating in 1897. John Junior immediately joined his father's business as a senior executive at Standard Oil (and also as a director of U.S. Steel). Despite the extraordinary opportunity to become a high-profile playboy, John Junior remained pious and extraordinarily shy throughout his life.

In 1901, tragedy again struck John Junior's family when his sister Edith's three-year-old son, John Rockefeller McCormick, died of scarlet fever on January 2, 1901. The family responded with the endowment of an institution dedicated to medical research to serve as a cornerstone in medical research throughout the 20th century, a period Edward Shorter has called "The Health Century."[8] Whereas John D. Rockefeller Sr. had intended the Rockefeller Institute would focus upon infectious diseases, such as scarlet fever, which claimed his grandson, John Junior was more inclined to avenge the disease responsible for the death of his childhood friend, Bessie Dashiell. This remarkable young lady had not only altered the future by inspiring the creation of a powerhouse of scientific research, but Bessie made an equally important contribution to inform and inspire therapeutics, which are just now showing promise to help end many different types of cancer.

Bessie's lasting presence continued to be felt not only by John Junior but by her attending physician, William Coley. Perhaps Coley was too inexperienced at the time to realize death was a mainstay of his profession. Alternatively, Coley may have not yet been disabused of the view held by many young physicians that no disease is insurmountable if only you try hard enough. Then again, Bessie's vivacious personality contributed to these feelings. Regardless, it is safe to say the memory of Ms. Dashiell continued to pester, inspire, and arguably obsess Coley for years. He often spent his little free time down at the archive room in the basement of the New York Cancer Hospital, poring over records of other round cell sarcoma patients, invariably finding each victim had succumbed to this devastating disease. All but one.

Fred K. Stein was a German immigrant who came to New York City and found employment as a housepainter. In 1880, the 31-year-old had been admitted to the New York Cancer Hospital with a diagnosis of round cell sarcoma on his neck. After four failed surgeries to remove the tumor, the doctor had scrawled "absolutely hopeless" on the case record and the only recourse was the dreaded "watchful waiting." Then something remarkable happened. Mr. Stein contracted an infection, known as *erysipelas*, which we now know to be caused by the same bacterium causative of scarlet fever. Barely surviving the infection, the doctors watched as the tumor miraculously shrank over the following days, disappearing altogether. Stein was later discharged in full health and disappeared back into the hubbub of New York.

William Coley was energized after reading Stein's case history and began a quest to find this one obscure immigrant who had disappeared in one of the world's largest and fastest growing cities in the world. It wasn't even clear if Stein was still residing in the United States, much less New York City. Coley took up the challenge of locating Stein, often by going door-to-door in neighborhoods with a large number of German immigrants. Remarkably, his diligence paid off within a few weeks, when Coley found Mr. Fred K. Stein alive and well in a tenement house in Lower Manhattan. Although he had not met the man, Coley knew all about his medical ordeals and verified this was the correct Fred Stein when he observed the faded scar on his neck, where the tumor had been growing prior to his encounter with scarlet fever.

Wading further into the medical literature, Coley found other examples of miraculous outcomes. One example was an 1868 report from Bonn, Germany, in which a Professor Busch noted the exact same effect: a bout of erysipelas had triggered a spontaneous regression of cancer.[9] Two different European clinicians, working separately in 1882 and 1844, had intentionally infected cancer patients with fetid and gangrenous discharges of pus or soiled bandages and witnessed tumor regressions.[10][11]

Coley was convinced to try a similar vein of investigation and looked to a strangely fated source for this work. The unsurprising part of the story is Coley sought funding from John D. Rockefeller Jr. and Sr. to help develop a treatment for the disease that killed Bessie Dashiell. The rather more complicated circumstance is Coley's cure would utilize the same bacteria responsible for the death of John Rockefeller McCormick in 1901 and so inspire the donation behind the Rockefeller Institute. Thus, the same bacterium would function as both a killer and as a tool for redemption.

Coley began his studies in 1891 with an Italian immigrant and drug addict, Signor Zola, who had been admitted to New York Hospital with a disfiguring sarcoma on his right cheek. The tumor had enlarged into his neck and threatened to close his pharynx and cause death by strangulation. He had been given only weeks to live and was discharged from the hospital to go home and die. What Zola didn't know until the knock on the door one evening was Coley had obtained a sample of pus from an erysipelas patient and had sought out Zola's apartment with the goal of injecting this toxic sludge into his face.[12] Having no other recourse, Zola agreed to the treatment. While the tumor shrank, it quickly rebounded. Although disappointed, Coley recognized the patient did not develop the high fever characteristic of a robust infection with erysipelas. Consequently, the young scientists was convinced his bacterial culture was not strong enough.

Refusing to give up, Coley had heard a rumor a German professor by the name of Robert Koch had isolated a more powerful version of the scarlet fever bacterium. Coley sent away to Berlin for a sample. As soon as it arrived, Coley returned to visit Zola at his home and encouraged the patient, who by this time was bedridden and nearing death, to accompany him back to the hospital. Coley then resumed his experiment with Zola and the deadly bacterium. This time, Coley's plan worked exactly as intended. Within an hour, Signor Zola had developed a 105 °F fever and began to display the red rash associated with scarlet fever. The infection was indeed more pronounced and caused the patient, already weakened by the consequences of end-stage cancer, to be febrile and miserable for a week and a half. Even within this short time span though, the tumor had shown signs it was beginning to shrink. Over the next week, the deadliest part of the tumor on his neck disappeared altogether and another tumor in his tonsil calcified but remained lodged in his throat, albeit much smaller than it had been before. The patient indeed was able to walk out of the same hospital, where a death sentence had been conveyed not long before. Zola remained healthy for the next eight years, eventually succumbing to a recurrence once the living cells of the hardened mass in his tonsil broke free and were once again able to metastasize throughout his body.

Over the following months, Coley repeated his experiment on as many as a dozen patients. A recurring problem was tumor regression would only arise in patients with full-blown fever.[13] More importantly, the fever itself often proved to be deadlier than the cancer (at least two patients died from the infection). Nonetheless, Coley persisted.

By 1899, Coley had realized dead bacteria could elicit a fever almost as powerful as a living pathogen but was not quite as dangerous (since the body did not have to simultaneously fight off a tumor and an infection). Coley experimented with the recipe to create an efficacious concoction, eventually deciding upon a witches' brew of dead scarlet fever bacteria and *Serratia marcescens* (a bacterium linked to urinary tract infections and many hospital-acquired infections). He found an interested partner in a Detroit, Michigan, pharmaceutical company. Parke, Davis & Company, which began manufacturing "Coley's toxin" in 1899.[14] Within months, this remedy would start to be used throughout the United States.

In 1902, Coley reached the apex of his career with the receipt of a large grant from the Huntington family, the first private endowment focused entirely to research new means to treat cancer. Over the following decade his clinical practice thrived, and his prestige worldwide continued ballooning upward. However, all of this was about to change, and Coley would fall from grace even more quickly than he had ascended.

Coley found himself undermined by his own institution and his own supervisor. In the same year Parke-Davis began marketing "Coley's toxin," New York Hospital was renamed General Memorial Hospital and began a partnership with the Medical College of Cornell University and its founding professor, Dr. James Stephen Ewing. Ewing was one of the world's leading pathologists and had a genius for organizing and fund-raising. In 1902, Ewing helped Coley to administer the Huntington Foundation grant and five years later founded the American Association for Cancer Research, a prominent professional society. In 1913, Ewing also cofounded the American Society for the Control of Cancer, which was renamed the American Cancer Society in 1944. In short, Ewing was a force to be reckoned and, much to Coley's chagrin, was not positively inclined toward Coley or his toxin.

By 1911, Ewing had displaced Coley as the brightest star in New York oncology. Ewing's fund-raising efforts were focused toward James Douglas, a Scottish-born immigrant and entrepreneur, who had amassed a fortune from copper mining and mining technologies. Douglas's daughter, Naomi, had been diagnosed with breast cancer and despite multiple surgeries, the cancer continued to recur. In desperation, Douglas took Naomi to London, where a new cancer treatment was being touted with great acclaim. Discovered only a few years before by Marie Curie, radium therapy was all the rage in Europe and Douglas hoped the new radioactive therapy would save or prolong Naomi's life. Although she did live a few years longer than expected, the disease eventually claimed Naomi as well. Upon her death in 1910, her father set his mind to dedicating the rest of his career, companies, and fortune to avenge her death.

Using his mining expertise, Douglas improved the methods to produce radium, a rare and prohibitively expensive metal. By the end of the decade, the new methodologies put forth by Douglas and his company had increased the availability of the radioactive element by more than fivefold. With encouragement from Ewing, Douglas also dedicated both cash and an enormous reserve of radium to Memorial Hospital. However, this donation had a catch: General Memorial Hospital would be required to focus its own energies solely to advance the use of radium to combat cancer.

As a consequence of this magnanimous and well-intended act, it can be argued the field of cancer therapy was paradoxically and unknowingly set back, perhaps by as much as a half century. This unexpected outcome arose because Ewing, knowing not to bite the hand feeding him, actively cut off Coley's experimentation with his toxins. This was possible because, by the time Douglas's gift had arrived, Ewing was Coley's boss. Radium ruled and toxins were toxic within New York's General Memorial Hospital.

Tensions between Coley and Ewing were inevitable and the two frequently squared off. However, Ewing held all the cards and Coley none. Ewing therefore eventually forbade any of Coley's toxins in the hospital and personally led attacks on Coley's methods in an effort extending well beyond the confines of the hospital, New York City, or even the United States. Over much of the remaining decades of the 20th century, Coley's remarkable advances using his toxin remained largely forgotten. Due to declining sales, Parke-Davis eventually abandoned his product.

Coley found himself increasingly alienated and eventually, in January 1925, was ejected from General Memorial Hospital. He landed on his feet as the surgeon-in-chief at the less prestigious Hospital for the Ruptured and Crippled.[15] Although out of Ewing's shadow and control, Coley by this time was sixty-three years old and elected to focus his energies on administrative activities rather than trying to revive work with his toxins. He remained at the hospital for eight years, retiring in 1933. He spent his remaining three years of life organizing his papers and looking over his life's work, perhaps contemplating an attempt to revisit his remarkable toxins. Upon his death in 1936, it seemed far more likely Coley's work was destined to fade into utter obscurity.

Among the few sparks keeping Coley's toxins alive were key actions by his daughter, Helen Coley Nauts. In the days after her father's death in 1936, Helen began sifting through his treasured papers, which were stored in a barn, and gained a new appreciation for how truly impactful his work had been and might still be.

Helen decided to write a biography and to begin a campaign to rebuild her father's sullied reputation. She approached Memorial Hospital (Ewing had stepped down in 1939) and was informed, for a reappraisal of her father's work, it would be necessary to obtain complete patient records for at least one hundred patients.[16] The administrators haughtily presumed this would be enough to dissuade her. To their considerable surprise, Helen delivered more than a thousand detailed patient reports. Although Helen herself had not been trained in medicine, the records she compiled from her father's notes were detailed, pristine, and were still utilized even after of her death in 2001. Indeed, her work bordered upon and occasionally crossed the point of obsession as exemplified by responding to a plea from her own daughter to play: "I can't play, because people are dying when I'm not working."

In 1953, Helen built further upon her father's work by founding the Cancer Research Institute, which was dedicated to preserving the work of her father and advancing the idea an active immune system could be used to battle cancer.[17] Resurrection would thus once again be intimately linked with Coley's toxins. Ironically, the rebirth of Coley's ideas and methods would occur within the walls of the very same Memorial Hospital over which Ewing had dominated and dismissed Coley's ideas with a wave of the hand a century earlier.

### *Vindication*

Before returning to Coley's toxins, our story once again requires a minor detour, five decades and fifty blocks from the site where William Coley's toxins were discovered. From Memorial Hospital's location at the corner of 67th Street and York Avenue in Manhattan, we travel down a bit to East

17th Street to the location of the New York University Medical Center. It is here a remarkable multinational scientist unexpectedly began the quest to revolutionize cancer immunology and build upon Coley's original work, setting the stage for its renaissance.

In 1920, almost four decades after Coley's encounter with Bessie Dashiell, Baruj Benacerraf was born in Caracas, Venezuela, to a Spanish Morrocan father and a French Algerian mother, both Sephardic Jews.[18] The family moved to Paris when Benacerraf was five years old but returned briefly to Caracas a decade later with the threat of impending war and ultimately landing in New York City. After obtaining his bachelor's degree at Columbia University, he applied to medical school but was repeatedly refused admittance, likely because of his ethnicity and religious affiliation. However, a family friend happened to be an administrator at the Medical College of Virginia and arranged for an interview, which secured for Benacerraf the final open slot for the incoming medical school class. After returning from France as an officer in the United States Army, Benacerraf again underwent basic training, this time in the Columbia University laboratory of Elvin Kabat, who introduced him to the field of immunology, which was just emerging in 1948. However, Benacerraf was drawn back to France a year later as both his and his wife's families were then living in Paris. He continued pursuing research and was also drawn into his father's banking business activities, but increasingly felt isolated from most Parisians, who considered him an outsider.

As these feelings were crystallizing, Benacerraf received an offer from Lewis Thomas (who we met in chapter 2) to join the faculty at New York University. His decision to move back to New York initiated an extraordinarily busy time in his life. Benacerraf found himself in the mid-1950s working four days a week at NYU while at the same time managing the Colonial Trust Company, a family bank owned by his family. Benacerraf knew this double duty could not last and agonized over what to let go. His family encouraged him to remain full time at the bank, which was far more lucrative than the poor wages to be earned as an academic. Likewise, Benacerraf knew his social status among the rich and powerful within New York City would be shattered were he to leave the Colonial Trust Company. Nonetheless, Benacerraf's passion for research won the day and he elected to dedicate his life to research. This decision to focus all his energies upon cancer research would have massive ramifications for millions of lives over the years and, in a more immediate sense, for the scientific development of another budding scientist, who likewise would face a critical decision, this between science and music, and would be equally impactful for resurrecting William Coley's life-saving research.

### An Old Story

Lloyd John Old was born on September 23, 1933, and grew up in the Bay Area of Northern California. The son of a middle-class construction engineer, Old was inculcated with a passion for classical music and for striving to become the best in his field of choice, whatever it may be. That instinct became problematic as the young Old was drawn to the violin and stood out among his high school orchestra. This talent led him to advance his studies by leaving California and training at a musical conservatory in Paris. Despite the fact Old's personality was reserved and quite private, he always drove himself to commit his utmost for each practice and performance and demanded no less from those around him. Given this ideal, it is not surprising Old walked away from a musical career after realizing that, while he was excellent at his art, he would never rank amongst the world's best violinists. Second fiddle just would not do.

Old returned to his hometown to attend college at the Berkeley campus of the University of California. Maintaining his constant drive for achievement, Old graduated from Berkeley Phi Beta Kappa. Unsurprisingly, he similarly placed at the top of his medical school class at the University of California, San Francisco four years later.

In 1958, Old left California for a second time, this time embarking upon a transcontinental relocation to New York City. More specifically, Old had accepted a residency at the Memorial Sloan Kettering Cancer Center, where he would remain a fixture for the rest of his life and be known simply as "LJO." Old departed California on this journey in rare form, driving a candy apple red Corvette the entire way from San Francisco to New York. Within weeks after his arrival, he began a collaboration with Baruj Benacerraf just as the latter was agonizing over whether to remain in academia or leave to join the family banking business. It is unclear whether Old's arrival impacted Benacerraf's decision, but it is safe to say these months proved pivotal for both men and to create the foundations of a series of breakthroughs, which would forever change cancer care.

The first breakthrough arose almost immediately after arriving in New York, when Old, Benacerraf, and Donald A. Clarke began reinvestigating the question of whether inflammation and fever might be used to combat cancer. With the exception of Benacerraf's laboratory farther downtown at NYU, this reappraisal was centered at Memorial Sloan Kettering, where such investigation had been banned by Ewing years before. Rather than using Coley's toxins, these studies utilized BCG, a vaccine to prevent tuberculosis and first made available for that use in 1921. As detailed in my earlier book, *Between Hope and Fear*, BCG is short for Bacillus Calmette-Guerin, so-named for the two French scientists who had discovered a bacterium responsible for tuberculosis. Starting in 1908, these investigators had serially cultured this new bacterium in a brew of bile and potato slices to create a less virulent variant of tuberculosis than the form of the bacterium in the wild. This weakened BCG variant was still capable of causing a rather nasty infection, conferring immunity by triggering an aggressive immune response associated with high fever and scarring at the site of injection. The vaccine was deployed widely in the years following its discovery, but its use had largely waned as increasing hygienic standards served to minimize the dangers arising from tuberculosis. Put another way, the likelihood of encountering tuberculosis had diminished so much the side effects of the vaccination were not deemed worthy of the risk of not being immunized. Sealing its fate, the advent of antibiotics meant tuberculosis could be treated with these new miracle drugs (although drug-resistant forms of the disease now threaten to reinvigorate the disease for future generations).

The Memorial Sloan Kettering-NYU team reasoned a vigorous immune response might create a hypervigilant immune and allow tumor cells to be unmasked as a foreign danger. This idea built not only upon the previous work by Coley at Memorial Hospital, but also invoked a controversial 1929 autopsy study that happened in Baltimore, Maryland.

Raymond Pearl was born on June 3, 1879, in Farmington, New Hampshire. Like Old, he was a musical prodigy as a child, reportedly able to play virtually all wind instruments by the time he entered Dartmouth College at the age of sixteen, the youngest in his class.[19] However, Pearl was not being cultivated for a life in music but rather as a classicist. This decision did not reflect a burning desire by the young Pearl but seems to have been imposed upon him by doting parents, who in turn were merely continuing a long tradition in the Pearl family. Consequently, Pearl wandered a bit as a college freshman and did not take his courses in Latin and Greek very seriously. However, a fire was lit one week into his second semester, when Pearl became utterly enamored with the subject of biology. Despite creating a rift with his parents (a wound requiring many years to heal), Pearl petitioned his professor to change his major to biology.

After graduating from Dartmouth, Pearl obtained his Ph.D. at the University of Michigan in 1902, where he also met his future wife and lifelong collaborator. Pearl's expertise was in genetics and statistics and he honed his skills in the subjects by bouncing around Europe and the East Coast of the United States over the next decade and a half, earning a reputation rising to the attention of no less than William Henry Welch. Welch was a pioneer in the creation of the modern research university and his foundation of Johns Hopkins University as a premier research institution was a subject of one of my earlier books.[20] Welch recruited Pearl to Johns Hopkins in early 1918, a year pivotal for Welch, who would oversee the outbreak of the Spanish flu in the United States just weeks later.

Over a career entirely spent thereafter at Johns Hopkins, Pearl published more than seven hundred scientific works, including seventeen books, a truly remarkable achievement. Many of these manuscripts were based upon Pearl's expertise in genetics and heredity. Reflecting his imperfect times in a way understandably uncomfortable to modern eyes, some of Pearl's early works advocated the burgeoning subject of eugenics and supported the ideas put forth by Sir Francis Galton, a Victorian English scientist who founded the field and whose ideas were hijacked and used to justify atrocities committed by Adolf Hitler and the Nazi party decades later (not to mention American ethical and medical malpractice arising from the Tuskegee studies of syphilis in the mid-20th century). However, in the late 1920s, prior to the launch of these miscarriages of humanity, Pearl renounced eugenics, arguing against widespread over-interpretation and implementation of practices favoring one race above another. It is another event in this timeframe to which we now turn.

Beyond the tragedy of the Spanish flu, tuberculosis had been a constant plague confronting the medical profession for millennia up to and through the first half of the 20th century. Unsurprisingly then, a handful of Pearl's papers focus on that subject. Of particular interest was a work on tuberculosis Pearl published in 1929.[21] In this work, Pearl summarized outcomes derived from studies of 7,500 autopsies conducted at The Johns Hopkins Hospital in Baltimore. A subset of these patients (816 in total) had suffered from tuberculosis and Pearl observed these patients had a markedly lower incidence of cancer than individuals not infected with tuberculosis. Even more striking was an observation those patients, who were actively fighting tuberculosis at their time of death, had the lowest incidence of cancer. Although Pearl did not cite Coley or his toxins, his findings were entirely consistent with the idea an active bacterial infection, in this case tuberculosis, had triggered an immune response with the ability to protect against cancer.

As the science and ethics of medicine had thankfully advanced considerably in the more than half century since Coley injected a drug addict with a syringe of bacteria and toxins, Old was not about to start injecting people with tuberculosis to see if it could shrink their tumors. Instead, he practiced the more rational approach of first testing his ideas on mice. Rather than employing infectious tuberculosis, Old opted to utilize the BCG vaccine. In a landmark 1959 scientific manuscript, his team showed BCG could stimulate the immune system of mice to redirect it to shrink or eliminate tumors altogether. This outcome was a clear validation and vindication of Coley's work and facilitated a lifelong friendship and professional partnership with Helen Coley Nauts, who was still seeking to restore the credibility of her father's seminal work. Perhaps unsurprisingly, Old's contributions would later be recognized with the first William B. Coley Award from the Cancer Research Institute, the nonprofit organization Helen had founded years before to rehabilitate her father's reputation. Despite this seeming opportunity for a comeback, Coley's toxins were officially abandoned by the FDA on November 9, 1965, and relegated by the American Cancer Society to its list of Unproven Methods of Cancer Management. However, BCG was here to stay.

For the rest of his long career, Old continued his work to determine how and why the body had responded to BCG (or Coley's toxins) and caused tumors to shrink. Within a decade, he propelled the field forward by identifying the seemingly magical substance induced by BCG responsible for killing cancer cells. This breakthrough blended chance with a well-prepared mind, to misquote Louis Pasteur. In these 1975 studies, Old had isolated a "factor" produced by mouse immune cells, which could selectively and quite aggressively kill cancer cells. The substance, termed *tumor necrosis factor* (TNF) by Old and his collaborators, could be generated by treating mice with BCG or with the same toxins used by Coley (derived from *Streptococcus pyogenes* and *Serratia marcescens*). His 1975 report emphasized TNF was "selectively toxic for malignant cells" and this began a race to isolate and manufacture this magical substance for potential use in the treatment of cancer. As related in an after-hours discussion between a budding scientist and a nonscientific executive founder at Genentech ("A Prescription for Change"), which was still struggling as a fledgling biotechnology company, this led to the isolation and cloning of the gene responsible for the effects of the mysterious "TNF." Within four years, the first clinical trials on TNF had begun.

Like the larger story surrounding immune oncology, the situation with TNF was one of "hurry up and stop" with regards to the race for a cure. The first, longest, and most devastating interregnum had transpired during the time between Coley's work in the early 20th century and Old's 1959 report of the efficacy of BCG against tumors in mice. During this time, most of the medical research community had drifted away or utterly abandoned the concept of immune-based oncology and instead adopted the approach of trying to directly kill cancer cells with toxic radioactive and/or chemotherapy regimens. Old restored Coley's vision and the first account of success with BCG in people with cancer was published in the year after the discovery of TNF. A team led by Alvaro Morales revealed the attenuated but live form of tuberculosis, when injected into the bladder, could kill tumor cells without the need for other chemotherapeutic agents. This finding led the FDA to approve BCG for the treatment of bladder cancer in 1990 and the drug is still in use today.

In clinical trials, TNF itself proved to be far more powerful and dangerous in its purified form than BCG, triggering uncontrollable fever and an exaggerated immune response. The massive inflammation caused by TNF treatment too closely mimicked the toxic effects of many dangerous autoimmune diseases but in an accelerated and more potent manner. Thus, investigators were soon demoralized by the fact TNF would not provide the much-needed drug for use in humans. Nonetheless, the excitement around the molecule did serve to reenergize the field of immune oncology. Although this strained the patience of many cancer patients, this new interregnum would be thankfully shorter until a next chapter would begin.

While TNF did not provide a panacea for cancer, a side effect of this therapy was nonetheless a tremendous breakthrough for advancing medicine. This unexpected outcome arose when investigators studying TNF therapy postulated the profound inflammation associated with TNF might suggest a way of combating autoimmune and inflammatory diseases, such as rheumatoid arthritis, Crohn's disease, and lupus. Specifically, researchers suggested the same biotechnology approaches used to generate TNF might be utilized to develop new medicines to block TNF in patients with autoimmune diseases. The first successful deployment of a medicine to block TNF for removal arose with the FDA approval of Enbrel® in November 1998. This landmark event triggered the development of a myriad TNF-based drugs, mostly monoclonal antibodies. Unsurprisingly, this class of drugs is designated with what is known as a *black box warning*, a strong cautionary note from the FDA indicating the elimination of TNF "may cause cancer" (or at least impair the body's ability to remain vigilant to combat the disease).

Although Enbrel and other TNF-based medicines have improved the lives of many suffering from various autoimmune maladies, we again return to the story of Old, as the discovery of TNF was but one of his many contributions to our understanding of the intimate connection between cancer and the immune system. While TNF disappointed by not being itself the much-desired remedy for cancer, the discovery of the mechanism utilized by the immune system to kill cancer following TNF treatment had rebuilt the field of immune-based oncology from the ashes of Coley's toxins, and Old's next steps would convey yet another giant leap toward the goal.

*Helpers, Killers & Suppressors, Oh My!*

In the days following the report by Lloyd J. Old and Baruj Benacerraf that BCG could block tumor growth in mice, the field of cancer biology began to explode. In 1960 (a year after the seminal BCG paper), a British junior scientist by the name of Edward Arthur Boyse was recruited to Benacerraf's team at NYU. By this time, Boyse had already lived a rather full life, having volunteered for the Royal Air Force in 1941 at the tender age of seventeen and, beating the odds, surviving the conflict as a flight lieutenant. At war's end, Boyse enrolled in college, graduating from the University of London in 1952 and earning a research-based doctorate degree in 1957 at the prestigious Guy's Hospital, also in London. Over the next three years, Boyse had remained at Guy's, conducting research in the laboratory of Peter Gorer, where he assisted in the discovery of key molecules of the immune system responsible for decisions as to whether the body would accept or reject transplanted tissues. In doing so, Boyse gained invaluable experience in mouse breeding and genetic research, all while continuing a friendly rivalry with Peter Medawar, another genial character, who resurfaces periodically throughout our story. Given the desire to utilize mice to study cancer, it should come as no surprise Boyse was aggressively recruited by Benacerraf to come to New York.

Upon his arrival, Boyse joined the Manhattan tumor immunology cabal, working with Benacerraf and Old (and later transferring from NYU to Memorial Sloan Kettering with the blessings of both). Within weeks, he had initiated a series of studies to exploit the fact there were many inbred mouse strains with subtle genetic differences. Their approach was to use the cells from one strain to elicit immunity (and generate antibodies) against others. The strategy soon identified a series of molecules, known as *Ly antigens* and showed these were enriched upon the surface of a subset lymphocytes.[22]

As we have already seen, a population of immune cells were known to be created in the thymus and were referred to as "T cells." The first two Ly antigens (Ly-1 and Ly-2) seemed to distinguish between two different sub-populations of T cells. Stated another way, antibodies binding Ly-1 recognized one population of cells and Ly-2 antibodies recognized a distinct set of cells. This discovery aligned nicely with the view the immune system had two primary ways of dealing with perceived invaders. In one case, the T cells were thought to first trigger and then continue to assist the production of antibodies by B-lymphocytes, the guided missiles of the immune system. These targeted projectiles could, in turn, paint a target for death, either by triggering a cascade of events allowing molecules in the serum to organize and kill a target and/or by soliciting help from other cells, which evolved to "eat" antibody-decorated cells.

Independent of these antibody-associated events, a second population of T cells were known to directly kill "foreign" cells (without the need for the serum proteins or participation of other cells). However, which population was which, or more specifically, did Ly-1 or Ly-2 distinguish between these helper and killer T cells?

As Boyse and Old discovered, a key property of the Ly antibodies, namely their ability to eliminate the cells to which they bind, helped out nicely in distinguishing between Ly-1 and Ly-2 cells. Specifically, the investigators realized they could inject mice with either Ly-1 or Ly-2 antibodies to remove the cells with Ly-1 or Ly-2 on their surface, respectively. Boyse and Old could then ask if or how the loss of these cells had changed the ability of mice to attack "foreign" cells. Such reasoning revealed cells with the Ly-1 antigen were needed to dispense help to B cells to produce antibodies, whereas the Ly-2-expressing cells were responsible for the direct killing of foreign cells. Over the years, the molecule originally identified as Ly-1 was renamed CD4 whereas Ly-2 became known as *CD8*. As we have already seen, and as is now widely known to many nonscientists as a result of the HIV pandemic, the CD4 T cells play a key role in providing the assistance needed for the entire immune system to function, and low T cell counts resulted in the incredible loss of life to AIDS. Whereas the CD4 cells gained the moniker of "helper T cells," the CD8 T cells were given the more insidious identifier of "killer cells."

The idea one type of cell could actively seek to kill another was quite a foreign idea when it was introduced in 1960 by a pioneering Belgian scientist by the name of Andre Govaerts. Working with dogs that had received kidney transplants, Govaerts discovered lymphocytes from the recipient animals were capable of killing the transplanted organs.[23] Up to this time, it had been well-established that antibodies found in the serum had such killing ability. Govaerts had demonstrated in this case, the sera was not the source of the killing but instead it had been caused by a subset of lymphocytes that recognized and eliminated the cells of the foreign organ. These killer cells were later determined to be T cells. Later still, the use of Ly-2 antibodies by Old and Boyse to eliminate what we now know as CD8 T cells revealed this particular population to be largely responsible for the cell-mediated killing.

With the discovery of killer T cells (also known as *cytotoxic T lymphocytes*, or CTLs), it was presumed such a powerful mechanism must be tightly regulated to prevent damage to normal cells and tissues. Though ultimately proven accurate, the means by which CTLs in particular and the immune system in general were regulated to prevent damage to "self" tissues confused and misled scientists for decades, thereby delaying the advent of new therapies with the ability to radically improve cancer therapy.

### *Teased by Ts*

Whereas the 1960s had begun with the Govaerts's discovery of cytotoxic T cells, it ended with the discovery of suppressor T cells. In 1969, two Japanese scientists, Yasuaki Nishizuka and Teruyo Sakakura, stumbled onto a discovery whose far-reaching significance would require years of additional research and would unexpectedly trigger an intercontinental controversy reflecting both the best and worst of the scientific process.[24] The study responsible for this row had been intended to determine if the thymus might serve as a hormone-producing gland that governs reproduction.

To address this question, Nishizuka and Sakakura removed the thymus (a procedure known as a *thymectomy*) from mouse pups at various times after birth. They then asked if these mice would be able to mate and produce progeny. The investigators were working on an assumption the removal of the hormones produced by the thymus would impair the ability of the thymectomized mice to reproduce.

To their delight, the studies revealed the removal of the thymus three days after birth did indeed prevent reproduction and the cause was attributed to a cessation in the development of the ovaries. In contrast, removal of the thymus seven days after birth did not alter the ovaries. This outcome seemed to provide conclusive evidence supporting the idea the thymus was indeed secreting vital hormones necessary for the development of ovaries. Hormones produced by the thymus were presumed to be needed at or around three days after birth in mice for ovarian development but were thought to be no longer needed by day seven (by which time the ovaries were fully developed).

While Nishizuka and Sakakura's findings with regards to ovarian development could be readily reproduced by other investigators (again, a hallmark of the scientific process), the explanation for this outcome was far more complicated. To the surprise of all involved, the loss of reproductive potential caused by the removal of the thymus on day three did not reflect the loss of a vital hormone necessary for ovarian development. Instead, the study by Nishizuka and Sakakura had revealed removal of the thymus at day three caused a set of killer T cells in the body (those produced before day three) to actively seek out and kill the cells of the ovary, thereby sterilizing the animals. In other words, the thymus had been producing something normally restrained by the immune system from killing the ovaries. However, this restraint would be lost if the thymus had been removed on day three. Even more strangely, the removal of the thymus either two or four days after birth did not cause the destruction of the ovaries. The immune suppression caused by the very early removal of the thymus (on day two) was quite straightforward, as this prevented any T cells from being produced. Since T cells were needed to support or mediate the attack on the ovaries, their absence in early thymectomized mice made sense. However, this fact did not explain the larger problem: Something was happening on day three to create killer cells and something else had happened on day four to silence these very same killer cells. These perplexing outcomes caused considerable head scratching for decades to come.

At roughly the same time Nishizuka and Sakakura were publishing their work linking thymic and ovarian function, a young investigator by the name of Richard K. Gershon was working at Yale University on a subject known as *tolerance*. This word does not reflect the more widely known social or psychological definition relating to opinion or behavior, but to decisions of whether or not the immune system will attack a particular cell or molecule. Specifically, Gershon was utilizing a well-established experimental system to assess the stimuli causing human B cells to decide to attack a foreign substance. These studies used radioactively labeled sheep red blood cells, which provided a simple way to assess immune attack. If the sheep cells within a test tube were "tolerated" by B cells, then they would remain intact and the radioactivity would follow the cells to the bottom of the test tube after being spun in a centrifuge. On the other hand, if B cells produced an antibody responsible for killing the sheep cells, then the radioactivity would be dispersed throughout the liquid media after centrifugation.

Prior to Gershon's work, it had been established T cells were needed to assist B cells in the production of antibodies. The induction of these antibodies would then proceed to kill the sheep red blood cells. This T cell support arose from the population we now know to be the CD4-expressing T helper cells and, returning to a familiar subject, molecules, such as interleukin-2, provide this support. It was also known that certain drugs, namely those with the ability to kill or prevent the T helper cells from providing support, would render a state of "tolerance." Such findings were the foundation for research into new therapies to prevent organ rejection following transplantation.

While these ideas were well-established, Gershon upset the understood consensus with a 1970 report. In this study, he revealed the presence of certain T cells was sufficient to prevent the B cells from killing the sheep red blood cells. Similar to the unexpected nature of findings from Nishizuka and Sakakura, Gershon had linked T cells to the active suppression of an immune response. This was in direct contradiction to the idea T cells functioned to support or amplify an immune response. Two years later, Gershon published a second study, which built upon his earlier findings and suggested these miscreant T cells had not only blocked B cells, but had also prevented other T cells from providing assistance necessary for the B cells to take action against foreign intruders. Gershon referred to this novel behavior as being mediated by a population he named "suppressor T cells."

For the next decade or so, the race was on to isolate and characterize these exciting and new suppressor T cells. Returning to the thymectomy studies from the earlier Japanese studies, it became apparent suppressor T cells were produced in mice on or around the fourth day after birth, a day after the killer and helper cells had been created. This finding suggested removal of this organ prior to the creation of the suppressor cells had removed a constraint upon the mouse immune system, thereby freeing it to destroy the ovaries.

A key feature propelling immunology in the second half of the 20th century was the widespread availability of the many different mouse strains, some of which we have discussed previously. This abundance facilitated studies using genetically similar (in some cases, almost clonal) mice, which could facilitate studies of tissue transplantation, rejection, and tolerance. In 1976, these models supported the publication of a paper on the suppressor T cell phenomenon that had seemingly mapped the genetic region and allowed these cells to suppress the immune response. This mysterious chunk of DNA, referred to as "I-J region," was the focus of much investigation by Gershon as well as by the extraordinary Baruj Benacerraf and other high-profile scientists.[25] This finding led many investigators on a quest to determine the identity of the I-J gene and how it functioned to suppress the body's host defense.

There was only one problem: I-J did not exist and was an experimental artifact. Although the work leading to the identification of this putative gene had been performed up to the highest standards of the time, the scientific precision and technical capabilities required to understand the suppression of the immune system simply did not exist. By the early 1980s, support for the I-J hypothesis was waning and there were many attempts to explain why investigators had not yet identified it or explained how suppressor T cells could function. The failure to explain the elusive I-J genes triggered a schism within the scientific community and led many to question the existence of anything related to the phenomenon of suppressor T cells. As the scientific process tends to rely heavily upon peer review, both to procure the funding necessary to underwrite studies as well as to publish their outcomes in reputable journals, anything smacking of controversy or pseudo-science can quickly render a subject untouchable. This was certainly the case for T suppressor cells. Curiously, the rejection of T suppressor cells was rather dependent upon geography.

The skepticism about T suppressor cells took on a global significance as defenders of suppressor cells tended to cluster in Europe whereas its detractors gained more and more of a foothold in the United States. American immunologists quickly washed their hands almost entirely of the subject, turning their attention in the 1980s to other areas of investigation (at a time when the rise of HIV/AIDS and its associated immune suppression soon captured the bulk of research funding). For much of the following decade and a half, proponents of either side would shake their heads and remark on the naiveté of partisans holding an opposing view. The divide created a bad taste on both sides of the Atlantic Ocean as summarized by the title of a November 2, 2007, blog post from Ian York, a scientist at the Centers for Disease Control.[26] In an article titled "How to embarrass an immunology: The I-J story," York shows the number of published scientific manuscripts citing "I-J" rose quickly in the mid-1970s and then fell equally fast in the years following 1984 as the "bubble popped." However, the fallacy of the I-J hypothesis was merely a bump in the road and would soon be forgotten by most.

As we will soon see, the phenomenon of immune suppression and suppressor T cells would return with the beginning of a new millennium. This new (and more accurate) assessment of immune tolerance and regulation of the immune system by T cells would quickly and vastly eclipse the premature and failed story around I-J. Before returning to the questions surrounding immune suppression, it is important to point out progress in the field of tumor immunology did not in any way halt in the late 1980s and 1990s, but instead was largely redirected toward new technologies launched as a new and much improved salvo in the war against cancer.

# 6

## *Smart Bombs and Payloads*

T he name of a man who would make medical history and inspire activities, who would save countless lives may never be known, was simply referred to with the initials "N.B." This 54-year-old white male first appeared as a patient at the Sidney Farber Cancer Institute in Boston on a warm August day in 1976.[1] Over the past year, he had experienced an increasing frequency of malaise and waking up in the middle of the night drenched in perspiration. As these complaints worsened, he began experiencing pain and swelling in his neck, armpits, and groin accompanied by the symptoms of a persistent cold, or even influenza, including a fever, sore throat, and runny nose. His primary physician diagnosed the likelihood the man was suffering from lymphoma and referred the patient to Boston's finest cancer center.

An institute eponymously named for its founder, Sidney Farber, who founded the Children's Cancer Research Foundation (CCRF) in 1947, the Dana-Farber Cancer Institute pioneered the use of conventional small molecule chemotherapies, many of which are still used today.[2] To provide some perspective, a diagnosis of childhood leukemia at the time the CCRF was founded was invariably fatal. The first publication by Farber and his coworkers of remissions and cures was met with skepticism bordering on accusations of academic misconduct.[3] Clearly, many thought Farber must have "cooked the books" as part of modern-day snake oil salesmanship to raise money for his new center.

Such critiques reflected a cynicism directed personally at Farber. He was quite adept at fund-raising as evidenced by the creation of The Jimmy Fund, named for a twelve-year-old patient who captured the hearts of America as he courageously fought a disease that was presumed to be his death sentence. Jimmy's fame began with a national radio program broadcast on May 22, 1948, by the Variety Children's Charity of New England and featuring the Boston Braves baseball team.[4] The nation was enraptured by the story of Jimmy's fight against childhood leukemia, and the inspiration he conveyed was matched by the joy he received during the broadcast in meeting his idols on the Boston Braves. In the following days, donations totaling almost a quarter million dollars poured into the CCRF, first to purchase a television set for young Jimmy to watch his beloved Braves and then to support the CCRF in its efforts to improve treatments for the dreaded childhood cancers. The CCRF fundraising activities became known as the Jimmy Fund, a moniker still recognizable today.

In reality, young "Jimmy" was actually Einar Gustafson, the son of a potato farmer in New Sweden, Maine.[5] His name had been changed to Jimmy, both to make it more relatable to American donors and to protect his privacy. One day in 1947, Einar began experiencing pain in his abdomen while walking to school. Two surgeries later, the boy had been diagnosed with non-Hodgkin's lymphoma and his abdominal distress was the result of swollen lymph nodes surrounding his bowel, which were engorged with tumor cells and pressing upon his intestines. Einar was transferred to Children's Hospital in Boston, where his doctor was Sidney Farber. The nation followed "Jimmy's" progress and were thrilled to listen to their radios as Jimmy continued to cling to life.

Over time, Jimmy faded from the public consciousness and most assumed he eventually had died from his struggle with childhood leukemia. However, the staff at The Jimmy Fund were surprised to open a letter penned by Einar's sister in 1997, indicating he was indeed still alive and well. Einar himself called officials from the charity days later to confirm his survival. He related how he had gone on to live a long life, operating an interstate trucking service and fathering three daughters. Einar eventually died in early 2001 at the age of sixty-five, with a cardiovascular event cited as the cause of death for this pioneering grandfather.

Despite this one-off success, skeptics still doubted Farber and many dismissed his claims, published in the June 3, 1948, edition of the *New England Journal of Medicine*, just two weeks after the radio broadcast.[6] In this landmark paper, Farber reported five children had experienced at least temporary remissions from acute leukemia following treatment with a drug known as *aminopterin*.[7] This may not seem impressive by today's standards, in which childhood leukemia is considered highly survivable, but such findings were extraordinary for the early days of modern cancer therapy.

In 1969, Farber broadened its mandate to include adults, such as the aforementioned "N.B." On the August 1976 day N.B. entered the cancer center, his oncologists noted a very high number of white cells in his blood. Pathology reports confirmed a diagnosis of diffuse, poorly differentiated lymphocyte lymphoma. N.B. responded well to an aggressive course of chemotherapy with the most advanced chemicals of the day and his spleen was later removed to eliminate as many tumor cells as possible. However, in 1979, the disease returned and proved refractory to additional rounds of chemotherapy. The only options remaining were experimental.

At this time, N.B. was introduced to a young physician by the name of Lee Marshall Nadler. Nadler was a stereotypical New Yorker: tough, aggressive, and as they say in his adopted Boston, "wicked smart." Born into a lower middle-class family in the Bronx, Nadler had largely taught himself to read at the late age of fourteen (with the help of a sympathetic librarian, who guided him to the best books to do so). Despite this deficit, Nadler graduated from Queens College in 1969 and was later accepted into Harvard Medical School, an extraordinary achievement for any person, much less one who had been unable to read just a handful of years before.

As he related in a 2007 interview with William Roberts at Baylor University Medical Center, Nadler's acceptance at Harvard was all the more remarkable given the unconventional happenstance of his interview.[8] His first meeting had been conducted at the Harvard Medical School and he was then informed the next meeting would take place at Massachusetts General Hospital. Unfamiliar with Boston and its subway system, the three-mile trek was executed on foot through sleet and snow. Upon his arrival at the office of his interviewer, Dr. Sanford Roth, Nadler was drenched to the bone and an awkward conversation ensued as Nadler began by noting Roth had a map of Vietnam, with pins indicating sites of ongoing battles. Roth admitted his fascination and strong support for the war. Nadler, frustrated and figuring his drenched clothing and lateness alone precluded gaining a positive review, proceeded to argue with Roth about the justification for the war. The argument continued for the entire interview, whereupon Roth informed Nadler he was the only interviewee ever to challenge Roth. Roth then shocked Nadler by telling him he would push hard to get him into Harvard.

As an aside, Nadler has developed a well-earned reputation for not being averse to a good argument or confrontation, traits learned on the streets of Queens. Nadler admitted in the same 2007 interview, "We spent more time stealing than studying and reading books." Indeed, one can argue this audaciousness and the ability to bluntly communicate his ideas, even at the expense of potential offense, propelled him forward. For example, Jeffrey Toobin reported in his 2008 book, *The Nine*, about a time when the then-president of United States asked Nadler to provide feedback on the health of a potential Supreme Court nominee, Richard Arnold, who had previously battled a type of cancer for which Nadler was an international expert.[9] Bill Clinton indicated he would send Nadler the medical records for the candidate but Nadler bluntly cut off his nation's commander-in-chief, replying succinctly, "Mr. President, you can ask me to do anything you want. But if somebody is going to ask me to look at this guy's records, it's got to be him. Then I would report to him, and he could share the report with you." When this series of events did transpire, Clinton called Nadler back to make sure he directly understood Nadler's view. Rather than immediately addressing the question at hand (which was sadly, a very dire prognosis), Nadler could hear Clinton chewing in the background and asked what he was eating. Clinton responded, "A Big Mac and fries," which compelled Nadler to volunteer to the president, "As an oncologist, I don't think that's so smart." From a less constructive standpoint, Nadler reportedly exploded in rage during a game between the perennial rivals, the Boston Red Sox and New York Yankees.[10]

Rooting for his adopted home team, Nadler was incensed by an equally vocal fan for the Yankees sitting nearby, Billy Crystal. Undeterred by the comedian's fame, Nadler launched into an expletive-laden tirade, shocking all within earshot.

Personality traits aside, Lee Nadler had been impressed and inspired by an early reading (after he had taught himself to do so) of Sinclair Lewis's book *Arrowsmith*.[11] The Pulitzer Prize–winning book was based on the life of the Franco-Canadian virologist Felix d'Herelle, and served as an inspiration for at least two generations of future scientists. Inspired by *Arrowsmith*, Nadler had entered medical school to become a medical researcher. He and another Harvard medical student, David Keith Lee, performed nonmentored research and identified a substance purified from Hodgkin's disease samples with the ability to suppress the activation of normal (i.e., Nadler and Lee's) lymphocytes (this may have been tumor necrosis factor). However, this work was utterly quashed when a committee consisting of Harvard faculty conveyed they did not believe Nadler and Lee's work was worthy of publication or further study. Utterly humiliated by the experience, Nadler swore off research and refused even to attend his graduation ceremony, returning instead to New York to leave Cambridge and academic research behind.

During a residency at Columbia University, Nadler had the opportunity to renew his passion for medicine and his retinue of patients included many celebrities, such as Charles Lindbergh and Duke Ellington.[12] During this time, his passion to perform research overcame the humiliation experienced years earlier at Harvard, and Nadler accepted a stint to hone his skills in medical research at the NIH in Bethesda, Maryland. Following two years as a mouse doctor, learning the science of immunology, Nadler had intended to return to start a lucrative human practice at Columbia. Instead, he found himself agreeing to return to Harvard, of all places, in 1977, for a clinical oncology fellowship at Sidney Farber Cancer Institute (the CCRF had been renamed in 1974 in recognition of its founder and would again be renamed Dana-Farber in 1983 after a sizeable financial contribution from the Charles A. Dana Foundation).

His mentor at Dana-Farber, Stuart Schlossman, would be no less of a critic than those earlier professors who had so thoroughly rubbished his work years before. Schlossman was a pioneer in immunology but had a reputation for collaborating and mentoring protégés in a style not always regarded as terribly constructive. This was not a hindrance to Nadler, who was no shrinking violet.

Nadler was determined to explore potential utility of a new technology, a risky venture for an upstart investigator. This "monoclonal antibody" technology had been developed just two years earlier in the laboratory of Dr. Cesar Milstein in the other Cambridge (England). As I have related in greater detail both in *A Prescription for Change* and *Between Hope & Fear*, monoclonal antibody technology originally grew out of a need for reliable sources of antibodies to conduct research.[13] [14] Keep in mind antibodies for this purpose had been generated by immunizing rabbits, goats, and other animals. Consequently, there was considerable variability from animal to animal. Working with his colleague, Georges Kohler, Cesar Milstein had utilized some ingenious but straightforward tricks to develop antibody-producing mouse cells with the ability to both live forever and synthesize only a single, defined antibody. These "monoclonal antibodies" conveyed both an improvement in quality control and the ability to define the precise molecule, or portion of a molecule, one might want to target.

In Nadler's case, he wanted to target a molecule on cancer cells and patient "N.B." provided an opportunity to do so. Executing upon a clinical protocol approved by the Harvard Human Protection Committee in April 1979, Nadler obtained a tumor sample from N.B. and used this material to immunize mice.[15] The immune systems of these mice responded to the tumor cells and generated a milieu of different antibodies, most of which were not relevant or unique to cancer. Consequently, sera obtained from animals would target virtually all human cells and this would create an obvious problem in terms of the likelihood these antibodies would harm benign and healthy tissues. However, as Nadler appreciated, the ability to generate a monoclonal antibody meant the negative consequences of targeting "human-ness" could be avoided and tumor-specific antibodies could arise.

Despite the strenuous objections of his scientific preceptor, Nadler proceeded to execute his plan. Over the next few months, Nadler led a team that generated monoclonal antibodies against molecules on the surface of N.B.'s cells. The team focused on one particular antibody, known as *Ab89*, which could recognize N.B.'s tumor cells in the laboratory but did not bind to nonmalignant cells from the same donor.[16] Nadler also conducted a variety of experiments to ask if the antibody could target N.B.'s tumor cells in the laboratory and found it capable of killing the tumor cells by processes relevant to events occurring in the body—namely, antibody-dependent cellular cytotoxicity (ADCC) and complement-mediated cytolysis (CDC).

The obvious question then became whether the antibody would similarly show efficacy if used to treat N.B. This question was challenging for multiple ethical and scientific reasons. First and foremost, no monoclonal antibody had ever been tested in a person. There was no evidence supporting or refuting whether such an antibody might cause more harm than good. Compounding this, it had been known from infusion studies with other animal-derived antibodies that the human immune system can react violently when confronted with animal antibodies. In other words, the rejection of the mouse-derived Ab89 antibodies could be mediated as a consequence of conventional immunity reacting against something perceived as foreign, or a process known as *hyperacute rejection,* either of which could be life-threatening. From a scientific standpoint, it wasn't even clear whether a monoclonal antibody administered to a patient could find a tumor in the body, much less bind to it and an immune response with sufficient gusto to have any meaningful clinical effect.

Despite and arguably even because of these unknowns, Nadler and the Dana-Farber team moved forward to treat N.B. with the antibody developed against his tumor. Enough material had been manufactured to perform six-hour infusions, once a day, for a total of three days. On day one, the antibody was infused into the patient as everyone held their breath, unaware of whether the patient might suddenly and violently reject the antibody through a process similar to the effects of an allergic bee sting. As the infusion began to drip twenty-five milligrams of antibody into N.B., nothing notable happened.[17] The patient had no complaints nor symptoms suggestive of any problems or efficacy (unlike the violent reactions experienced following treatment with Coley's toxins or TNF). After collecting some blood from the patient, no antibody was seen on the tumor cells nor could any antibody be found in the patient's blood. This perplexing finding could be explained by the fact the tumor had produced so much free antigen (a type of decoy not attached to a tumor cells but instead to protein floating in the blood) that not enough Ab89 could get past this decoy to find its antigen on the tumor cell and kill it.

On the second day, three times the amount of Ab89 (a total of 75 mg) was infused into N.B. This larger dose was impactful. Whereas the patient had 388,000 tumor cells per milliliter of blood on the day before, the antibody caused a rapid decrease to 240,000 circulating tumor cells per milliliter. Stated another way, more than a third of the tumor cells in the blood were gone. Moreover, whereas only 4% of the tumor cells in N.B.'s blood were dead at the beginning of the day, the fraction dead, or more accurately killed by Ab89, had increased to 30%. Coincident with the killing of tumor cells, the patient began complaining of discomfort in his lymph nodes and liver, two anatomical sites where the tumor cells were hiding. These complaints were promising signs the antibody was performing its intended job of finding and eliminating the tumor. Despite these encouraging findings, tumor cells obtained from the patient at this time suggested there was still not enough Ab89 in the patient's blood to fully occupy the tumor cells (known as *saturating*). Indeed, the amount of free material shed by tumor cells continued to provide unwanted decoys precluding the full potential efficacy of the treatment. This meant an even higher dose might be needed to improve the outcome. Worse still, the number of tumor cells in N.B.'s blood quickly rebounded as reserves of tumor residing in other organs in the patient's body had emerged into the blood.

On the third and final day allowed by the study's protocol, 150 mg of antibody was infused into N.B., twice the amount administered on day two. The number of tumor cells circulating in his blood again declined, but only temporarily as even more malignant cells left his tissues to take up residence in the blood. In theory, this game of hide and seek could have continued for days or weeks until all tumor had been cleared from his body. The problem was the clinical protocol had been approved to allow for only three days of treatment. A more positive clinical outcome was also frustrated by the continued blocking of the antibody by "decoy" antigen, a fact that again had minimized the amount of achievable tumor killing.

Fortunately, the protocol did allow for a large dose to be given a month later, if only the patient could survive this long. Thankfully, N.B. did survive (though it would be impossible to say whether the earlier treatments had prolonged his life, as there was simply no precedent). On this date, he received a whopping 1,500 mg infusion. Even at this high dose (ten times the amount received on day three), the amount of free material circulating in the blood was still sufficiently high to serve as a decoy (as it had been given a month to replenish). While the number of tumor cells in the patient's blood did decrease for a time after treatment, this was only transient and N.B.'s disease continued to progress, eventually proving to be fatal.

Although the final outcome was tragic, N.B.'s contributions to science were nonetheless extraordinarily heroic and durable. His courage in volunteering provided the first evidence monoclonal antibodies could be tolerated in the body and could be used to kill tumor cells in patients. These studies, both the creation of the Ab89 and the experiences gained in its clinical experience, were published in August and September 1980, respectively.[18] [19]

The lessons learned from this experience also taught Nadler an invaluable lesson: It is virtually impossible to impact a cancer with an antibody when the tumor is constantly shedding material, which acts as a decoy and binds up the antibody before it can reach the tumor cells themselves. The key would be to identify a target on a tumor but not shed into the blood. As the evidence would later show, the remarkable Lee Nadler had already done so.

## B Cells & Antibodies

The broad term *cancer* encompasses countless maladies, as each person's disease is unique and individualized. Nonetheless, one can distinguish major groupings of cancer based on the type of cells that go awry and/or where they are located. The terms *lymphoma* and *leukemia* both share the fact they are derived from blood or bone marrow cells, mostly lymphocytes. For reasons not entirely clear, malignant B cells encompass the vast majority of these blood cancers. This knowledge motivated Lee Nadler to ask whether this cell lineage might provide an opportunity to selectively target B cells while minimizing damage to other blood cell types.

In a bit of irony, Nadler's idea was to use the product of one form of malignant B cell, monoclonal antibodies, to seek out and betray other malignant B cells. This was accomplished and reported in a scientific paper appearing in October 1980, just one month after the publication of Nadler's studies with N.B.

In this second landmark paper in just under a month, the same team that had developed Ab89 reported the creation of an antibody with the ability to selectively recognize B lymphocytes. This antibody recognized a new molecule, "B1," different than any other B cell marker. Specifically, B1 antibodies appeared to recognize all B cells (whereas previous B cell markers were more limited in their ability to do so). Moreover, experiments with the B1 antibody in the laboratory revealed it had the potential to eliminate all B cells by harnessing the killing capacity of complement and cell-based means the body's defenses have evolved to cope with a constant onslaught of infectious invaders (and cancers). Having achieved their milestones in the optimized and sterile conditions of the laboratory, the question then pivoted to asking if these antibody-based cancer drugs could realistically do the same in the bodies of patients with B cell cancers.

Over the next few years, Nadler continued using monoclonal antibodies to characterize B cell tumors and to identify opportunities for deploying the rapidly evolving technology. Although three additional B cell–specific targets were identified (now known as *CD19, CD21,* and *CD22*), the B1 molecule continued to shine as the best potential for targeting B cell cancer. While the laboratory results with B1 antibody was very promising, the greater challenge was to identify what the B1 antibody was binding.

The identification of B1's target required expertise in protein biochemistry provided by additional partners who worked with Nadler and Schlossman. By 1983, the protein recognized by the B1 antibody had begun to be characterized and, by 1985, it had been revealed a protein, soon be renamed CD20.[20][21] As predicted by Nadler's studies, CD20 was found on the surface of all B cells, thus minimizing the possibility some B cell tumor cells might escape detection. While the science surrounding CD20 came into greater focus, the race was on to test antibodies against CD20 for their potential utility in treating B cell cancers. This contest would include many practical obstacles associated with the new monoclonal antibody technology and the competitors in this challenge comprised an unlikely group of biotechnology entrepreneurs.

## Of Mice & Men

An early advocate of monoclonal antibody technology was a Brooklyn-born Manhattan stockbroker. In 1980, a 24-year-old David Blech was working on Wall Street while his older brother, Isaac, was employed in public relations.[22] The two gambled all their savings in technology stocks at a lucrative time when semiconductors and computers had begun to emerge and reshape modern society. In the late summer of 1980, David purchased an edition of *The Sciences,* a now-defunct science magazine, and read with considerable interest an article titled "Immortalizing immunity: Taming cancer cells to mass-produce antibodies," by Lloyd Henry Schloen.[23] In this article, Schloen likened the potential impact on medicine of the new monoclonal antibody technology to the revolutionary power of the transistor to restructure electronics. This idea resonated with an investor, who was realizing the gains from a semiconductor market, where returns were beginning to "mature" (i.e., end their extraordinary growth rates).

Despite knowing nothing about antibodies, David quickly reached the conclusion he must become a pioneer in biotechnology, a nonexistent sector just a few years before. The idea propelled David into action when on October 14, 1980, he watched in amazement as the initial public offering (IPO) of one of the first biotechnology companies, Genentech, doubled during its first day of trading. The gambler's instincts in David caused him to place a large bet on the nascent biotechnology industry.

The Blechs used the monies gained in traditional technology first to hire the writer of the impactful magazine article (Schloen), along with a handful of additional advisors, to help identify emerging leaders in the coming field of monoclonal antibodies. This team soon zeroed in on another Brooklyn native, Robert Nowinski, who was across the continent working at the Fred Hutchinson Cancer Research Center in Seattle. Nowinski had an entrepreneurial instinct and had already been approached by more sophisticated venture capitalists the year before. At the time, Nowinski had hesitated, unsure of how best to interface with institutional investors, a class of professional known for their suits and conservative approaches (in terms of thinking style, if not politics). This stereotypical view contrasted with the small subset of scientific researchers on the leading edge of their fields, who tend to be more iconoclastic and originators in terms of their thinking styles.

The Blechs approached Nowinski and assured him they were similarly aggressive in their pursuit of shared goals and would be better partners than more staid investment houses. Nowinski countered he would agree only if the Blechs could raise at least a million dollars by the end of the year and three to six more million dollars within six months. If not, Nowinski wanted to retain the ability to walk away. With those agreed-upon terms, along with an extraordinary compensation plan gifting Nowinski with a sizeable portion of the new venture, the partnership launched. This company, which was formed in Delaware (but based in Seattle), on November 18, 1980, a mere month after the Genetech IPO was named Genetic Systems.[24]

Within six months and with virtually nothing to show other than a snazzy name, the Blechs were able to raise the requisite amounts of money from institutional investors and a large Mexican pharmaceutical company by the name of Syntex (which was later purchased by Roche). Genetics Systems filed for an IPO in June 1981, pricing shares worth nothing, or at most a few pennies just months before, into an enterprise worth six dollars a share. With capital raised, Genetics Systems began to develop products, the first of which was a monoclonal antibody-based diagnostic test for chlamydia. This product was approved for sale in the United States by the FDA in January 1983. A second diagnostic product to detect herpes was approved by FDA later in the year. Although these products generated much-needed revenue, they were products only to diagnose disease, not to treat or prevent it. Treatment was where the real money resided.

In the same year Genetics Systems's first two diagnostic products were approved for sale, the company spun out a new therapeutics enterprise. The new organization, to be known as Oncogen, was a joint venture between Genetic Systems and Syntex dedicated to the development of monoclonal antibody therapeutics. The company launched operations in 1983 and was led by two additional researchers from the Fred Hutchinson Cancer Research Center, Ingegerd Hellstrom and her husband, Karl. The Hellstroms were Swedish-born immigrants to the United States, arriving in 1966. The couple became early pioneers in making the connection between the immune system and cancer (quite an iconoclastic view in the mid-to-late-20th century) and during their studies, the Hellstroms had collaborated with Nowinski to discover a variety of monoclonal antibodies.

In 1986, the scientific team at Oncogen reported the creation of a CD20 monoclonal antibody known as *1F5*.[25] The Hellstroms had already shown certain types of mouse monoclonal antibodies, those of a type known as *IgG2a*, would engage best with human killer cells to allow the killer cells to kill malignant B cells. Not coincidentally then, 1F5 happened to be the first CD20 antibody to be tested in patients with B cell lymphoma.[26]

In 1987, Oncogen scientists partnered with their old colleagues at the Fred Hutchinson Cancer Research Center to begin human testing with 1F5. The original study allowed 1F5 to be administered to four patients with incurable lymphoma.[27] None of the patients experienced untoward effects, indicating the drug was safe, which is always the first goal of testing a new experimental medicine. Two of the four patients had measurable numbers of tumor cells circulating in their blood and, in both cases, 1F5 eliminated 90% of them within a few hours of infusion. In another promising finding, the patients receiving the highest doses of 1F5 showed the greatest magnitude of efficacy in terms of the extent and duration of disease remission. Unfortunately for all involved, this initial trial was limited to a short duration of treatment. Consequently, the remission was short-lived, and the disease returned, eventually claiming three of four of the patients over the following weeks. Despite these heartbreaking outcomes, the main takeaway was the CD20 antibody might show promise if only the drug could be given more frequently, longer, and at higher doses.

The immune system will invariably recognize a mouse antibody, such as 1F5, as foreign and work actively to eliminate it. In the best case, the outcome is the patient's body defense system will eliminate the antibody as soon as it is encountered. At the other extreme, this anti-antibody response can become so vigorous it triggers responses comparable to the experiences following a bee sting or nut allergy in sensitized individuals. Because this response can take days or even weeks to make itself known, the patients in the Oncogen-sponsored study of 1F5 did not experience this extreme effect as the original patients had been dosed with the drug for only five to ten days. A longer duration of treatment would inevitably have caused harm.

In recognition of this concern, scientists around the world began asking if and how to eliminate the reaction against the mouse portions of the antibody. This hurdle proved quite the challenge and it was widely recognized overcoming it would require new thinking and significant resources. To this end, it may come as no surprise Oncogen elected to first align and then sell itself in 1986 to Bristol-Myers, a large pharmaceutical company with ample ideas and resources.[28]

With access to the funding and expertise available following the acquisition of Oncogen by Bristol-Myers, a decision was made to attempt a novel procedure known as *chimerization*. The reader may know the term *chimera* refers to a monster with mixed traits of species, such as a creature with a human head upon an equine body. A more familiar and applicable example is the mythical Egyptian sphinx, which features a human head upon the body of a lion. Reflecting the latter, a chimeric antibody portrayed the idea of starting with a mouse antibody and swapping the murine backbone for a human variant. To this end, the investigators at Oncogen elected not to proceed with 1F5 but rather a better-behaved CD20 antibody named 2H7.[29] About 90% of the mouse portions of the 2H7 antibody protein were then replaced with their human counterparts. The antibody was then tested to ensure it could still recognize and eliminate CD20-bearing B cells in the laboratory and a report of the existence of this chimeric antibody was published by the Oncogen (now Bristol-Myers) team in 1987. Although the chimeric 2H7 antibody proved to be quite promising in the laboratory, the transition from Oncogen to Bristol-Myers gobbled up valuable time in the development of it (as often occurs when a team dedicated to a single project has to give way to a larger bureaucracy). Compounding this, the Oncogen/Brisol-Myers team may not have been aware they were in a footrace with other competitors seeking to develop a CD20 monoclonal antibody. Like the proverbial hare, the presumably faster team gave up the lead to a hungry upstart, who happened not to be a tortoise but an even faster hare who won the race to target successfully CD20 on B cell tumors.

Before changing gears, it is important to close out the Genetic Systems story. As we have seen, David Blech gambled on the creation of both companies and their acquisition by Bristol-Myers paid off nicely. Unfortunately, Blech's brilliance in backing biotechnology was a side effect of a far darker gambling addiction. Rather than betting on cards or dice, Blech's obsession was with shares of start-up companies. The constructive instincts behind the foundation of Genetic Systems, Oncogen, and a handful of other companies eventually gave way to less rational bets upon more reckless companies. As he admitted in a story first reported by Andrew Pollack of the *New York Times*, Blech was one of the wealthiest Americans in the 1990s.[30]

By 2013, David Blech had squandered all his wealth and more and was $11 million in debt and preparing to enter prison under a conviction of securities fraud. According to Blech himself, "There's no question that if I had been in a coma for the last twenty years, I would wake up a billionaire today." Instead, within days of making this statement, he would wake up in a federal prison in Fort Dix, New Jersey, and would not regain his freedom until he had served four years in jail. This outcome was the result of viewing biotechnology investments as something akin to placing random bets on a blackjack table. As the tables turned on Blech, it wiped out his fortune. At one court visit, he pleaded with the judge to consider his diagnosis of bipolar disease and the fact his early investments had been in companies dedicated to improving healthcare. However, this excuse fell on deaf ears when tried again after being convicted for a second time of securities fraud as Blech continued to double down on these bets. Eventually, David Blech had no choice but to utilize illegal means to back those losing bets by defrauding investors, and these actions expedited his relocation from the penthouse to the workhouse.

## The Idea for IDEC

Twelve hundred miles south of Seattle and more than twice the distance southwest of Manhattan, another start-up biotechnology company had been founded in San Diego two years before the founding of Genetic Systems. Hybritech began as the result of an unusual negotiation in the early days after publication of the Kohler and Milstein article on monoclonal antibodies. The negotiators on one side were Ivor Royston, a young assistant professor at the University of Californa, San Diego (UCSD), and his postdoctoral student, Howard Birndorf. On the other side was one of the most accomplished biotechnology investors in history.

Howard Birndorf had largely grown up in or around Detroit and, being a mediocre student, was surprised to be accepted into a start-up college by the name of Michigan State University-Oakland.[31] Now Oakland University, the campus is situated on a large estate formerly owned by John Francis Dodge (one of the two Dodge brothers who started the eponymous automobile maker) and his wife, Matilda Dodge Wilson.[32] Matilda Rausch, as she had been formerly known, graduated from business college and began working in 1902 at Dodge Motor Company, later falling in love with and marrying the company's founder. Upon John's death in 1920, Matilda had become one of the wealthiest women in the United States and five years later, she was remarried to a lumber magnate by the name of Alfred G. Wilson.

Matilda was very active in statewide politics and was appointed lieutenant governor for the State of Michigan in 1940 (the first woman to do so) by

Luren Dickinson, who was the only person to be appointed governor following the death of an incumbent. Matilda could very well have been the second as Dickinson was seventy-nine when he entered office, though he did indeed remain alive for the remaining two years of his appointment. Voted out of office (in part because of Dickinson's age), Matilda Dodge Wilson returned to high society, but her stint of public service had left an indelible impression. Five years prior to the death of her second husband, Matilda found an outlet for this need (and some of her wealth) by founding Oakland University through the donation of $2 million and the entire 1,443-acre estate (and its buildings) Matilda had shared with John Francis Dodge.

Birndorf enrolled at the start-up university in 1967, being one of its earliest students.[33] His classmates during his tenure at Oakland, though it is unclear if they ever crossed paths, included two relatively famous actors, David Hasselhoff (of *Knight Rider* and *Baywatch* fame) and Robert Englund (better known as Freddie Krueger from *Nightmare on Elm Street*). Like many of his fellow students who were motivated by the ongoing Vietnam War, Birndorf majored in political science. He later changed his major to biology after becoming enamored with science following an independent study project working with algae.

Birndorf again found himself enrolling in another start-up, this time being in the first class of the Wayne State University College of Medicine. Remaining intrigued by research, he ended up dropping medicine and instead earned a master's degree in research, while working at the Michigan Cancer Foundation (now the Karmanos Cancer Center) at night. Eventually, the stress of leading this double life, compounded by health concerns with his father, forced a change in scenery and life plans. Birndorf left the bitter winters of Detroit behind and moved to the Bay Area, where he sought to earn a Ph.D. at Stanford.

It was during this time Birndorf first became exposed to monoclonal antibody technology, being one of the first people in the United States to practice the technology. While at Stanford, Birndorf first met Ivor Royston, an English-born doctor who obtained his medical degree from Johns Hopkins before choosing Stanford for his residency.[34] Royston's passion also was centered in research, and he ended up in the laboratory of a junior professor by the name of Ronald Levy. Levy had earned his medical degree in 1968 and was starting down a path leading him to become one of the most respected experts in lymphoma. Royston was interested in immunology and was recruited to UCSD in 1977, bringing along his newly credentialed friend, Howard Birndorf, to join him as a postdoctoral fellow.

A year later, the pair found themselves entertaining a pair of famous venture capitalists at their San Diego laboratory. Fate seemed to have destined Birndorf to enter a third start-up (after Michigan State-Oakland and Wayne State University), this one being an organization of his own making. Over the intervening year since arriving in San Deigo, Birndorf and Royston had not only built an academic laboratory at UCSD, but also had strategized a start-up company to market monoclonal antibody products. The pair determined $178,000 would be needed to initiate this venture.[35] However, the two scientists could not gain interest from investors until fate intervened in a quite unusual way.

After their arrival in San Diego, Birndorf had befriended an oncology nurse working on the wards of the UCSD hospital and introduced her to Royston. Collette Carson and Ivor Royston became a couple and later married. In the course of establishing a relationship, one often tends to avoid mentioning prior affairs. This was not the case with Carson and Royston as Carson admitted having dated a venture capitalist by the name of Brooks Byers. Byers worked at the legendary investment firm of Kleiner, Perkins, Caufield, and Byers. The Menlo Park, California-based venture capital organization had or would seed the creation of many legendary Silicon Valley companies, including America Online, Amazon, Compaq, Netscape, and Google, to name but a few.

Byers's focus was upon a different technology sector, namely life sciences. One of the firm's early investments included Genentech, which as we have already seen, paid off with huge dividends, including the largest biotechnology IPO up to then. Byers had been hired to expand the number of biotechnology investments and in light of this mandate, was receptive to a phone call from a past relationship. During this interaction, Carson asked Byers if he would meet Royston in Menlo Park. Despite the potential for a disaster, the meeting went quite well and prompted a follow-up visit by Byers and Tom Perkins to San Diego a few weeks later.

At the end of a productive day of discussions about the commercial promise of monoclonal antibodies, Royston was driving Byers and Perkins to the airport, when Byers asked how much money would be needed to start the company Royston had envisioned.[36] Having strategized this question with Birndorf weeks before, he was ready for the question and considered responding with the very exact number of $178,000. Upon second thought, Royston wanted to give himself a cushion and instead stated, "$200,000." In a rare occurrence for a venture capitalist, Byers countered this would not be enough and instead offered "$300,000."

With funds in hand, a biotechnology company was founded on September 18, 1978, in the sleepy San Diego suburb of La Jolla. This new entity was given the name of Hybritech (reflecting a combination of technology with hybridomas, the unique type of engineered cancer cell, which can produce monoclonal antibodies). Over the next five years, the investment in Hybritech paid off nicely with the development of multiple monoclonal antibody–based products to improve the diagnosis and tracking of disease. Indeed, the formation of Hybritech was the nucleating event in the creation of a thriving biotechnology community in La Jolla, and entrepreneurs from Hybritech alone are credited with the creation of at least forty follow-on biotechnology organizations.[37] Hybritech, and its attendant monoclonal antibody technology, was to become so successful, Eli Lilly and Company acquired the company in September 1985 for $300 million, seven years and one day after its founding and at a price one thousand times higher than Kleiner, Perkins, Caufield, and Byers's original investment.

By the time of the Lilly acquisition, Birndorf had left Hybritech to start another La Jolla-based monoclonal antibody company. This company was founded in 1985 by the same duo behind Hybritech (Royston and Birndorf) and would also include their former Stanford colleague, Ron Levy, and a UCSD colleague by the name of Robert Sobel. The company was financed by a superstar consortium of investors led again by Brook Byers of Kleiner Perkins. The new company's name was IDEC Pharmaceuticals.[38]

Whereas Hybritech had been quite successful in proving the application of monoclonal antibodies to diagnostics could be impactful (and profitable), IDEC would seek to develop antibodies to be used for therapy. The initial scientific approach for IDEC had been intended to develop what are known as *anti-idiotype antibodies*. Without going into too much detail, this was an ambitious idea to create personalized therapies for a set of B cell cancers and certain autoimmune indications. However, like many other highly ambitious and cutting-edge ideas, executing this plan would prove to be a bit too complicated, even for relative veterans like Birndorf and Royston.

In August 1990, IDEC scientists pivoted and initiated a rather simple but extraordinarily crucial experiment that would forever change cancer therapy: A mouse was immunized with a human B cell tumor cell line. As one might expect, the mouse rejected the tumor cells because the cell line was from a different species and the immune system has evolved over billions of years for this exact purpose. In doing so, the mouse produced an array of antibodies targeted at the foreign intruder. The investigators performing the study anticipated the mouse antibodies would be directed primarily against proteins distinguishing human cells from their mouse counterparts. This would entail proteins mostly irrelevant to tumor biology but maybe, just maybe, they might get lucky and find something else. To hedge their bet in their favor, the IDEC scientists used a trick. Multiple mice were immunized with this cell line. Before going through the laborious undertaking of making monoclonal antibodies, they only selected mice that showed a strong predilection for generating antibodies against CD20 (which you may recall was the molecule identified by Ratner and had shown some promise in the treatment of B cell leukemia/lymphoma). This trick dramatically increased their luck.

The monoclonal antibodies arising from the mouse immunized with human B cells included one particular clone known as *2B8*. This clone bound nicely to CD20 and likewise showed promising behavior in terms of killing tumor cells via multiple laboratory measures (techniques known as *complement and antibody-dependent cellular cytotoxicity*, or ADCC).

Recognizing the limitations in advancing a mouse antibody, the IDEC team subjected 2B8 to a similar chimeric strategy their competitors at Oncogen/Bristol-Myers had adopted. The IDEC team isolated the DNA that produced the 2B8 antibody and, using molecular genetic techniques still evolving at the time, they were able to create a mouse-human chimera. As you may recall, this chimeric antibody had been designed to minimize the likelihood that, once injected into a patient, their immune systems would recognize it as foreign and reject the therapeutic antibody before it could perform its intended function to seek out and kill tumor cells.

Recognizing the competition with the Oncogen/Bristol-Myers team, the IDEC scientists kept their findings rather secretive until after the clinical investigation was well underway. The first description of this new experimental therapeutic IDEC-C2B8 (the "C" indicating it was a chimeric antibody) would not be released until January 1994.[39] Just as this publication was appearing, the IDEC team was in the process of submitting for publication a paper reporting the outcome of the first clinical trials, which appeared later in October.[40]

In December 1992, IDEC had filed paperwork with the FDA as necessary to initiate clinical trials of IDEC-C2B8.[41] This investigation had commenced in February 1993 with a single-dose study in patients with non-Hodgkin's lymphoma, a B cell cancer known to have abundant amounts of CD20 on the surface of the malignant cells that could be targeted by their antibody. After receiving a single dose of IDEC-C2B8, the results were striking: Of fifteen patients treated, six had shown signs of tumor shrinkage. Remaining nimble, secretive, and driven, by the time the report of this trial had been published in October 1994, IDEC had already completed what is known as a *phase II clinical trial* to verify the efficacy of their product. These results were needed to identify the dose to be used for the pivotal phase III clinical studies necessary to receive a nod from FDA for marketing. This key phase III clinical study had already been largely designed (often a process requiring months or years) and was preparing for a launch in March 1995. Keeping up this relentless pace, the IDEC team would not only efficiently complete the phase III trial but submit the entire package of information needed by the FDA (thousands upon thousands of pages), all within two years. In November 1997, the FDA had reviewed the outcomes and approved the product, now known as Rituxan (rituximab). By this time, IDEC had also taken an aggressive business strategy approach and licensed the marketing rights for rituximab to Genentech, keeping the product within the stable of companies created by Brook Byers. The strategy of partnering with Genentech also allowed the IDEC team to utilize the existing sales and marketing engine of the more established company, Genentech, to maximize sales of their B cell leukemia product while IDEC went back to developing more cancer drugs.

These dates and timeline may not seem remarkable to most readers, but it truly was extraordinary, especially since rituximab was a different beast than had ever been considered previously for use in humans. In 1985, the FDA had approved the first monoclonal antibody therapeutic, a mouse antibody named Muromonab-CD3. This antibody targeted and killed T cells in organ transplant patients. By essentially shutting down the immune system (by depriving it of T cell help), Muromonab-CD3 had the beneficial side effect of decreasing the likelihood the mouse origin of the drug itself would cause it to be rejected by the human immune system. However, the utter destruction of the body's defense network, as evidenced by maladies like AIDS, is not a preferred way of addressing any disease for a prolonged time.

In 1994, another antibody product, known as *abciximab* (or ReoPro®) was another pioneer. ReoPro had been engineered to be chimeric (thereby decreasing the likelihood it would be rejected) but the product was only a fragment of an antibody.[42] It had been developed for short-term use in protecting or treating patients from ischemia (a blood clotting disease) by blocking platelets, the small cell-like fragments responsible for blood clotting. The developers of ReoPro had themselves minimized the risk their product might elicit protective immunity by chopping away the bulk of the antibody, thereby removing much of the mouse portions that might betray the antibody therapeutic as foreign. Such an approach was not an option for IDEC since these very regions were necessary for the efficacy of rituximab.

What distinguished rituximab from these earlier products was its design to optimize the active elimination of diseased cells by utilizing the natural killing capacity of the human immune system. Let's unpack this rather ambitious sentence a bit. Beyond the beneficial effects of decreasing the likelihood rituximab might itself be recognized as foreign, the product was innovative, as rituximab had been engineered to deploy the human portions of antibodies essential for tumor cell killing by the complement cascade or by antibody-dependent cellular cytotoxicity.[43] Muromonab-CD3 had not met this goal because the mouse portions of the antibody worked relatively inefficiently with human killing mechanisms. Likewise, ReoPro had not accomplished this task as it was designed simply to block its target (platelets) rather than to kill them.

Given the novelty of the product and efficiency for killing, the regulators at FDA were understandably concerned about the potential for unwanted toxicities arising in patients after rituximab treatment. For example, if the drug bound to other cells in the body (other than the intended B cells targets), the greater efficiency in killing might be imparted upon normal tissues, causing collateral side effects or even death. Another problem with

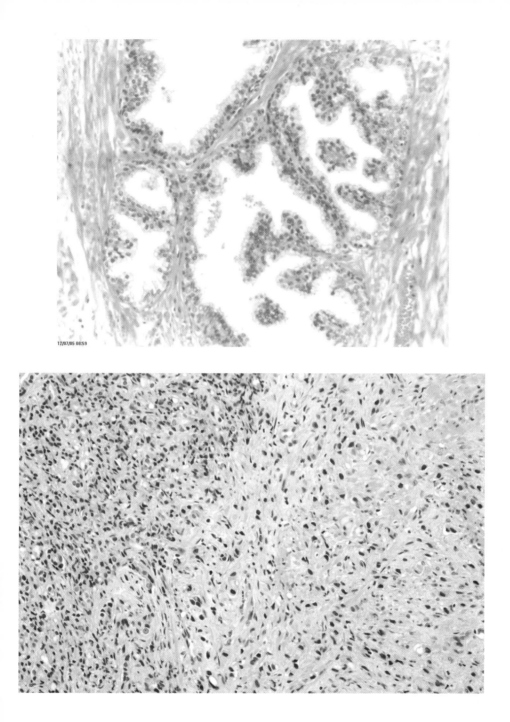

**FIGURES 1A and B. WHAT IS CANCER?** At a fundamental level, cancer is a disease of inappropriate cell growth or survival. Contrast the open spaces and organized structure of a benign prostate (A) with the crowded and muddled architecture of an individual diagnosed with prostate cancer (B). These samples were prepared using special dyes that stain the DNA-containing nucleus (violet) and proteins (pink) to allow a pathologist to assess the shape and number of cells in a specimen.

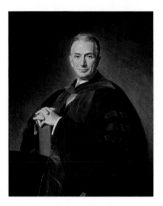

**FIGURE 2 (LEFT). SURPRISINGLY HIGH FREQUENCY OF CANCER.** By analyzing prostate specimens (see above) under the microscope, Arnold Rice Rich of Johns Hopkins University revealed in 1934 a disconcertingly high frequency of prostate cancer in men displaying no symptoms of diseases. This finding would be periodically rediscovered and raises questions about the definition of "disease" and when and how to intervene.

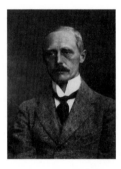

**FIGURE 3 (RIGHT). SPREADING LIKE A VIRUS.** The Danish scientist Vilhelm Ellerman was amongst the first to realize that some cancer could spread like an infection. Ironically, a deadly infection, contracted while shaving with a cut-rate shaving brush, killed Ellerman in 1924.

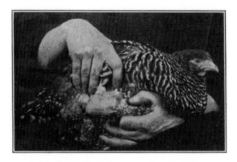

**FIGURE 4 (LEFT). NOT A BIRD-BRAINED IDEA.** A photograph of one of oncology's most important contributors. A chicken, brought to the Rockefeller Institute laboratory of Peyton Rous and Simon Flexner in October 1909, sported a tumor with the ability to be spread to other birds, ultimately revealing certain viruses contribute to cancer.

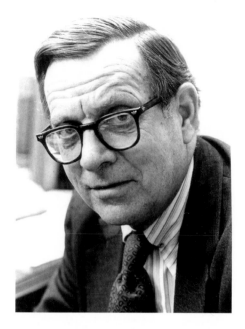

**FIGURES 5 A AND B. RABBIT EAR EPIPHANY. (A)** Lewis Thomas (1913–1993) was a polymath biologist, who became fascinated with the dynamism in the body, based in large part based upon the observation that injection of the meat tenderizer, papain, into the ears of rabbits caused them to flop and, over time, to rebound to normal. **(B)** Thomas appreciated that the ability of cells and tissues to grow and repair might also explain cancer as a disease of inappropriate growth.

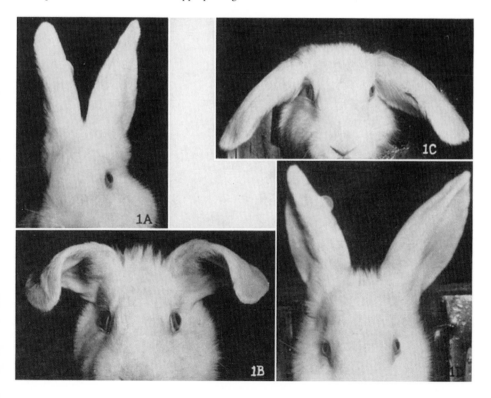

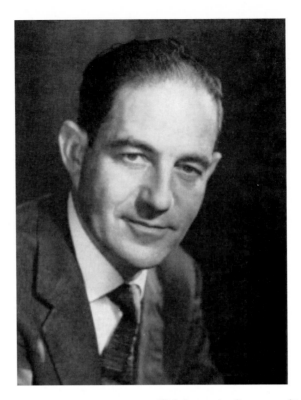

**FIGURES 6 A AND B. DISCOVERY OF INTERFERON. (A)** Alick Isaacs, the discoverer of interferon, based his work in part on understanding how infection with one virus can protect the body from other viruses. **(B)** The potential use of interferon for viral infection, cancer, and presumably many other diseases captured public attention, as evidenced by a Flash Gordon cartoon relating the miraculous (most which were speculative) properties of Isaacs's discovery.

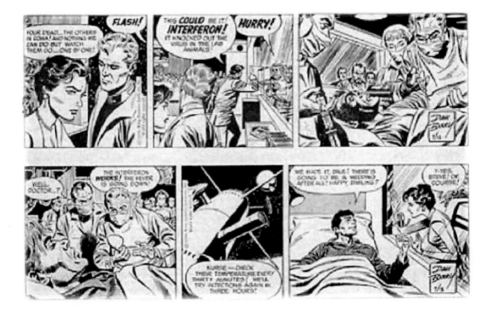

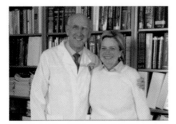

**FIGURE 7. A NEW WONDER DRUG?** In the latter quarter of the twentieth century, much excitement surrounded interleukin-2, a chemical the immune system utilizes to stimulate its activity. One example of the potential of immune therapy was conveyed by Linda Taylor, a US Navy officer diagnosed with incurable melanoma but who was successfully treated with interleukin-2 by a National Cancer Institute investigator, Steven Rosenberg.

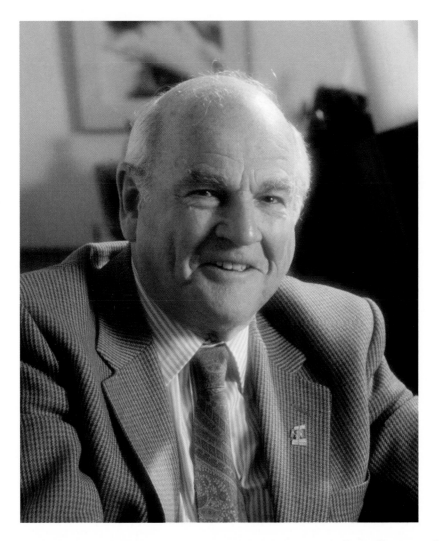

**FIGURE 8. SEARCH AND DESTROYING A VIRAL CAUSE OF HUMAN CANCER.** Originally motivated to analyze the differences between the genetics of different individuals, Baruch Blumberg chanced upon a finding that led him to discover hepatitis b virus (HBV), the cause of many liver and other cancers. Moreover, Blumberg led a team that soon thereafter introduced a vaccine with the potential to utterly eliminate HBV-mediated cancers.

**FIGURES 9 A, B, AND C. A MYTHICAL CREATURE CAUSES THE ELIMINATION OF DEADLY CANCERS.** Shown are photographs of mythical and real-life jackelopes, rabbits sporting large "horns." The studies of Richard Shope revealed a family of papilloma viruses that cause these benign tumors and provided the foundations for later vaccines to prevent cancers caused by human papillomavirus, most notably cervical cancer.

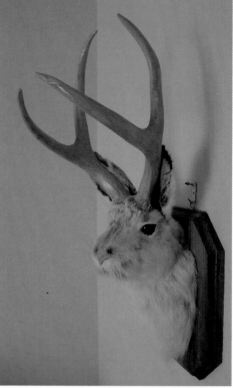

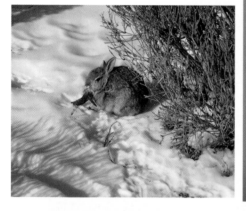

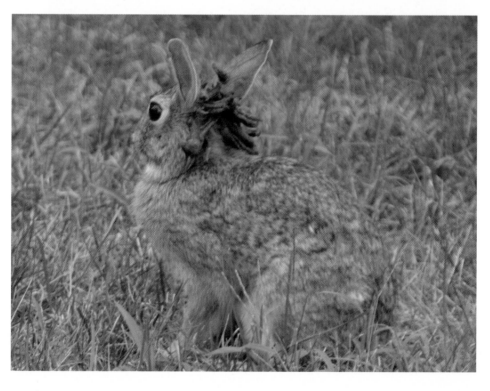

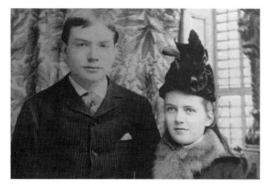

**FIGURE 10 (LEFT). A TRAGIC FRIENDSHIP THAT IGNITED A REVOLUTION.** A young woman, Elizabeth (Bessie) Dashiell (right), whose best friend happened to be John David Rockefeller, Jr. (left), would soon die after an agonizing bout of cancer, an event that inspired both her physician and Rockefeller.

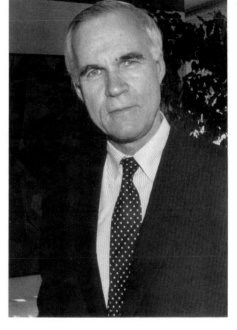

**FIGURE 11 (RIGHT). AN OLD STORY.** Supported by William Coley's daughter and the non-profit organization she created, William Old pioneered a rediscovery of Coley's concepts for provoking the immune system to target cancer.

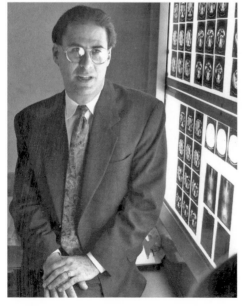

**FIGURE 12 (LEFT). PROFANE AND PROFOUND.** The outspoken personality of Lee Nadler helped propel him to international fame, pioneering the clinical application of a new type of targeted medicine, known as monoclonal antibodies, designed to selectively target cancer cells and recruit the immune system for their elimination.

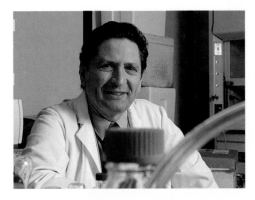

**FIGURE 13 (LEFT). LAUNCHING AN ENTERPRISE.** The biotechnology pioneer Howard Bierndorf founded a series of companies that helped transform the esoteric science of monoclonal antibodies into a commercially-viable enterprise that would soon revolutionize cancer care.

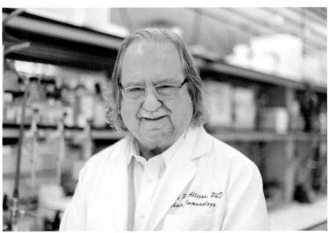

**FIGURES 14 A AND B. DRIVING THROUGH A CHECKPOINT.** The decisive discoveries leading to a new generation of so-called "checkpoint therapies" for cancer, which re-sensitize cells of the immune system to target cancer was made by a pair of immunologists, (A) James (Jim) P. Allison and (B) Tasuku Honjo, both of whom were recognized with the 2018 Nobel Prize in Physiology or Medicine.

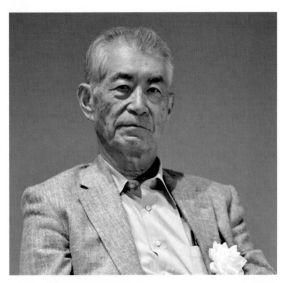

the human-mouse chimeric approach was the antibody could remain in treated subjects for days, weeks, and even months. This is different than a conventional small molecule, which tends to be eliminated within a few hours. Consequently, any unwanted toxicity imparted by rituximab might be expected to last for prolonged periods and this fear triggered proportional worries on the part of FDA regulators.

Another obvious problem was rituximab could recognize and kill all B cells. This meant not only would malignant cells be eliminated, but normal B cells, which provide a service in fighting infection, would likewise be killed. However, such concerns paled in comparison with the morbidity and mortality arising from non-Hodgkin's lymphoma and other deadly B cell cancers.

Any or all of these concerns might easily have been predicted to impede the ability of IDEC even to begin human testing, much less to gain a blanket approval for its sales and marketing within a handful of years. The rituximab experience is remarkable as, despite or perhaps because of these concerns, IDEC and the FDA were able to work together efficiently to allay potential fears surrounding a new medicine that would break ground in terms of the mechanism, efficacy, and safety of this experimental medicine. Consequently, the success in approving rituximab so efficiently should be noted by advocates and critics of both the biopharmaceutical enterprise and its regulators (the FDA) as one of many instances where the public interest was best served by a close communication and partnership and demonstrated courage needed to gain approval for a new type of medicine with extraordinary potential and equally daunting risks.

### Ending with a Bang

As the results from clinical trials of rituximab began to look more and more promising, the FDA, as well as other biotechnology companies, became more enthusiastic about the potential for monoclonal antibody therapeutics. Indeed, one can make a strong argument the approval of rituximab opened a new era for cancer therapy, the limits of which have yet to be realized.

In an unexpected way, the technology conveyed by monoclonal antibodies captured the imagination of both investors and the public from a most unusual source: the 1991 Gulf War. During the operation to oust

Iraq from its occupation of neighboring Kuwait, the world stood in awe of the firepower and accuracy of new missiles with the ability to home in on targets, seemingly down to the inch, and then pulverize them into dust. The specificity of monoclonal antibodies and their ability to recognize a target and then destroy it provided a useful analogy for countless presentations by entrepreneurs pitching investors to elicit their support for a new monoclonal antibody company to target cancer.

As a consequence of the pioneering product represented by rituximab, waves of antibody-based therapies were tested and many approved. Overall, monoclonal antibodies grew to represent almost a third of all new medicines approved by the FDA by the end of the century and at least half of these antibodies were directed against cancer. Virtually all were inspired or impacted by the experience of rituximab.[44][45]

A rather dirty secret about rituximab, however, was its clinical efficacy was not really spectacular. It was closer to mediocre. While the drug was certainly less toxic than conventional cancer chemotherapy, which tends tended to kill virtually all growing cells, rituximab targeted only B cells. However, not all patients responded robustly to treatment with the drug and in many, the disease would return. One drug's weaknesses inspires the creation of a potential usurper. In a phrase, the field needed to "go nuclear."

In *A Prescription for Change*, I detail the rationale behind and the fate of two later monoclonal antibody products, Zevalin® and Bexxar®, but some points warrant repeating. The developers of both drugs (Zevalin® was developed by IDEC and Bexxar® by Corixa, a Seattle-based company, partnered with GlaxoSmithKline) recognized the deficiencies offered by rituximab and addressed these by making a radioactive form of a CD20 antibody. The idea was the radioactivity would not only destroy the tumor cell bound by the antibody but also other tumors cells in the vicinity. Using molecules on hand, the antibody developed by Lee Nadler (which you may recall was named "B1") was licensed to Coulter Pharmaceuticals and then to GlaxoSmithKline and formed the backbone of Bexxar®. The potency of this "hot" drug derived from the fact it had been creating and linked to iodine-131, a powerful gamma ray-emitting radioactive element. The radiation from Bexxar® kills surrounding cells in intimate contact with the malignant B cell, which usually includes other tumor cells and a network of supporting cells.[46] Likewise, Zevalin® was a CD20 antibody from IDEC (though not rituximab, as this molecule, you may recall, had been licensed to Genentech). This drug used as its warhead Yttrium-90, a highly radioactive decay product of strontium-90, which in turn is a byproduct of radioactive uranium from spent nuclear reactor fuel (in some cases, another energetic isotope, Indium-111, is used for Zevalin®).

The addition of a radioactive warhead to a CD20 antibody did indeed prove far more effective in rooting out tumors and demonstrated clear superiority for the treatment of B cell cancer. However, much inconvenience resulted from having a patient loaded with radioactive material, whose bodily fluids and feces had to be collected, documented, and stored as radioactive waste. These encumbrances combined with a profound disconnect between the different types of oncologists, who prescribe or are reimbursed by insurance companies for chemotherapy. Specifically, most chemotherapeutics are prescribed by a cancer specialist, or a medical oncologist, whereas the radioactive drugs required a prescription from a radiation oncologist. The field of radiation oncology is dominated by the use of x-ray and other radioactive devices and antibody therapeutics were outside the normal boundaries of the field. Consequently, both drugs showed great potential in the clinic but failed in the marketplace. Nonetheless a lesson had been learned: Good antibody products might be made great if given a bit more of a "kick."

The experiences with the superior efficacy, though failed, commercial prospects effectively destroyed the future for radioactively labeled antibodies. However, biotechnology advances meant a number of other killing properties of antibodies might be improved. One distinct advantage of a chimeric antibody over a mouse monoclonal antibody was the utilization of ADCC and complement killing mechanisms. These killing pathways were enhanced further by tweaking antibody products to perform each function more efficiently. Unsurprisingly, CD20 was the target for the first of these products with the 2013 FDA approval of obinutuzumab, which had been developed by Genentech (subsequently acquired by Roche) and a Swiss company, Glycart Biotechnology (also acquired by Roche).

Further improvements could be achieved by linking the antibody to a deadly toxin. The idea here was to use drugs so toxic they could not be given alone. These toxins were so powerful they could kill virtually any cell with which they interacted. By linking the toxin to an antibody, the toxin could act as a type of warhead with the antibody providing the guidance mechanism. In doing so, very little toxin would be needed, and the antibody homing system would prevent the toxin from encountering friendly or benign cells.

The first antibody-drug toxin to receive an approval from the FDA was gemtuzumab ozogamicin (commercial name: Mylotarg™). The landmark drug was developed by Wyeth (later acquired by Pfizer) and received an approval for the treatment of acute myeloid leukemia in 2000. The product combined a monoclonal antibody with the ability to recognize a molecule on the surface of the Acute Myeloid Leukemia (AML) tumor cells—a particularly nasty little molecule known as *calicheamicin*. This toxin is produced by a bacterium known as *Micromonospora echinospora* and is famous in part because is it believed to have contributed to the poisoning death of Alexander the Great in the 4th century B.C.E.[47] High levels of calicheamicin in certain bodies of waters in the Middle East are also believed to have spawned the myth of the River Styx, the river of death separating Earth from Hades.

The downside of using Mylotarg has been that calicheamicin continues to live up to its nasty reputation. Even when given at the very low levels as when attached to antibodies, the antibody-drug toxin has a frustrating tendency to fall apart. The detachment of the toxin from the antibody released microscopic amounts of calicheamicin, but the toxin was so powerful that even these small amounts released from the antibody were sufficient to cause side effects, ranging from a bad fever to failure of the bone marrow, lungs, or often blood vessels, sometimes resulting in death.[48] Indeed, the drug was withdrawn from the market in 2010 due to this bad reputation. However, like a mythic hero able to return from Hades, Mylotarg came back from the dead in 2017 when the FDA determined the dangers from AML sufficiently outweighed the potential for damage from Mylotarg and allowed Pfizer to resume sales.

The experiences with Mylotarg (and its tendency to release the toxin from the antibody) prompted technological improvements, which have indeed proven utility as evidenced by recent successes in the clinic. A prominent example is provided by the antibody-drug toxin conjugates produced by Seattle Genetics (a company founded by survivors of the Oncogen/Bristol-Myers team following the decision by Bristol-Myers Squibb to close its Seattle research site). In November 2017, Seattle Genetics gained an approval for brentuximab vedotin for the treatment of certain blood cancers. This product entailed improvements in both the choice of toxin (derived from a toxic mollusk from the Indian Ocean and western portions of the Pacific Ocean) and a rather clever linker, which was engineered to remain highly stable outside of cells but once internalized into cancer cells, is cast aside to allow the toxin to kill the tumor. These improvements conveyed a product far more sophisticated, safe and effective than Mylotarg.

Although promising, antibody drug conjugate technology can still be quite dangerous as was learned by Seattle Genetics itself. Despite having what is considered some of the best technology for developing these unique types of medicines, another drug the company had developed for the treatment of acute myeloid leukemia, vadastuximab talirine, was withdrawn after it was implicated in the deaths of four volunteers during clinical trials.[49] Such toxicities can arise if or when the toxin happens to disengage from the antibody and thereby gain access to normal cells where it commences to inflict damage. These types of events have proven challenging but at the same time have incentivized constant improvements in toxin technology, which will enhance the safety and efficacy of future guided missiles to fight future battles against cancer.

## BiTE Me

From reading this book, you might come away thinking I have a really annoying habit of popping out of my chair in excitement from time to time. You would actually be mostly accurate in this assessment. In my defense, this has only happened on a handful of occasions, perhaps a half dozen or so, and to my knowledge, there have not yet been any restraining orders issued by the court due to this unfortunate tendency. One of the times this has happened (beyond my popping out of my seat at the revelation of the high frequency of prostate cancer) arose with the technology now being highlighted. Undoubtedly, my writing of this section will induce at least a few instances of bounding off my chair but, thankfully, the reader will not witness this from your vantage point.

In late 2002, roughly a year after I had "turned to the dark side" by leaving an academic career to head cancer biology at a biopharmaceutical company, I was asked to attend a presentation from a small Munich, Germany, based start-up company. This company named Micromet AG was pioneering an approach to manipulate the types of standard advantages afforded by antibodies, namely their specificity, into products with the potential to revolutionize medicine. The resultant technology, known as a *BiTE*, was so-named for being a bispecific T cell engager. Taking this mouthful of a name apart, what it represents is fairly straightforward. The Micromet team had built upon a well-known technology known as *scFvs*, which deserves a quick introduction.

As the promise of monoclonal antibody technology began to come into focus in the 1980s, many questions arose as to how these molecules might be manipulated were springing forth in the early years of the biotechnology revolution. The biotechnology revolution started quite small, literally, focusing on molecules that could be created and produced by bacteria (and then purified for use in people). Unlike relatively straightforward molecules, such as insulin, which tend to live in the real world as a single protein, antibodies are a complex and frustrating combinations of four different proteins (you may recall them being a dimer of dimers). Like the most complex jigsaw puzzle imaginable, even a slight variation in how the pieces come together can destroy the entire structure. This fact created an extraordinary challenge to investigators seeking to modify and improve upon nature (to improve safety, efficacy, or even the ability to grow the antibody and at a scale sufficient to manufacture product to sell). In the mid-1980s, two investigators at the Max Planck Institute of Biochemistry in Martinsried, Germany, found a way to reliably deconstruct an existing antibody, say in a mouse or person, and rebuild the "business end" (the portion binding to the foreign substance) in a bacterium.[50] This single-chain variable fragment (or scFv) could then allow investigators to deploy the array of tricks to improve how the antibody interacts with the rest of the world. For example, one could modify the antibody so it maximizes the binding to a viral protein while minimizing its potential to interact with (and potentially harm) human cells.

One person immersed in such technologies was Patrick Baeuerle. Born in Friedrichshafen, (West) Germany, in 1957, Baeuerle first studied at the University of Konstanz before receiving a Ph.D. in biochemistry from the Ludwig Maximillian University of Munich. After postdoctoral training with a Nobel laureate at MIT, Baeuerle returned to Germany, and led a research team in Martinsried. In the same year I started as a professor in academia, Patrick was leaving to join the private sector, where he further honed his skills in drug discovery in general and monoclonal antibody technology (especially scFvs) in particular, eventually ending up as the head of research at Micromet.

The team Baeuerle led was extending the ideas behind scFvs and essentially "gluing" two scFv molecules together. Rather than using an actual adhesive, the Micromet team genetically engineered the DNA of scFvs so a single molecule could be produced with two antibody-like ends, each of which recognized a different molecule. The idea behind Micromet's success was one end could recognize and stimulate the T cell receptor complex in such a way that it provoked the T cell to kill whatever was recognized by the other side of the BiTE molecule. Their strategy was therefore to identify molecules to selectively betray the identity of cancer cells so nearby T cells could kill it.

Given the high frequency of cancer, one might surmise cancer cells actively seek to stay as far away as possible from T cells (the constables of the body whose job it is to seek and destroy them). Actually, quite the opposite is true. Oftentimes, a tumor may be virtually bathed in T cells but the key here is these T cells either have lost their ability to kill cancer cells (a subject to which we will return) or recognize virtually anything other than the tumor. For example, the T cells surrounding a tumor may recognize the outcome of the flu shot you received last autumn or the cold you had as a child. Most of these T cells may not specifically recognize molecules displayed on the surface of tumor cells. Thus, one ends up in an almost comical situation, where the prisoners readily walk among the guards and even shout their exploits for all to hear. An extreme analogy is the predominance of irrelevant T cells surrounding a tumor may reflect something akin to the "human shields" deployed by Saddam Hussein during the Gulf Wars in which the purpose of the T cells (from the tumor's perspective) is to prevent those capable of lethal force from getting to the cancer cells.

Therein lies the clever trick of the BiTE technology. These small Janus-like warheads are designed to seek out and engage a tumor-specific molecule and then to interact with surrounding T cells in such a way that an immune cell will override its limitation in targeting only an influenza virus and instead attack the cell bound by the other end of the BiTE molecule.

Returning to autumn 2002, as I was sitting through a description of this idea by Patrick Baeuerle, its significance was immediate and extraordinary, hence the popping from my seat. Within months, we had not only confirmed the value of this technology to projects for which we were engaged at MedImmune, but also licensed Micromet's lead program. This BiTE, known as *MT-103*, was directed to target CD19, a molecule you may recall from earlier is found on every B cell, including the large number of B cell cancers. In the laboratory, MT-103 could bind to a malignant B cell and within minutes recruit a bystander T cell to kill the tumor cell. Moreover, we confirmed Micromet's finding that a T cell could kill and kill again, converting a peaceful bystander into a serial killer.

In clinical trials, the molecule also worked like a charm. In fact, it worked too well. In thinking through how it was designed to be used, MT-103 would co-opt one type of immune cell (a T cell) to kill another (a malignant B cell). Many T cells would be activated, a byproduct of which is the dumping of molecules known as *cytokines*, which evolved to help alert the body to the threat of a foreign invader. One impact of these cytokines is to loosen the blood vessels, a response that evolved to allow immune cells in the blood to gain access to tissues. These actions explain why wounds tend to rapidly swell with excess cells and bodily fluids. When amplified and accelerated by a vigorous dose of cytokines, the same response can dramatically decrease blood pressure and quickly starve critical organs, such as the kidneys, of much-needed oxygen, essentially asphyxiating the victim from within. Worse still, the target of MT-103 was another type of lymphocyte, which itself would shed its own cytokines in its final throes of life as it was being killed. As a consequence, we predicted and found MT-103 treatment would cause a rapid escalation in symptoms worse than one might encounter in all but the worst cases of influenza infection, caused by the cytokines. Indeed, if left unregulated, MT-103 could cause a cytokine storm more acutely lethal than the cancer itself.

The solution to this problem was found by again by exploiting a weakness of the BiTE itself. The BiTEs tended to fall apart rather quickly after being administered. For this reason, they were given *via* an intravenous line (slowly through a needle in a vein). If the drug was too effective in killing tumor cells and causing too much fever and other symptoms of a cytokine storm, the rate of delivery could be slowed and any undesired effects would resolve themselves fairly quickly since excess molecules would quickly break down in the body. On the other hand, if higher amounts of tumor killing were needed, the amount and rate of the drug could be increased.

In the clinic and the laboratory, the results were remarkable. One morning, I was asked to witness a cohort of mice with large tumors on their backs. These animals then received BiTE therapy. By the time I left for home, the tumors had all but disappeared. With one other exception (another immune-based therapy), I have never witnessed anything like this. Similar results were being registered in the clinic. Once the rate of delivery of the drug had been optimized (which could present a challenge given how quickly and efficiently the BiTEs killed tumor cells), patient responses were equally remarkable.

Ultimately, the MT-103 project did gain an FDA approval and is sold as blinatumomab (trade name: Blincyto®). However, the purveyor of the product would turn out to be Amgen, a rival to MedImmune. The reasoning for this switch is complex and to this day still largely baffles me, but MedImmune elected to abandon MT-103 out of concerns the drug would require a "backpack" for its administration. The term *backpack* is an intentionally derogatory term to signify the long, slow delivery of the drug would require the patient to have an intravenous line in place for up to two weeks. Although this device was readily available and used to treat other indications, the marketing team at MedImmune wanted a single injection and claimed the patient would balk at having to lug around a "backpack" for half a month. One of the counterarguments made by my clinical colleagues and myself was that the size of the device was actually more reminiscent of a "fanny pack" and patients would embrace the temporary distraction of the fanny pack if the alternative was death. Although it still pains me to write this (more than a decade later), it is nonetheless clear the marketing department is tasked with ensuring revenues and, consequently, revenue trumps science or medicine. The marketing group decided to abandon the BiTE technology and within months, I made a decision to leave MedImmune. As a postscript, Blincyto generated $46 million worldwide in the fourth quarter of 2017 (which translates to about $190 million per year) and was growing by 59% year on year. So much for backpacks not selling . . .

Beyond BiTEs, antibody drug conjugates and naked antibodies (those lacking any tricks), along with the use of monoclonal antibodies and the exquisite targeting opportunities they conveyed, inspired the creation of a series of next-generation medicines, which sought to more fully harness the killing capacity of the immune system to target cancer. Inspired in part by the results with BiTEs, these newer medicines sought to unleash the extraordinary power of the most lethal cells in the body: killer T cells.

# 7

# *Designer Drugs*

You may recall this book kicked off with a description of my work studying prostate cancer, a disease perhaps inevitable in any male still alive after retirement age. Despite its prevalence, many scholarly reports claim prostate cancer had never been described in medical literature until 1853. These views cite a paper in the prestigious British medical journal, *The Lancet*, from a pathologist at the Royal London Hospital named John Adams (not to be confused with the second or sixth U.S. president of the same name), who described the disease as he analyzed a specimen removed from a patient under a microscope.[1] Adams described the features of the cancer in microscopic detail (literally) and claimed the disease was "very rare" and, regarding therapy, "unfortunately, little of a satisfactory nature can be said." A closer look at the scientific literature reveals that Adams neither sought nor deserves the credit for discovering the disease, although the geography was fairly close. Rather, the earliest known description of the disease was recorded by William Lawrence in 1817 (when Adams was eleven years old), based on observations by his colleague, George Langstaff, a physician at St. Giles's Cripplegate workhouse, a debtor's prison in London.[2]

Although Adams had inaccurately claimed the disease was rare, he was spot-on in claiming treatment of the disease was particularly challenging. In what may seem rather paradoxical, the fastest growing forms of cancer often tend to be the most amenable to therapy. These tumors tend to consist of rapidly growing cells and in their frenzy to obtain nutrients to support their growth, they will ingest practically anything they are given. Exploiting this rabid appetite, researchers devised poisonous versions of the components of DNA and proteins. In their haste to acquire nutrients, tumor cells tend to be far more likely to ingest these toxins and die.

This feeding frenzy is the basis supporting most chemotherapeutic break-throughs of the second half of the 20th century. However, this strategy does expose its own problems as some normal cells, particularly fast-growing ones, also tend to dine on these poisons and are thus responsible for the nausea, anemia, and hair loss frequently associated with cancer chemo-therapy. Despite these considerable side effects, in the early years of the war against cancer, massive strides were made against fast-growing tumors. A very different outcome faces patients with slow-growing cancers. These tumor cells can be quite picky about their nutrients, which precludes effec-tive therapy with conventional antitumor drugs. And among the slowest growing tumors of them all is prostate cancer.

It may be unsurprising, then, that prostate cancer is not often a candidate for conventional chemotherapy. The exceptions, of course, are the minority of patients with fast-growing prostate cancers. However, in general, other than surgery or ablation with implanted radioactive "seeds," or the optimis-tically termed option of *watchful waiting* (doing nothing), the alternatives are fairly sparse.

Watchful waiting is not quite the utter inertia the name implies. The idea is the physician should monitor the levels of various markers that betray the presence of malignant cells. The most famous of these is a molecule known as *prostate-specific antigen* (PSA), a protein produced by the prostate, which can find its way into the blood at a level more or less proportional to the number of prostate cells. Thus, changes in the levels of PSA provide an estimate as to the size and growth of malignant cells of the prostate over time. The relevance of PSA as a means to diagnose or predict the outcome of prostate cancer has been the source of quite vociferous arguments within the medical community and is likely to be an issue truly never resolved. However, we will not focus too much attention upon PSA but instead will introduce another marker of prostate cancer, whose utility goes far beyond the mere diagnosis of disease and may harken its potential eradication in some patients.

### Mansplaining the Prostate

Taking a step back, the prostate gland is a rather remarkable and mysterious organ. The name for the organ is derived from the ancient Greek term, *prostates*, which loosely translates into "protector" or "guardian." Indeed, one might argue this is an appropriate name for the walnut-sized organ nestled between the bladder and the rectum, as its guards the entire human species—absent its function, our reproductive capabilities would cease.

The function of the prostate is to secrete a milky-white fluid accounting for about a third of the volume of a male ejaculate (much of the rest being from sperm created in the testicles). This is not simply a space filler—the prostate manufactures a handful of proteins whose job it is to clean the "plumbing" in a manner facilitating the survival and mobility of the sperm upon ejaculation. This essential role has evolved, as nature has repurposed certain parts of our anatomy to do entirely different things. Specifically, the same reproductive site responsible for producing and dispensing semen is used to eliminate liquid wastes from the bladder. Urine tends to be rather acidic and these acids are quite harmful to sperm, often causing them to coagulate and form globules, which could impede their ability to swim upstream in search of an egg to be fertilized. Thus, the prostate manufactures proteins and fluids that cleanse and neutralize the acidic environment and render it suitable for the safe passage of sperm. One molecule involved in this process is known as *prostatic acid phosphatase* (or PAP).[3]

In 1938, a husband-and-wife team of Columbia University oncology researchers described the presence of a particular enzyme, known as a *phosphatase*, in the blood of men with metastatic prostate cancer.[4] Alexander and Ethel Gutman had followed up on seminal work from the University of Heidelberg, Germany, that described an acid phosphatase, produced in the prostate, whose activity was optimal under acidic conditions.[5] What made the Gutmans' work stand out was the potential to measure PAP levels in the blood to predict the metastatic spread of prostate cancer.[6] This idea was confirmed by later researchers, who further delineated PAP levels in serum to the likelihood prostate cancer had spread to the bone. Given the high frequency and yet slow growth of prostate cancer, a reliable marker would provide a crucial means to track progression of the disease. This outcome led PAP to become a widely used diagnostic marker (though the acronym was sometimes modified to "PAcP" to avoid confusion with the diagnostic test for cervical cancer, which had been developed by the Greco-American Georgios Papanicoloau; or Pap for short [see chapter 4]). The diagnostic PAP test for prostate cancer was later supplanted by PSA due to certain technical advantages, and PAP might have faded into oblivion had it not been for two Stanford University professors.

At first glance, one might consider the extraordinary specificity of monoclonal antibodies to be an ideal way to target a tumor-specific molecule, such as PAP. As we saw with early antibody therapies, the presence of a target floating in the blood often conveys an insurmountable obstacle, which blockades an antibody therapy before it can reach the tumor. An alternative opportunity might be realized if one could direct the cells of the immune system to become sensitized to a tumor. This strategy is analogous to a vaccine used to prevent an infectious disease, such as measles or mumps, with two distinct differences. First, the vaccine would be used in a therapeutic setting to treat, rather than prevent, disease. More crucially, the vaccine would have to target a molecule considered "self" and thus the immune system may tolerate the target in an effort to avoid autoimmune damage. Overcoming this latter effect requires the reader to tolerate a bit of basic immunological science.

### Even More Mansplaining

The thymus-derived lymphocytes (or T cells) in the body can become activated to recognize and kill a foreign intruder. This killing is the outcome of an intricate dance between the T cells and a specialized blood component known as an *antigen-presenting cell*. The first example of an antigen-presenting cell was unknowingly put forward by a German prodigy with an extraordinary capacity to see what others could not. Paul Langerhans was born on July 25, 1847, to an upper-class family in Berlin, a time and place of increasing economic hardships. The region had suffered from a series of crop failures as well as surges in immigration and the use of child labor in factories, both of which drove down wages at the same time the price of basic foodstuffs had begun to skyrocket.

This combination of stressors triggered a peasant-led *Kartoffelrevolution* (potato revolution) just three months before Langerhans's birth.[7] A relatively minor outbreak of violence was sparked when a potato merchant responded to customers' grousing about high costs by stating perhaps she should just sell them hay to eat (an insult accurately interpreted by her customers that they were no better than livestock). This unseemly comment prompted a riot in which the market stalls were torn asunder and much produce was stolen. The unrest was quickly suppressed by the Prussian military but resurged months later in the form of the Revolutions of 1848, which engulfed Prussia and indeed most of Europe in the spring and summer. These uprisings were particularly pronounced within the German Confederation, a loose organization of thirty-nine separate German-speaking states. The rise of German nationalism at this time conveyed both the public's dissatisfaction with the status quo and the desire for the creation of a single German state. In particular, this period ushered in the launch of the political career of a young Junker by the name of Otto von Bismarck.

Unlike the tumult on the streets of his birth, Langerhans's childhood was spent not toiling in the factories but immersed in a classical education at Berlin's most prominent private school, Evangelisches Gymnasium zum Grauen Kloster. Among its many alumni, the school had educated no less than von Bismarck himself. Langerhans was precocious, and his experience at Grauen Kloster revealed a particular talent for medicine, the chosen vocation of his father. His education moved quickly and Langerhans not only finished his secondary education, but had become a medical doctor and defended his thesis by February 1869, at only twenty-one years old. By this time, Langerhans had also already made two discoveries, which would immortalize him in two entirely separate medical fields.

During his medical school training, Langerhans had demonstrated a particular talent for observation using a fairly obscure technology known as *light microscopy*. Although the microscope had been first pioneered in the 17th century, its use had been largely confined to a handful of secretive aficionados, who closely guarded the techniques needed to construct and use these crude instruments. That would change in the mid-to-late-18th century, and largely in the German states, through the pioneering work of Karl Zeiss, an optician who founded a company in Jena devoted to the manufacture of microscopes a year before Langerhans was born. Consequently, there was still much to be learned about the microscopic world two decades later.

It may be no coincidence that Langerhans first encountered a microscope during his studies of medicine in Zeiss's Jena. History does not record whether Zeiss and Langerhans, arguably one of microscopy's most successful early advocates, ever crossed paths, nor is it clear whether Langerhans used a Zeiss instrument. We do know that in 1868, Langerhans's most well-known discovery occurred in the midst of a medical course in what we would today call histology, the study of cells and tissues in the body. Langerhans had been studying the pancreas and noted small islets of cells throughout the organ and asked his instructor about them. The existence of the pancreas had been known since its discovery by Herophilus in the 4th century B.C.E., but its function in the body, if any, was largely a source speculation.[8] Most scientists of the day presumed it had something to do with the digestion of food due to its location behind the stomach. To commemorate this finding, the scientific world referred to these clusters of cells as "Islets of Langerhans" and the product these islets produced would likewise be named for the Anglicized Latin term for island: *insulin*.

Although most closely linked with providing the foundation for the modern understanding of insulin and diabetes, Langerhans's relevance to our story comes from a discovery made at least a year before his first viewing of the pancreas, while Langerhans was still an undergraduate student. In this case, Langerhans was examining a sample of human skin under the microscope and was the first person to note a spindle-shaped cell, which he drew in his notebook.[9] Given its shape, with tentacle-like projections in all directions, the young Langerhans presumed the cell was part of the nervous system and responsible for conveying sensory input from the skin to the brain. Although a good guess, Langerhans can be forgiven his mistake (after all, he was still just an undergraduate). For, almost a century and a half thereafter, other scientists would likewise remain flummoxed by the identity and function of the eponymous "Langerhans cells." All this would change with the assistance of a new technology over which Langerhans undoubtedly would have salivated.

As for Langerhans, his story soon took a tragic turn. After graduation, Langerhans began a rather risky expedition to Syria and Palestine but returned to Europe to serve in the Prussian army during the Bismarck-provoked 1870 Franco-Prussian War. Having survived two potentially perilous adventures, Langerhans settled down to a faculty appointment at the University of Freiburg, becoming a full professor within two years. Although Langerhans remained largely at the microscope and did not interact much with patients, he was exposed to infectious agents within the samples he was examining. One night in 1874, Langerhans began experiencing bouts of fever, night sweats, and pulmonary distress. He was soon diagnosed with tuberculosis, a death sentence in a time before antibiotics. His only hope was a more hospitable climate, which he found in Funchal, the capital of Madeira, off the Portuguese coast. This story sadly concludes with the notable fact the great discoverer of pancreatic islets died on the island of Madeira at the young age of forty.

Although the legacy of Langerhans would forever be linked with the discovery of insulin and the role of the pancreas in diabetes, an entirely different group of researchers would come to appreciate his discovery of Langerhans cells, though this would take more time to coalesce. In 1973, another breakthrough in the field of microscopy would again be needed to elucidate the function of these mysterious cells. In Langerhans's day, a typical microscope had the ability to magnify tissue specimens from ten- to about two-hundred-fold. Although this allowed Langerhans to identify and sketch out the cells in the skin named for him, their function was assessed by a scientist working in New York with a microscope with the ability to magnify samples up to ten thousand times their original size.

Inga Silberberg was a dermatologist at the New York University School of Medicine, who solved the mystery of Langerhans cells in a talk given to a meeting of the American Federation for Clinical Research in Atlantic City, New Jersey, on April 30, 1972.[10] Rather than conveying a study of nerve cells, as might have been anticipated by Langerhans, the topic of Silberberg's lecture was allergy. Specifically, Silberberg had turned the extraordinary power of the electron microscope onto the study of skin samples obtained from patients suffering from contact dermatitis (the itchy outcome suffered by some people following contact with irritants, such as poison ivy, cosmetics, soaps, or other environmental chemicals). As the allergic reaction progressed, Silberberg found Langerhans cells reorganized their subcellular milieu and became "activated." Soon thereafter, these cells were found to engage and remain in contact with these lymphocytes throughout the inflammatory process. In short, Silberberg had found the job of the Langerhans cells was to activate the local immune response and, in doing so, engaged intimately with the lymphocytes tasked with the command and control of the body's defenses.

Long in the shadow of the islets of Langerhans, the cells named for the same Prussian scientist soon rose to the fore. Subsequent studies of these cells followed quickly and emerged with a better understanding of the immune system. The Langerhans cells were found to be a core element in a larger population known collectively as dendritic cells. These cells were in turn part of an even larger grouping of cells known as *antigen-presenting cells*. We now know whereas T cells are widely regarded as "the generals" guiding the immune response, the dendritic cells are more like the intelligence agents that feed the generals with the data needed to decide whether or not to attack. As we will see for the rest of this book, such decisions are the outcome of a complex interplay between intelligence arising from the body and counterintelligence from attacking enemies. In particular, cancer utilizes strategies akin to the "fake news" propagated by Russian trolls in an effort to convince the immune system not to attack. Although we will build upon this surprisingly relevant analogy in the next chapter, it suffices to state that absent active intervention, the purveyors of "fake news" can allow the cancer to metastasize under the noses of the defense mechanisms meant to stop it.

### *When It Absolutely, Positively Has to Be There Overnight*

Edgar Engleman had developed an extraordinary pedigree by the time he was recruited to Stanford University in 1978.[11] He followed an undergraduate degree from Harvard with medical school at Columbia University and postdoctoral stints at the NIH and the University of California, San Francisco. He had come to Stanford to work with Hugh McDevitt, a geneticist credited with discovering how the body utilizes the major histocompatibility

complex (MHC) as the means to distinguish friend from foe, greatly facilitating the birth of widespread organ transplantation. With such credentials,
Engleman likely could have written his ticket for an academic position virtually anywhere in the world but elected to remain at Stanford. His reasoning
was rather unconventional: He wanted to run a blood bank.[12]

This motivation could wrongly be confused with a tendency toward vam-
pirism but instead reflected a more mundane and highly practical rationale
to gain access to rare blood components. As an immunologist, Engleman
was always in need of white blood cells for his research endeavors. These
cells are often removed from the blood given to patients because if present
in transfused blood, they might see the tissues of the recipient as "foreign"
and attack. In the spirit of one person's junk being another's treasure, the
white cells discarded from the blood bank could be a treasure trove of rare
immune cells. Among the rarest and most coveted were Langerhans and
other dendritic cells. Engleman was determined not only to isolate these
rare cells but to determine how dendritic cells could be propagated in the
laboratory.

This ambition would require a lot of blood, sweat, and tears. However,
just over a decade after starting at the helm of the blood center, Engleman's
team reported the isolation of human dendritic cells and the means to
grow them in the laboratory.[13] With a supply of these elusive cells in hand,
Engleman followed up on Inga Silberberg's pioneering studies and began
demonstrating how dendritic cells (such as Paul Langerhans eponymous
cells) regulated T cell activation. Pushing the envelope, Engleman won-
dered whether a pure source of dendritic cells might be exploited to train
T cells in the body to recognize and kill tumor cells. Immersed within
the entrepreneurial core of Silicon Valley roughly two years after this
pivotal paper on dendritic cell isolation had been published, Engleman
had partnered with another Stanford luminary, Samuel Strober (who had
previously developed understanding of how to optimize therapy for organ
transplant recipients), to start a company called Activated Cell Therapy,
Inc. Strober, whose specialties include leukemia, worked with Engleman
to develop an idea for isolating dendritic cells from patient samples and
stimulating them in the laboratory with proteins unique to or enriched
on leukemia cells. These dendritic cells might then be reintroduced into
a patient, primed and ready to stimulate the patient's own T cells to

recognize malignant cells. In this way, they might deliver a therapeutic vaccine to treat certain blood cancers.

By the mid-1990s, a steady stream of advances arising from Engelman's laboratories at Stanford and Activated Cell Therapy, Inc., had progressed to a point where the ideas were ready to test in people. To do so, they approached another Stanford colleague, Ronald Levy (who you may recall was also a founder of IDEC), and planned a clinical trial to test their intended dendritic cell therapies in patients with B cell lymphoma. A 1996 manuscript revealed promising results for the therapy, demonstrating measurable shrinkage in the tumors of all four patients treated. Remarkably, in one patient, their tumor utterly disappeared. A larger study, published in 2002, again supported the promise of dendritic cell therapy for the treatment of lymphoma.

At this point, a combination of hope and fear broke the growing momentum pushing dendritic cell therapy. The fear stemmed from concerns that long-lived T cell recognition of malignant B cells might eventually clear out the tumor cells and then turn on the normal B components of the blood. Such an outcome would thereby effectively destroy the ability of the patients to protect themselves against myriad infectious diseases, which are kept in check by antibodies produced by nonmalignant B cells. To minimize such a negative outcome, the team at Activated Cell Therapy, Inc. (which by then had changed its name to Dendreon, a name reflective of their use of dendritic cells) brainstormed how their technology might be used to treat other types of cancer, where loss of benign cells bearing an antigen of interest would not be so problematic.

The scientists at Dendreon concluded prostate cancer provided a perfect venue.[14] Patients with prostate cancer generally have the entire gland removed. Consequently, a long-lived T cell response would either not have anything to attack or would simply mop up a small number of cells left behind after surgery. As the most common disease in men (in this case, the word is intentionally gender-specific), prostate cancer also offered a hope to tap into a lucrative and growing market. The Dendreon team selected as its target the prostatic acid phosphatase. The name of the dendritic cell product would be Provenge®.

The paperwork to initiate clinical trials for a prostate-specific, dendritic cell therapy was filed by Dendreon with the FDA on December 22, 1996.

A major and consistent hurdle with the FDA pertained to how the drug would be manufactured and distributed. For most medicines, a pill, tablet, or injectable substance is produced by the manufacturer, packaged in a standardized box, and then shipped to the hospital or pharmacy, where it is recognizable as such. For Provenge, one hurdle pertained to the complexity of the manufacturing. For each patient, blood must be collected and this material is then subjected to a process known as *apheresis* to isolate the white blood cells. These white cells are then shipped to Dendreon's processing facility, which isolates the dendritic cells and stimulates them with a specially engineered form of prostatic acid phosphatase. The stimulating entity is another example of a chimera, in which part of PAP is fused with molecule known as *granulocyte-macrophage colony stimulating factor* (GM-CSF). GM-CSF is known to stimulate the growth of dendritic cells. Consequently, the growth stimulatory properties of Provenge would both stimulate the growth of dendritic cells and load these cells with the molecule used to excite the T cells of the patient's immune system. After growing the dendritic cells in laboratory incubators and ensuring they remained viable, the dendritic cells are shipped back to the hospital and infused into the patient through an intravenous line. Once back in the body of their donors, the dendritic cells perform their normal function of stimulating T cells, which, in turn, gain renewed motivation to seek out and kill tumor cells.

Given the complexity of what you have just read, the process developed by Dendreon was more than a bit more complicated than simply taking a pill or receiving an injection. This multistep procedure requires logistical mastery of different parts of a medical and commercial establishment that often do not interact. For example, apheresis is relatively routine for entities like the American Red Cross, which may be seeking concentrated platelets or red blood cells, but can be viewed as an exotic endeavor for a run-of-the-mill hospital laboratory. Likewise, the idea of shipping a blood sample across the country (via FedEx) and ensuring the sample remain under appropriately guarded conditions (temperature, humidity, etc.) provided additional obstacles, which were compounded by questions of liability. For example, who would be to blame if a shipment is not collected at the appropriate time, not handled properly during transit, or is lost (a process known to pharmaceutical industry professionals as interruptions in the *chain of custody*)?

Ensuring product quality in the face of such scrutiny is essential for the development of any new medicine but is particularly challenging for regulators of personalized medicines, such as Provenge. Last but certainly not least was the question, seemingly simple, of the hospital pharmacy. Most pharmacies consist of benches and shelves overflowing with bottles of pills and capsules. A pharmacy to support Provenge would require specialized equipment to store and maintain the cells, both outbound to and inbound from Dendreon. As hospitals tend toward being large and complex bureaucracies, the proposition of setting aside specialized facilities simply to service one product and for one particular patient population proved quite the challenge. Consequently, although the paperwork had been filed with the FDA to start clinical trials in late 1996, the first patient did not receive treatment until 1998.[15]

Were these hurdles not enough, the commercial success of Provenge required parameters well beyond the control of Dendreon. As is true for all medicine, the first requirement is to demonstrate a product is safe and effective. Regarding safety, Provenge sailed through clinical trials without any major red flags. Indeed, an independent scientific advisory panel the FDA had convened in late 2007 to assess Provenge voted 17-0 to support for Provenge on the basis of safety.[16] A different story arose in this same panel regarding efficacy. The prostate cancer experts on the panel were asked to answer a question of whether there was "substantial evidence of effectiveness" for Provenge. The seventeen panelists split, with thirteen agreeing and four dissensions. This is not a particularly surprising outcome because experts frequently disagree on whether a potential new drug rises to the level required for FDA approval.

What was surprising was that officials at the FDA chose to ignore the advice of its advisors. Admittedly, the word *advice* reflects the fact it is simply a recommendation. However, the officials at the FDA overrode the recommendation of their advisors and instead asked Dendreon to provide additional evidence the drug was effective and could be manufactured in a consistent manner. Again, such an action is rare but not unheard of. What distinguished this decision was that three individuals, including one member of the advisory panel, wrote letters to FDA officials, attacking Dendreon and Provenge.[17] Moreover, these three letters were leaked to an industry newsletter. Some of these letters had been ghostwritten by FDA staff as part of something akin to a smear campaign. Compounding the problem, a dissenting advisory panel member had failed to disclose he was also a scientific advisor to a venture capital fund with a substantial investment in a company developing a competitor product to Provenge.

In the political environment of the American capital, these events were incendiary. Charges were leveled by elected officials and patient advocacy groups in all directions, claiming "ethical violations" for or against the FDA, and the little extant consensus agreed the procedure the FDA used to evaluate Provenge looked and felt debauched. In the twenty-four hours after the leaking of the advisory panel documents, Dendreon's stock value collapsed and shareholder lawsuits bloomed amid questions of culpability.

Part of the blame for the mess surrounding the Provenge controversy could be placed clearly in the lap of Dendreon officials. Corporate executives had made the decision to target prostate cancer because of the large market opportunity but seemingly failed to appreciate that the disease is, in actuality, a large number of subsets of different diseases. Not only is it easily defensible to state prostate cancer is not a single disease but it is equally safe to state each man's disease is different from every other man's disease. While this is true for many cancers, it is even more so for prostate cancer as the disease tends to be *multi-focal*—a term reflecting a patient often has multiple and independent cancers within a single prostate gland. Such facts dramatically increase the difficulty in determining whether a particular therapy is effective because if a patient has three different cancers at the same time and two are eliminated, the third may end up being fatal. Worse still, and as reiterated many times throughout this book, prostate cancer growth tends to be very slow and this can confound clinical trials designed to reach an answer as quickly and efficiently as possible.

Despite calls for congressional hearings and the removal of key FDA officials, the kerfuffle around Provenge quieted for a time and the therapy was finally approved on April 29, 2010, becoming the first "designer therapy" consisting of cells manipulated in the laboratory. Ed Engleman recalls being at a medical conference in Washington, D.C., when word of the Provenge approval was first announced, fully two decades after he had commenced his initial studies of dendritic cells. Referring to this memory, he is quoted as saying, "I remember where I was when Kennedy got shot. I remember where I was in the '89 earthquake. And that is about it, those three things."[18]

By this time, Engleman had largely left Dendreon to its own devices and was focused on his research at Stanford.

Nonetheless, the Dendreon roller coaster still had more hills to climb and fall. Given the extensive manipulations required for this customized vaccine, it was clearly going to be expensive. Dendreon executives shocked the medical and insurance communities with news the drug would list for $93,000 per course of treatment. Unlike the results obtained with leukemia/lymphoma, the efficacy of Provenge was modest, in part reflecting the fact prostate cancer is segmented into many different diseases, each of which behaves differently from the others. Given the high price and modest clinical outcomes, the expected arguments began, invoking reminiscences of Clinton-era "Death Panels" about whether a $100,000 price tag was worth an average of four months of extended survival. The volume and rancor of these discussions grew in 2015 when the United Kingdom's Institute for Health and Care Excellence balked at the price as too expensive relative to the value conveyed (even though the cost for British consumers was equivalent to $73,000).[19]

Ultimately, Dendreon seemed to have been put out of its misery when the company was acquired by the Canadian pharmaceutical giant Valeant. Yet this action only increased the magnitude of the problem, as Valeant's business plan had been to acquire companies with marketed medicines at a premium, and to pay for this premium by hiking the price of its products. Consequently, the price of Provenge was raised to $105,536 and an economic assessment published in 2015 concluded, with a 96.5% certainty, this price tag was too high to justify its benefits.[20] As of this writing, the fate of the medicine is as doubtful as ever since Valeant, whose business model came under state and federal scrutiny after accusations of price gouging and distribution violations, sold the rights for Provenge to a Chinese holding company in January 2017.

### CARrying On

Despite a lack of commercial success, the experiences with Provenge conveyed valuable lessons, both to the private sector and regulators, about the opportunities to engineer immune system cells to sensitize them toward cancer. In the case of Provenge, the approach was rather indirect, as the product modified dendritic cells to stimulate T cells, which in turn would begin to seek out and kill tumor cells. A more direct approach would be to directly engineer the T cells themselves. The ideal circumstance, it logically followed, would be to couple to exquisite specificity of monoclonal antibodies with the killing ability of a cytotoxic T cell. This approach is exactly what was done.

Zelig Eshhar was born in 1941 to Polish immigrants in the Tel Aviv suburb town of Petah Tikva (a center of high technology and the site where the pharmaceutical company Teva had been founded in 1901) and mostly grew up in Rehovot, the birthplace of Chaim Weizmann. Weizmann first earned fame as an extraordinary chemist who pioneered the field of industrial fermentation and later served as the first president of Israel. In acknowledgement of both sources of distinction, the Israeli government renamed an institute Weizmann had helped cofound in Rehovot (originally named for the Zionist English businessman, Baron Isreal Sieff) to be the Weizmann Institute of Science. This public university is widely recognized as the premier graduate school for scientists in Israel and has hosted three Nobel Prize winners (Eshhar could be the fourth).

Despite the benefits this geography might have been expected to play a leading role driving Eshhar to a scientific career, it was in fact bees that primed this outcome.[21] As a child, Eshhar took a strong interest in all things associated with these flying insects: how they developed from an egg into pupa as well as the elaborate interplay among workers, drones, and the queen necessary to sustain the hive and generate honey. He credits his interest in bees not only to his inherent curiosity but to the fact he was not afraid to get stung, a discipline undoubtedly helpful to steel him for travails to come.

During his mandatory military service, Eshhar was stationed at the Yad Mordehai, near the border with Gaza. He became an expert beekeeper after being placed in charge of the apiary within the army base. The installation was at a flashpoint amid a hive of geopolitical unrest after the tumultuous Suez Crisis of 1956, which pitted a cabal of Israel, the United Kingdom, and France against an unlikely political (though not military) coalition of Egypt, the United States, and the Soviet Union. During his time at Yad Mordehai, Eshhar recalls being transfixed by a talk from a visitor from his hometown of Rehovot who spoke of the scientific achievements in biology occurring at the Weizmann Institute. He stated in a November 2017 interview, "My jaw dropped. Immediately I wanted to translate all the wonders I'd come to know [about biology] into molecules. I enrolled for an undergraduate degree."

After earning a bachelor's and master's degree from the Hebrew University in Jerusalem, Eshhar realized his newfound dream to work at the Weizmann Institute, earning his Ph.D. under David Givol and Michael Sela on studies of the basic biology of the T cells receptor, the key determinant of whether and how a T cell will respond to the presence of a foreign antigen. This work provided him with insight as to the structural components allowing the T cell receptor to convey the signals to alert the immune system for action. In particular, Eshhar had identified portions of the T cell receptor on the inside of the cell responsible for transmitting signals to stimulate T cell growth. These signals, of course, were tightly regulated and required a complex arrangement of interactions of the T cell receptor on the inside and outside of the cell. Through this elaborate and highly regulated dance, key decisions are made to optimize the recognition and elimination of "foreign" invaders while preventing unwanted collateral damage to the "self" cells of the body.

As his doctoral studies were nearing their end, Eshhar had a conversation with Michael Sela about what he should do next. In the middle of this conversation, Sela spontaneously picked up the phone and called a friend in Boston, who agreed at once to host Eshhar in his lab. The friend was Baruj Benacerraf, and under the great scientist, Eshhar's interests in cancer grew and then metastasized to include thoughts about how the immune system might be adapted to kill tumor cells. As he was concluding his studies at Harvard in 1976, he learned about the new monoclonal antibody technology, which being developed and refined by Georges Kohler and Cesar Milstein, the first report on which had been conveyed in a May 1975 article to *Nature* magazine.[22]

During his trip home from Boston to accept a position at the Weizmann Institute, this time as a member of the faculty, Eshhar was inspired to take a spontaneous side trip to Cambridge, England, to visit Milstein. Literally walking into the lab one day unannounced, he asked Milstein if he could work in his laboratory to learn more about monoclonal antibody technology. Despite the unexpected intrusion, Milstein was surprisingly accommodating, but informed him the laboratory was full. Undeterred, Eshhar returned to Rehovot but persisted in contacting Georges Kohler, who had by this time returned from his postdoctoral stint at Cambridge to a permanent position the Basel Institute of Immunology. Kohler was therefore still staffing up his own laboratory and this afforded an opportunity for Esshar to work side-by-side with Kohler for a few months and soon after transfer the new monoclonal antibody technology to his nascent laboratory in Israel.

Eshhar generated a variety of monoclonal antibodies for more than a decade within his laboratory at the Weizmann Institute, often writing patents to be licensed to support his laboratory with the royalties earned from these patents. This supplemental funding was essential given the paucity of grant funding available to young academics.

In the mid-1980s, Eshhar was on sabbatical at Stanford University, when he conceived of an idea to marry the specificity of antibodies with the killing capacity of T cells.[23] Upon his return to the Weizmann Institute, he accepted a doctoral student into his laboratory who would put this idea into practice. In doing so, this project and the student would be sources of both considerable fame and angst. The student, Gideon Gross, had signed onto a project ingeniously blending the work of Esshar's own experiences during and after his Ph.D. studies that would forever define the academic and monetary fortunes of both men.

The fundamental idea Esshar, Gross, and their technician, Tova Waks, tested was to tether the signaling portion of the T cell receptor to a monoclonal antibody. This chimeric molecule would then be embedded on the surface of the T cell and span the membrane so it could trigger signals to promote T cell growth and killing capacity. The intended approach required the design of an artificial molecule grafted to a key portion of the signaling component of the T cell receptor gene (known as the *CD3 zeta chain*). This signaling motif, within in the interior of the T cells, would be fused to a part of a monoclonal antibody specific for CD19 (which you may recall is a molecule found exclusively on all B cells and B cell tumors). When this chimera was expressed in a T cell using conventional molecular biology techniques, the Frankenstein-like T cell gained the ability to kill targets as directed by the chimeric receptor. The Weizmann team revealed in a 1989 report this "chimeric antigen receptor"-bearing T cell (or CAR-T) could serve as a means to kill cancer cells in the laboratory.[24]

As often occurs in science, another team led by the renowned American biologist Leroy Hood had in parallel come up with the same idea. Hood had grown up in Missoula, Montana, and was recognized at an early age as a rising star, being a finalist for the 1956 Westinghouse Science Talent Search, a prestigious high school competition President George H. W. Bush described as "the Super Bowl of Science."[25] From then onward, Hood has been a force to be reckoned wit—producing more than seven hundred scientific publications, pioneering complex and emerging fields like genomics, and excelling in cross-disciplinary approaches to rethink human health.

My first recollection of Hood was immediately cemented into my brain upon squeezing into the back of a conference room at Duke University in the late 1980s. I was there to witness a fast-paced seminar by Hood in which the inspiring content predicting the potential for unlocking the mysteries of the human genome was exceeded only by his use of two sets of slide projectors, each of which contained a distinct set of slides. My disappointment at being wedged at the far back of the room proved to be a blessing as I became transfixed as the dueling projectors caused the entire audience to continuously pivot their heads back and forth as if witnessing volleys at Wimbledon.

Returning to the matter at hand, despite being outgunned by the "big science" conducted with the multimillion-dollar budgets available to Leroy Hood, Eshhar's lean three-person Israeli team beat the Americans to publication.[26] Furthermore, Eshhar advanced his technology during another sabbatical, this time with the NCI in Bethesda, Maryland, where he initiated a partnership with Steven Rosenberg. You may recall Rosenberg had gained international fame for his pioneering work on recruiting the immune system to target cancer by stimulating patients with IL-2 and other modulators of the immune system. Although IL-2 did not become the much-hoped-for panacea for cancer, Rosenberg was still intent upon exploiting the immune system to kill cancer, and recognized the value of Esshar's pioneering approach. As the CAR-T technology began to show promise, the patents developed by Eshhar's team were licensed to a Santa Monica, California, start-up by the name of Kite Pharma. This company had been founded in 2009 by an Israeli-American oncologist turned serial entrepreneur, Arie Belldegrun, who had studied at the Weizmann Institute and was well aware of Eshhar's groundbreaking work. Belldegrun was therefore intent upon translating Eshhar's academic work into a therapeutic product with extraordinary medical and commercial potential.

Although the early work performed in the Rosenberg laboratory with Eshhar's approach was promising, further understanding of T cell biology informed improvements to Eshhar's original idea by the time Kite began clinical trials. As has been emphasized throughout the entire book, the body has placed many constraints upon T cells to prevent them from causing unwanted damage to normal cells. Simply triggering the T cell receptor is generally insufficient to fully stimulate a T cell to begin its destructive rampage. Indeed, triggering the T cell receptor alone causes the opposite outcome, rendering the T cell a type of living dead zombie unable to respond to further signaling. This process is known as *anergy* (a Greco-German term loosely translating into "no allergy") and can provide a means to prevent unwanted autoimmunity.

Starting in the late 1980s, a series of reports emerged, largely out of the Seattle biomedical community, revealing productive T cell activation required simultaneous activation of both the TCR and a "co-stimulatory" molecule. Many of these reports emerged from the Bristol-Myers (formerly Oncogen) team led by Ingegerd and Karl Hellstrom, whom we met earlier. In particular, two scientists on their team, Jeffrey Ledbetter and Peter Linsley, had revealed CD28 was a key regulator of the decision of whether a T cell would become activated or anergic. As we saw in an earlier story, these scientists had demonstrated CD28 must bind to a molecule known as *B7* on the surface of an antigen-presenting cell (e.g., a dendritic cell) simultaneous with TCR signaling to fully activate a T cell.[27] Indeed, this signaling by CD28 would be the basis of TGN-1412 (a subject detailed in chapter 9). Ledbetter and Linsley's work on CD28 would convey monumental breakthroughs requiring two decades to begin fully realizing its clinical potential.

In a case of short-sighted cost savings, Bristol-Myers Squibb (BMS) had disbanded the Seattle research team in April 1997, causing the dispersal of an immensely talented group of people and unintentionally delaying BMS from fully exploiting its lead in a race to discover breakthrough immune oncology products (and an event particularly ironic for BMS in later years as we will soon see). The primary winner from this most unfortunate decision turned out to be the University of Washington and its affiliated Fred Hutchinson Cancer Center, which landed Ledbetter, Ingegerd, and Karl

Hellstrom. Another unintended consequence of closing the BMS Seattle site was the release of entrepreneurial founders and the creation of waves of biopharmaceutical companies, including Seattle Genetics (which we met in the last chapter) and Juno Therapeutics, which will play into this story momentarily.

The discovery of CD28 in particular had an impact on the work at Kite Pharma. The therapeutic construct to be expressed in T cells, as originally envisioned by Eshhar, had coupled antibody recognition of CD19 to the CD3 zeta chain. However, this construct would lack the crucial co-stimulatory signaling activity of CD28 and run the risk of actually being counterproductive by inducing T cell anergy rather than stimulation of tumor cell killing. To correct this, the Kite team modified their intended product to include a portion of the CD28 signaling machinery. This adjustment allowed the T cells expressing this CAR-T molecule to become fully activated when they encountered a CD19-bearing tumor cell.

This tweak worked as intended, as evidenced by the extraordinary efficacy of the resulting product, axicabtagene ciloleucel, in clinical trials. Early work showed an overall response rate (a clinical descriptor indicating the ability of a drug to shrink tumors) in 82% of patients treated, all who had previously failed prior treatments.[28] In other words, four of five patients, who were deemed hopeless and had failed all prior therapies, witnessed a miraculous shrinkage of their tumors. Based on such outstanding potential, Kite Pharma was acquired by Gilead Sciences in November 2017 for almost $12 billion. This purchase coincided with an FDA approval for axicabtagene ciloleucel a month earlier.

Although this should have been a time of utter satisfaction and comfort (both professionally and financially) for Eshhar, it instead marked a low point. For at the same time, Esshar was immersed within an ugly imbroglio of finger-pointing and greed. Hours before Eshhar would have been able to sell his stock in Kite, he was sued by his former student, Gideon Gross, who claimed misdeeds regarding payments and credit Gross asserted he was owed. Just months before Gross filed the lawsuit, the colleagues had maintained a cordial relationship, publishing a manuscript detailing the therapeutic potential of the CAR-T technology they had developed.[29] Although Gross had already received $1.5 million for work he conducted as a graduate student, he claimed he was owed ten times as much.[30] This uncomfortable situation turned even more ugly for Eshhar when his ex-wife likewise sought a portion of the windfall, which was estimated to be approximately $73 million. Eshhar now faced two separate lawsuits and months of future charges and countercharges of greed and ungratefulness. These legal proceedings sullied the reputations of all involved and the final resolution of these disputes will likely require years in Israeli courts.

Nor were these lawsuits to be the only ones surrounding the new chimeric antigen receptor (CAR-) T cells. Indeed, the Kite Pharma product approved by the FDA in 2017 was not the first, but the second CAR-T product approved by the FDA. As we will now see, the Kite product had been upstaged as the pioneer in CAR-T by a few weeks, prompting a cascade of other lawsuits and admissions.

### Two Sailors Walk Into a CAR

In his January 1971 State of the Union Address, President Richard Millhouse Nixon declared a "war on cancer." At roughly the same time, a high school senior contemplating his future was concerned about a very different war occurring in Southeast Asia. Carl June had drawn a draft number of 50, which was particularly problematic as all numbers below 195 would fate their holders to be drafted into military service.[31] To circumvent the potential he would end up as a private slogging through the jungles of Vietnam, June instead opted to apply to the United States Naval Academy in Annapolis, Maryland.[32] This decision came with the added bonus that Annapolis had just initiated a premed program, which was particularly attractive for a promising student fascinated with biology.

After graduating from the Naval Academy, June immediately began clinical training at the Baylor College of Medicine and completed his studies in three (rather than the standard four) years. Seattle again enters the story as June spent three years at the Fred Hutchinson Cancer Center as an oncology fellow, where he worked for a time with Jeffrey Ledbetter on CD28 function in T cells, among other activities.[33] June returned to the East Coast in 1986 to begin repaying the twelve years of service he owed the navy to compensate for his extensive educational costs.

Rather than being stationed in a faraway land or relegated to a backwater stateside, June received a dream assignment and ended up at the prestigious

Naval Medical Research Hospital, just across the street from the NIH. This place and time coincided with the nation's awakening to the raging HIV/AIDS crisis and June's experience studying T cells proved invaluable. June began experimenting with the idea of obtaining T cells from AIDS patients, who were severely lacking since the virus targets the elimination of T cells.[34] The idea was to stimulate these cells in the laboratory and grow enough so they could be given back to the patient to restore immune system function. The donor's cells were incubated with small iron beads coated with antibodies, which stimulate CD28 and CD3 and would thereby mimic the effects of a foreign intruder and cause the T cells to proliferate rapidly in the laboratory. Once a large number of these laboratory-derived T cells had been grown, they would be reinfused into the AIDS patient to help restore their immune functions. Although expensive and time consuming, the early preclinical results of these adoptive T cell transfer studies were promising.

As these studies began to progress, a prominent immunologist at the University of California, San Francisco, Art Weiss, was developing his own CAR-T strategy. Weiss's approach coupled the extracellular portion of the CD4 molecule (which is the target HIV uses to hijack T cells) to the CD3 zeta chain. Building on the same rationale Eshhar had invoked for the CD19-based CAR for B cell cancers, Weiss considered the CAR-T he had designed might allow T cells to kill HIV-infected cells. After verifying this concept in the laboratory, he sought out a collaboration with June's team in Bethesda to begin tests in people.

The concept proved successful and found financial backing from Cell Genesys, a San Francisco-based biotechnology company. While the clinical responses in HIV patients were promising, they were insufficiently so in the rough and tumble world of biotechnology. Consequently, Cell Genesys cancelled the program and the company itself later went defunct. However, June had seen enough to appreciate the potential behind CAR-T therapy and decided to return to his primary expertise: oncology.

Upon completion of his obligations to the navy in 1996, June accepted a position in academia at the University of Pennsylvania, bringing much of his team from Bethesda up to Philadelphia. Over the following decade and a half, June continued studies of CAR-T-based strategies to stimulate T cells. He was not alone for, as we have seen, Eshhar and others were moving forward with their own work. To this end, two other groups enter the story.

By this time, it was well-established T cell activation required co-stimulation by the T cell receptor as well as a second signal. This second signal most often included one or more of a set of so-called co-stimulatory molecules, which included CD28, CTLA-4, and 4-1-BB (also known as *CD137*). Regarding the latter molecule, the inclusion of a signaling domain from 4-1-BB had been demonstrated to dramatically improve the function of CAR-T cells in the laboratory by two groups: Helen Finney's team at Celltech Therapeutics, a London-based biotechnology company, and Michael Sadelain at Memorial Sloan Kettering. Based on these reports, June was sure to include 4-1-BB in the CAR-T experiments he was conducting at Penn.

The lead project in June's program was a CAR-T design quite similar to Kite's approach. The construct targeted CD19 on B cell cancers and signaled through both CD3 zeta and 4-1-BB (denoting a subtle difference from the Kite product, which signaled through CD3 zeta and CD28). The first patients to be treated with June's experimental medicine, named CART19 at first and later changed to axicabtagene ciloleucal, received their therapy in the summer of 2010. June's team had received grants totaling $350,000, which was enough to treat just three patients. This trio of volunteers was all men with leukemia, whose prior therapies had all failed them.

June's team, led by David Porter and Bruce Levine, obtained blood from the three patients and used techniques they had honed over the prior fifteen years (Levine had joined June's team in Bethesda as his first postdoctoral fellow) to express the CAR-T gene in their T cells. In two of three cases, there were ample numbers of engineered cells available to reinfuse back into the patients. However, the cells from the third patient had largely failed to grow.

This unlucky patient, Douglas Olson, was a 68-year-old grandfather who loved sailing but was preparing for death after a two-decade fight against chronic lymphocytic leukemia.[35] Almost half of Olson's bone marrow had been replaced by tumor cells. The disease had likewise swamped his blood and was threatening to trigger a full collapse of his immune system, which would render the patient susceptible to a massive and invariably final infection. Olson had stubbornly battled his disease for twenty years, but his body had become overwhelmed by early 2010. Equaling Olson's stubbornness in fighting the disease were his T cells, which refused to grow in June's laboratory. June's team concluded there were barely enough cells to treat even a rodent-sized subject.

Nonetheless, the Penn team moved forward, even with Olson. After the five-minute infusion of the cells into each patient, all held their breath. For days, nothing meaningful happened. Then, approximately two weeks later, the patients began experiencing chills, nausea, and fever. This could have been quite bad news, perhaps indicating the feared infection triggered by the collapse of the immune system (due either to the cancer or the therapy). To test for this possibility, additional blood was drawn for analysis by Porter, who searched for signs of infection. Instead, Porter found T cells, many engineered T cells, which indicated the immune system was fighting back. Over the following weeks, the number of modified T cells had expanded at least a thousandfold and began killing B cells. The clinicians later estimated more than two pounds of tumor cells were eliminated in each patient.

Of greatest concern, of course, was Olson, who had received barely enough cells to treat a mouse. Although unwilling to grow in the laboratory, these cells had gone berserk in Olson's body, expanding in number and attacking the cancer wherever it could be found. A month after the infusion, Olson was informed by Porter, "Doug, we can't find a single cancer cell in your body. Not in your bone marrow. In your blood. Not anywhere."[36] Within weeks, Olson had resumed his love for nautical adventures, so confident in his recovery that he bought an eighteen-foot sailboat.

## Fame, Fortune & Foibles

Although Carl June's team had hit the proverbial home run, it was with a small number of patients, and they were out of money. The three patients had cost the entire expenditure of $350,000 and they needed more resources. With nothing to lose, they took the risky approach of writing a paper for submission to the scientific community, hopeful it might trigger sufficient interest to help pry loose additional funding. Much to their surprise, the small number of patients did not deter the reviewers from accepting their publication, and their clinical study appeared in the prestigious journal *Science Translational Medicine* on August 10, 2011.[37] Accompanying this manuscript was an aggressive public relations campaign by Penn's medical school, spearheaded with headlines like "Genetically modified 'serial killer' T cells obliterate tumors in patients with chronic lymphocytic leukemia, Penn researchers report."[38]

Over the following months, June's research gained considerable publicity. Within a year, the NCI funded June to the tune of $2 million and Novartis had licensed the technology and provided additional millions in funding. The publicity engine driving Penn also benefitted, for example, the 2015 Ken Burns documentary *The Emperor of All Maladies* based on the 2010 book of the same name by Siddhartha Mukherjee, featured Penn and a particularly photogenic little girl, Emily Whitehead, whose disease had been sent into long-term remission by June's breakthroughs. Likewise, the sitting U.S. vice president, Joe Biden, who had months before lost his son Beau to brain cancer in May 2015, would announce the creation of a highly visible Cancer Moonshot program during a January 2016 visit to Philadelphia and the Penn Medical Center.[39] During the speech at Penn, Biden derided "cancer politics" for holding back cures, a cryptic comment to which we will return. Three months later, the Internet billionaire Sean Parker, who had founded Napster and served as the first president of Facebook, pledged a quarter billion dollars toward a cancer immunotherapy project, singling out Penn as one of its intended primary recipients.

Looking back at those heady days, there is an interesting statement in the August 10, 2011, "serial killer" press release that would haunt Penn in the years to come. In the document, it is stated that June thought there were several "secret ingredients" distinguishing the lackluster results from previous trials with modified T cells and the remarkable responses seen in his current trial.[40] Although certainly not intended to convey any dark motives or actions, these words would become uncomfortably accurate.

A CBS News report of Joe Biden's 2016 launch of the Cancer Moonshot program during his visit to Penn (where he would later accept a professorship), included the following statement: "Biden recalled his grandfather's adage that the world has three kinds of politics: church politics, labor politics, and regular politics."[41] He continued, "I hope you're not offended, but there are four kinds of politics in America. There's cancer politics."

Like many paradigm shifts rocking the scientific world over the past few centuries, the release of the 2011 study wrinkled more than a few noses in scientific and medical establishments. While scientists are often portrayed in the media as objective human thinkers, the key word in this descriptor is *human*. Being human, scientists are often just as susceptible to politics and resisting the changes that inevitably arise as one group of ideas and their advocates are pushed aside in favor of a successor. Although this can be painful and subject to considerable resistance, a key part of the scientific process is to acknowledge past lessons, both positive and negative, and interrogate all ideas and necessarily reproduce any questionable work.

Applying this idea to the 2011 report from June, one obvious concern pertained to the small number of patients and the possibility that the data from three volunteers might have been over-interpreted. This was to be expected and, indeed, had even been anticipated by June and his colleagues in planning their strategy for moving the program forward. Yet these same investigators were shocked when another wave of criticism arose from an unlikely source: Steven Rosenberg at the NCI. You may recall Rosenberg had published a study the year before on the success of a larger clinical trial of the Kite CAR-T product. This work had not been cited by June and the oversight triggered Rosenberg to deliver a blistering attack on June, in a November 2011 letter to the *New England Journal of Medicine*, not only pointing out the professional slight but questioning whether the three patients' remarkable responses might have been due to chemotherapy administered before June's CAR-T intervention.[42]

Another source of criticism had nothing to do with paradigm shifts but instead surrounded the use of the 4-1-BB signaling domain. The report from the Penn group was the first to test this particular motif in people (recall Rosenberg's clinical studies had utilized a CD28 signaling motif). However, the concerns did not pertain to the science or even politics so much as the law.

It seems the failure to cite Rosenberg's predecessor studies on CAR-T cells was not the only omission in the seminal 2010 paper from June's team at Penn. The authors had also neglected to reveal that the DNA construct used in their clinical studies had been "designed, developed and provided by a collaborator at the St. Jude Children's Research Hospital in Memphis, Tennessee." This omission, which was finally acknowledged in March 2016, left out a key verb as the St. Jude team had also "patented" this invention.

Tracing the story from its beginning, it seems Dario Campana and Chihaya Imai at St. Jude's had created the gene modification used in the Penn studies. Campana had sent June the key DNA in 2003 through a formal process known as a *material transfer agreement,* which stipulates, among other things, assurances regarding the proper credit for work using the material and the intellectual property rights and restrictions. In the 2011 paper, not only was the contribution by the St. Jude team not acknowledged, but the Novartis partnership likewise was based upon intellectual property Penn did not actually own.

These facts triggered a flap, which included a lawsuit from St. Jude and countersuits from Penn. The acrimony was driven by a combination of correcting the record to convey proper attribution, pride, and, of course, the large amount of royalties potentially derived from the work at St. Jude's and/or Penn. These allegations were the subject of Joe Biden's comments regarding politics and were finally resolved in 2016 with two actions. In April 2015, Novartis agreed to an initial payout of at least $12 million to Juno Therapeutics, a Seattle-based biopharmaceutical company that had licensed the intellectual property from St. Jude to develop a competing product (with additional future revenues arising from the sales of Novartis products using the St. Jude technology).[43] Then, in March 2016, the Penn team wrote articles to correct the record and to appropriately cite the contributions from the St. Jude team.[44]

Despite these setbacks, the future remained exceedingly bright for all involved, most importantly the patients. The Novartis product licensed from Penn (and indirectly from St. Jude/Juno) continued to show strong clinical efficacy in larger clinical trials (overriding Steven Rosenberg's early concerns). Indeed, the Novartis CAR-T product for B cell cancers was approved by the FDA on August 30, 2017, roughly six weeks before the approval of the Kite's CAR-T product, which received a similar nod two months later, on October 18. Beyond these two CAR-T treatments, both of which targeted B cell cancers, Novartis and Kite had been joined by Juno (which itself had been acquired by a larger biopharmaceutical powerhouse, Celgene, in January 2018). Buoyed by such results, a host of other established and start-up biotechnology companies began to pursue the use of CAR-T therapy to treat a far wider array of both immunological and solid tumors, including prostate cancer, which arguably helped resurrect the idea of cell-based immune therapy via the scientific (if not commercial) success of Provenge. The lessons learned in the creation of these cell-based CAR-T immune therapies seem to be a mere preview of an even more promising future to come.

Perhaps even more importantly, the experiences gained in the development of the cell-based adoptive transfer products developed by Eshhar, June, and others would unexpectedly herald the beginning of a new and potentially more exciting means to provide safer and more effective immune-based cancer therapies, and it is to this subject we now return.

# 8

# *Checkmate!*

The beauty of science is conveyed is its ability to humble even the most pretentious assumption of knowledge with the revelation of a seemingly minor piece of data. Such a finding can trigger an ignition of the stereotypical "lightbulb" in the brain, leading to greater understanding and this metaphor is quite apt in providing a real-world example of such illumination.

Max Planck was born in the northern German Duchy of Holstein on April 23, 1858. As a child, he took a liking to physics but was cautioned away from the profession during an 1874 course on the subject taught by Philipp von Jolly at the University of Munich, who advised: "In this field, almost everything is already discovered and all that remains is to fill a few holes."[1] Appropriately ignoring this device, Planck continued in the field, and was eventually hired as a professor at the Friedrich-Wilhelms Universität in Berlin, where, in 1894, he was enlightened by the surprisingly complex question of how to make a better incandescent lamp.

The researcher had been commissioned by the rapidly growing lightbulb industry to explain a paradox: Why does a lightbulb give off a yellow glow (indicative of a longer wave of radiation) when the radiation powering it is shorter-wave electrical energy. Planck solved the dilemma, eventually known as the *blackbody radiation problem*, in a seminar given on December 14, 1900, to the German Physical Society, in which he introduced the first ideas behind quantum mechanics, which, combined with Einstein's theories of relativity, upended the field of physics von Jolly had considered so passé a quarter century before.[2] Indeed, the unification of these ideas from Planck and Einstein still remains to be solved by future generations of hole-fillers.

Similar to the world of physics in 1874, our understanding of the regulation of the immune system was utterly turned on its head by a series of unexpected findings in the final years of the twentieth century. As you may recall, a fundamental assumption of immunology presumed activities in the thymus *in utero* had eliminated self-reactive T cells. These events prevented otherwise devastating damage in the form of autoimmune diseases. T cells hold extraordinary potential to wreak havoc. Unsurprisingly then, the thymus does not work alone during gestation to protect the body from potential autoimmune damage. Indeed, we now know the body has developed redundant and overlapping mechanisms functioning all throughout our lifetimes to minimize self-inflicted damage.

Despite these layered security measures, common sense tells us the system is imperfect, as evidenced by the existence of autoimmune maladies, such as rheumatoid arthritis, Type 1 diabetes, and ulcerative colitis. These particular illnesses would prove to be exceptionally illustrative for the discovery and creation of a new generation of cancer therapeutics with the potential to finally invoke the much-longed-for cure for many malignant diseases.

### Not What You Were Expecting

You may recall from chapter 3 that interleukin-2 (IL-2) was known to stimulate the immune system and, overlooking its side effects, had been deployed by Steven Rosenberg at the NCI to successfully treat a handful of patients with otherwise incurable metastatic melanoma. Such findings were consistent with evidence that IL-2 and its primary receptor (a molecule with the not-so-catchy name of CD25) were essential for stimulating the immune system in response to a perceived attack upon the body. This notion was entirely consistent with our understanding of how the immune system functioned until, yet again, two colonies of rather freakish mice utterly upended these notions and triggered much head-scratching.

In 1990, a German team at the University of Wurzburg in Germany led by Ivan Horak was studying the potential for IL-2 therapy and initiated what was presumed to be a relatively straightforward study. Using new genetic engineering technologies, they sought to create a mouse lacking IL-2 (a so-called IL-2 "knockout mouse"). In an age dominated by headlines about the rampaging HIV/AIDS pandemic, a mouse lacking IL-2 might provide a platform to study other ways to bolster the immune system or to understand the implications of profound immune suppression. With this in mind, the presumed outcome was the knockout mouse would exhibit a profound failure of the immune system needed to thrive.

In an August 1991 paper in the prestigious journal *Nature*, Horak's team reported these knockout mice were mostly fine at four weeks of age with ample numbers of T cells.[3] Although these T cells were a bit sluggish in terms of their ability to respond to stimulation in the laboratory, the differences were fairly trivial. Indeed, the only remarkable finding was a pronounced increase in the levels of circulating antibodies (suggesting heightened activity of B cells). The results with the IL-2 knockout mice were largely dismissed by the larger scientific community, which generally presumed something else must have been the counterweight for the loss of IL-2. For example, they reasoned, another known or unknown interleukin must have been produced to compensate for the loss of IL-2. Following up on this idea, the elevated B cell counts might have been a sign of this compensatory response.

The absence of a demonstrable defect in mice lacking IL-2 was consistent with many other studies of knockout animals of the day, which revealed layers of such compensatory changes. Indeed, the literature of the time was quickly filling with a lack of any dramatic outcome in knockout mice and this frequently confounded biologists utilizing the new technology.[4] In such a scenario, the only way of observing an outcome would arise when all the backup pathways were simultaneously obliterated. Thus, the IL-2 knockout mice experiment, like these others, might have just been an expensive waste of time. Later studies would show this was not at all accurate.

In October 1993, Horak's team published a follow-on study, which proved to be a real puzzle.[5] Although the IL-2-lacking mice were frustratingly normal for the four weeks after birth, as Horak had published earlier, roughly half of the animals had unexpectedly died within the following month.[*] Autopsies revealed gross manifestations contributed to the death of these older mice and included enlarged lymph nodes and spleens, all of which were engorged with lymphocytes. The surviving animals also displayed swollen lymph nodes and severe symptoms consistent with ulcerative colitis, a well-known autoimmune disease. Rather than too few T cells, as had been anticipated, mice lacking IL-2 had far *too many* T cells. Moreover, these cells were disproportionately autoreactive. Invoking the same ideas as before, some investigators put forth explanations for this unforeseen phenomenon suggesting some unknown compensatory mechanism might have first corrected for the lack of IL-2. The idea continued that the mechanism later went too far and caused autoimmune damage. For the most part though, the finding was stultifying to many of the most experienced scientists in the field.

Compounding the mystery, a study published by a team led by Frederick Alt from Harvard in October 1995 reported a similar phenomenon using CD25 knockout mice. CD25 is a key receptor engaged by IL-2 (and not by other interleukins).[6] Just as Horak's team had observed, mice lacking the receptor for CD25 appeared normal until later in life, when they spontaneously developed a massive engorgement of their lymphoid organs. The disease then progressed into a full-blown autoimmune reaction. As CD25 was known only to interact with IL-2, this finding seemed to preclude that an induction of another interleukin had compensated for the loss of IL-2 (matching the thoughts on Horak's mice). What was going on here?

## Rats!

As you may recall, the concept of suppressor T cells had been effectively refuted with the failure to identify the elusive "I-J molecule," in mice or in

---

[*]    As it generally takes longer than a month to prepare a scientific manuscript, one is further confused by the failure to report the unusual results in older mice by Horak and his team.

humans. Indeed, the burgeoning immunology community in the United States had moved on from this quaint idea, relegating it to the dustbin of old-world thinking. Although largely dismissed in North America, the concept of a regulatory T cell persisted in the European immunology community and was supported by information arising from a rodent a bit larger than a mouse and with a worse reputation.

Unlike the high-precision use of cutting-edge genetic engineering of mice favored by American scientists but seemingly generating more questions than answers, a more brute force and classical form of biology research was being deployed elsewhere. Building on reports throughout the latter quarter of the 20th century, a loose association of European, Australian, and Asian immunologists kept the fire of suppressor cells lit. For example, a Scottish team led by William J. Penhale in 1973 at the Royal Infirmary of Edinburgh utilized rats to show a combination of removal of the thymus and irradiation could trigger waves of autoimmunity against the thyroid gland.[7] Almost two decades later, Penhale and an Australian team further demonstrated these same techniques could cause rats to develop type 1 diabetes, a well-established autoimmune disease.[8] Three years later, investigators at the University of Oxford identified a population of CD4 T cells in rats responsible for conferring this rise in autoimmunity.[9]

In 1985, a newly minted Ph.D. by the name of Shimon Sakaguchi was building upon Penhale's early work by trying to identify the cells in the body responsible for suppressing the immune system. Much to the surprise of all involved, his work linked a population of CD4 T cells (which you may recall had been generally regarded as "helper" cells) with the phenomenon of immune suppression.[10] This concept flew in the face of the conventional wisdom of the 1970s, which extolled the idea CD8 T cells (and not their CD4 counterparts) mediated immune suppression.

Over the following decade, Sakaguchi narrowed the definition of T-cell-mediated immune suppression. Beyond CD4, these cells also expressed CD25, the IL-2 receptor—another shock since IL-2 had long been considered to be an activator of host defenses. As proof, Sakaguchi verified his findings in both rats and mice (which many readers may be shocked to learn are genetically further apart from one another than either species is to man). Consistent findings revealed while IL-2 deficient mice generally had large numbers of T cells (and a greater risk of autoimmune diseases), these same animals had fewer T cells with both CD4 and CD25. Moreover, a replenishment of these CD4/CD25 T cells (e.g., via transfusion) could correct the autoimmune defect in the IL-2 deficient knockout mice.[11]

As additional proof of Sakaguchi's concept, treatment of normal mice with IL-2 antibodies (which deplete the amount of IL-2 in the blood) was shown to be sufficient to depress the number of CD4/CD25 T cells and to trigger autoimmunity.[12] By the mid-1990s, the idea that certain T cells negatively regulated the immune system had even been verified by American investigators, most notably Ethan Shevach of the NIH.[13] This was indeed a watershed moment as many immunologists in the United States had long-since dismissed the idea of suppressor T cells. This thawing of animosities between new and old world immunologists introduced a new era and, perhaps as a means to bury the hatchet, these cells were described as regulatory T cells (rather than suppressor T cells). Within a few short years, much effort was invested to characterize these regulatory T cells (known as *Treg cells* for short). For example, Treg cells generally expressed not just CD4 and CD25, but other molecules such CTLA-4 (a cell surface molecule) and Foxp33 (a molecule in the nucleus of T cells controlling what genes are expressed by a unique population of T cells). Altogether, this unique assemblage of proteins caused Treg cells to restrain, rather than promote, T cell killing.

As the recognition of the existence and characterization of Treg cells widened, their biology and applications to diseases likewise expanded. An obvious clinical implication dominating these early years centered upon whether Treg cells govern decisions about autoimmunity. This association was confirmed when multiple studies demonstrated that a decline in the number of Treg cells was sufficient to promote the occurrence of autoimmune diseases, both in animal models and in people.[14] [15]

Taking the opposite approach, the oncology community questioned whether cancer might reflect a disease in which Treg cells had been manipulated to avoid killing tumor cells. To get some perspective on this question, it is important to realize normal T cells could be converted into Treg cells under just the right conditions. Specifically, two studies published in 2007, one from the NIH and the other from the La Jolla Institute for Allergy and Immunology, demonstrated dendritic cells could promote such conversion in the presence of substances known as *transforming growth factor beta* (TGF-beta) and retinoic acid (a form of vitamin A).[16] [17] TGF-beta had been known to be elevated in cancer (the name *transforming* is a scientific term reflecting the transition of a normal cell towards cancerous behavior) and this change suggested a direct link to how cancer was able to subvert the immune system.

From our earlier discussion underlying the rationale of BiTE therapeutics in chapter 6, you may recall the paradoxical finding repeatedly observed over many years indicating many tumors are bathed in components of the body's defenses (including both T cells and dendritic cells). The primary implication was Treg cells could essentially put tumor-specific T cells to sleep, thereby blocking the ability of the body reject tumors. Nonetheless, the efficacy of BiTEs also revealed that these sleeping cells could be awakened to regain the capacity to kill the tumor cells. Such findings held extraordinary potential if only one could find a way to block the Treg cells.

To summarize, the discovery of Treg cells provided a new means to explain observations confounding pathologists, immunologists, and oncologists for more than a century: Tumors are bathed in immune cells and yet the body's defenses don't seem to recognize the malignant cells all around them. In effect, T cells, which might otherwise kill the cancer, were being turned into Treg cells—reminiscent of a scene from *Night of the Living Dead*, where potential protagonists were being transformed into zombies—protecting the tumor from themselves and preventing any other cells it encounters from attacking the tumor.

The question quickly evolved to determine whether the zombification of these Treg cells might be prevented or reversed. Studies with the aforementioned BiTE molecules and CAR-T cells had conclusively demonstrated even the quiescent T cells surrounding a tumor could be reenergized to kill tumor cells. In both cases, this reversion required a rather extraordinary (and expensive) requirement to generate convoluted cells or molecules via equally complex protein and engineering technologies. Might there be another way?

*Everything New Is Old Again*

While the work was leading up to the discovery of Treg cells and BiTE molecules, some characters, old and new, were reshaping our understanding of how the immune system interfaces with cancer. As you may recall from chapter 5, Lloyd Old had consistently advocated for the concept of immune surveillance, a hypothesis largely discounted by many based on findings with immune deficient (nude) mice. However, Old had appreciated that these hairless mice did not lack an immune response; while they did not have T cells, this outcome was compensated by increased vigilance from dendritic cells and other innate immunological defense mechanisms. Old gained a valuable ally in the form of an emerging immunological pioneer in St. Louis.

Robert Schreiber was born in 1946 in Buffalo, New York, and received his bachelor's and doctoral degrees from the State University of New York in (relatively) nearby Rochester and stayed on further to perform his first postdoctoral fellowship. After postdoctoral training in immunology at the prestigious Scripps Clinic in San Diego, he remained on the faculty, where he developed expertise in understanding a dynamic interplay between the immune system and tumor cells. This work continued after Schreiber was recruited to Washington University in St. Louis, where he rose to become an internationally recognized expert in understanding the exquisite dance between cancer cells and the immune system meant to track and destroy them.

As Schreiber was building this expertise, the scientific field's view of cancer was also changing. As a brief overview, the 1980s and '90s were a time of unprecedented progress in the accretion of tools to study cancer and changes in the genetic events typifying the disease. The environment in St. Louis, where Schreiber performed most of his pioneering immunology research, was strongly influenced by its role as an epicenter for DNA sequencing (e.g., Washington University was one of the handful of sites leading the Human Genome Project) and medical imaging (e.g., PET scanning was invented at the institution).

These technological improvements revealed volumes of information about how the changes in DNA presage and characterize cancer progression. As a tumor matures, it increasingly accumulates individual mutations, which reveal themselves as small incremental changes in the tumor's DNA. As these mutations accumulate, the process continuously accelerates, particularly when these mutations arise in key genes tasked with maintaining the fidelity of DNA (e.g., DNA repair enzymes). The process continues to speed up, reaching a point where entire portions of chromosomes are either duplicated, shifted around to other chromosomes, or are lost altogether.

These massive changes cause a Darwinian selection for cells able to survive the hostile environment where the cancer resides and can also facilitate metastasis to distant and foreign sites in the body.

The culmination of Schreiber's major contributions to science was a demonstration that these changes do not occur in a vacuum but are intimately linked with parallel changes in the interaction of the tumor with the immune system. Schreiber cites "three E's" to summarize these altering interactions.[18] The first "E" arises as malignant cells are selectively seen as foreign and *eliminated* by the cells of the immune system. This idea conforms nicely to Old's original concept of immune surveillance. Schreiber built upon this and added the concept of "neo-antigens," in which the mutations characteristic of cancer generate waves of subtle differences distinguishing "self" and "diseased" cells and allow the immune system to discriminate between these distinctions.

Schreiber and Old began a long-term collaboration to build upon this idea that cancer is mostly kept in check by immune targeting of neo-antigens, keeping in mind the many negative critiques constantly highlighting the flaws in the immune surveillance theory. Clearly, their concept was incomplete, as betrayed by the prevalence of cancer in society (and, recalling the results of prostate cancer biopsies, arguably within most of us). Incorporating this valid criticism into their new theory, Old and Schreiber postulated a second "E," in this case representing the word *equilibrium*, reflecting the fact cancer is far from a static disease. The mutations allowing malignancy to arise in the first place are persistent. The resulting constant change resembles a game of whack-a-mole in which the rate of tumor mutation changes dynamically and bidirectionally with the immune system.

A high rate of mutation means the tumor is constantly experimenting with changes in order to potentially render the cancer cell resistant to killing by immune cells. Although most of these modifications are in vain, the tumor is in parallel utilizing its interactions with the immune system cells to secrete factors, including molecules like TGF-beta, to expand the number of Treg cells. Eventually, this combination of mutation and subversion defenestrates host defense pathways, rendering the tumor virtually invisible to the immune system. At this point, the third "E," which stands for *escape*, can begin. Escape is a process whereby a localized tumor has gained the ability to de-fang the immune system and gains the ability to spread throughout the body. At this point, the disease transitions from a local annoyance to a systemic killer, as metastatic cells migrate to and disrupt the function of organs throughout the body (e.g., the lungs, liver, or brain).

Schreiber and Old's new model, which they termed *cancer immunoediting*, was groundbreaking in part by implicating the immune system as an active participant in the promotion of cancer. This unexpected outcome arises as the immune system helps weed out less aggressive tumor cells, unintentionally selecting the metastatic variants with the potential to escape and form dangerous metastatic lesions throughout the body. Schreiber and Old's new model demonstrated how the process works to silence the immune system through the creation of Treg cells, which in turn follow the spreading cancer cells and shut down immune responses against these invaders.

The theory of immunoediting was a paradigm shift incorporated understanding, new and old, which had confounded scientists struggling to understand the dynamic interplay between tumor cells and the body's defenses. However, the question remained: Could this knowledge presage useful approaches to combating the disease? In particular, might targeting the mechanisms responsible for the creation of Treg cells provide an opportunity to restore the tumor-killing capacity of the immune system? Despite such awakenings, a shocking early setback nearly scuttled the entire Treg cell enterprise.

### Bloated Ideas

As monoclonal antibody therapeutics, the subject of chapter 6, began to flourish, they were generally presumed to be safe. All this changed on a specific date and place: March 13, 2006, in London, England.

Dr. Daniel Bradford had anticipated a routine day. Bradford received his secondary education at the prestigious Dulwich College. With this strong beginning, Bradford was accepted at Cambridge University and received medical training at Manchester University. In 1999, he returned to medicine and to London, where he became interested in clinical trials research. He accepted a private sector opportunity to work with Quintiles, a large contract research organization (CRO) specializing in human testing of new medicines. This experience ignited an interest in pharmaceutical research and, after a brief stint with another London CRO, took a position as an associate medical director at Parexel, a prestigious London-based CRO, where is specialties included oversight of safety and ethical reports. During this time, he also enrolled in a program at the University of Surrey to obtain a postgraduate diploma to demonstrate his expertise in pharmaceutical medicine.

At the start of Bradford's routine day on March 13, 2006, he clocked in at Parexel—which was tucked into a private wing of the Northwick Park Hospital in north London, two floors above the intensive care wing—where he had conducted more than three hundred different clinical trials.[19] He had a rather unique perspective, participating in ten or so trials himself to earn a little money on the side. He had intended to spend his morning overseeing a study with eight volunteers, who had agreed to be treated with an experimental medicine known only as TGN-1412. These volunteers had been attracted by a £2,000 inducement, and most had also expressed comfort in knowing they would be helping to advance medical science. Indeed, much would be learned from this clinical trial.

In counseling the small troupe of men as to what they might expect, Bradford repeated a process he had performed hundreds of times before using the guidelines provided by the sponsoring organization, TeGenero, and approved by the British (and European) medical regulators, which included relating to each volunteer the potential risks associated with this particular drug. The drug to be tested, TGN-1412, had been intended to treat blood cancers by altering their regulatory T cells and thereby allowing the immune system to naturally control the disease. The animal trials had not raised any concerns about safety, but to be cautious, the drug would be infused at one five-hundredth (0.2%) of the highest safe level tested in primates.[20] Bradford read through the potential side effects that were possible since the drug targeted immune cells, which included a potential for hives or, in the extreme, an anaphylactic response comparable to a response when allergic individuals are stung by a bee or consume shellfish. Such responses are easily recognized and manageable with a dose of steroids, Benadryl, or, in extreme cases, a shot of adrenaline. Having finished this required instruction, the volunteers signed the voluminous paperwork to inform them of their rights as first systemized in the 1947 Nuremberg Code (a direct outcome of the actions by Joseph Mengele and other Nazi atrocities during the Second World War) and improved by numerous updates in the intervening half century to minimize the ethical and personal risks to clinical trial volunteers.

In *A Prescription for Change*, I provided a moment-by-moment overview of the events of the day.[21] Since that time, additional details have since come to light, particularly with the release of an outstanding BBC documentary, *The Drug Trial: Emergency at the Hospital*, which first aired in February 2017 and is particularly relevant to the present story.[22]

The trial was designed to slowly infuse TGN-1412 into six of the eight men, with the remaining two serving as sham controls (to preclude potential psychosomatic effects). Even before the eighth volunteer had begun to receive drug, the first of the volunteers began to complain about a constellation of rapidly worsening symptoms. A minor headache quickly progressed into a migraine pulsing in increasingly powerful waves. This presaged uncontrollable shaking and severe pain in the back and extremities followed within the hour by involuntary vomiting and diarrhea. One patient became so distressed he tried to escape the ward, believing this would alleviate his distress, but collapsed before completing his flight.

The medical staff had been blinded as to who had received the placebo but this was obvious as two men were terrified at the events around them but were otherwise healthy.[23] They were dismissed and did not tarry in leaving the ward, where the noise, smells, and extraordinary sights of the crisis continued to worsen.

Bradford was at a loss for what was causing these dramatic problems, as one by one his patients began to fade in and out of consciousness. He tried phoning the intensive care unit (ICU) ward but could not get an answer, so he bolted down the two floors to grab any ICU physicians he could find.[24] By the time reinforcements arrived, the six volunteers had, in Bradford's words, "tumbled like dominos" and became the newest patients of the ICU of the Northwick Park Hospital. Within twelve hours, one patient's lung had begun to fail and the domino analogy soon applied to the collapse of other organ systems (lung, kidney, heart) until extreme intervention (e.g., ventilators, dialysis, etc.) was necessary to keep these men alive.

The ICU doctors were similarly perplexed by the sudden and extraordinary medical calamity taking place all around them and suspected sepsis, a bacterial infection of the blood.[25] This diagnosis was consistent with an idea that the TGN-1412 drug under investigation might have unknowingly been contaminated. Consequently, the police arrived and cordoned off the Parexel ward, questioning whether such contamination might have been intentional, looking for signs of a crime or even terrorism. During this time, Bradford had run back to his office and pored over the paperwork provided by TeGenero, eventually finding a statement that the drug, in the extreme, might cause a cytokine storm. Bradford again raced back into the ICU, informing the doctors of this alternative hypothesis.

The ICU physicians were forced to make a snap judgment. If the symptoms were caused by a cytokine storm, then the proper course of action would be to administer massive doses of steroids and other powerful medicines meant to drastically tamp down the immune system response. On the other hand, if the volunteers were suffering from sepsis, this action would undermine the immune mechanisms needed to fight the bacteria and would ensure the battle against the infection would be lost. In the end, the doctors chose to administer the steroids as well as daclizumab, a monoclonal antibody therapeutic designed to block IL-2 (which you may recall is one of the most powerful cytokines in the immune arsenal).

Everyone involved then held their breath, questioning whether they had just saved or killed the six volunteers.

The next of kin for the six men were notified to come to the hospital as soon as possible. Upon her arrival at Northwick Park Hospital, the fiancée of one volunteer, David Oakley, was informed her partner might look a bit different. In an interview for the BBC documentary, the fiancée related David's head had swollen so much his head looked like a massive ball with two slits, where his eyes were. The other patients were in the same shape, giving rise to a tag the British tabloids used to label the volunteers: The Elephant Men. Likewise, their stomachs were distended and appendages so swollen some fingers and toes would die and fall off (or have to be surgically removed).

The physiological explanation for these grisly effects resides in the fact one effect of cytokines is to loosen the blood vessels and allow fluids and cells to more readily move in and out of these tissues. Such a response is quite similar to the swelling often arising in the minutes following a simple cut or puncture. This inflammation both allows immune cells into the wound and cordons off the site to localize any freeloading infectious agents away from the rest of the body. However, a cytokine storm is a situation where the swelling occurs in all organs and thus fluids from the blood stream invade tissues everywhere, disrupting organ function and causing dangerous decreases in blood pressure (since much of the fluid and cells from the blood have left the vessels). Indeed, a patient enduring a cytokine storm will soon undergo a form of shock (akin to extreme blood loss) and the only response is for physicians to replenish these fluids, which in turn starts a new cycle of fluid movement into the tissues and organs, and this vicious cycle continues. One outcome is the horrific disfigurement associated with "the elephant men."

Thankfully, the timely and bold intervention by the staff at Northwick Park Hospital had indeed saved the day and all six men survived (though one remained hospitalized for four months and has effectively lost the use of his hands due to irreversible tissue damage). As each volunteer was discharged from the hospital, he was warned of a high likelihood that cancer or autoimmune diseases might arise as a consequence of their experience with TGN-1412.

As a postscript just over a decade later, none of the more dreaded outcomes has yet occurred. All six men remain alive, though their future prognoses remain unknown. Based on the events on the fateful day, Bradford decided the TGN-1412 event would be his last trial and though he has remained dedicated to developing new medicine, his work is now supportive, with no activity directly in the wards. Looking back, the unwitting volunteers of the TGN-1412 experiment may eventually be seen as the first pioneers of a growing population of survivors, as we will soon see.

Having related this horrific incident, I conveniently neglected to explain what TGN-1412 had been intended to do. The rationale behind the drug, which had never before been tested on people, was to override the roadblocks preventing Treg cells from killing cancer. As you may recall, Treg cells and/or the process of anergy can arise due to insufficient stimulation of the T cell receptor combined with a co-stimulatory receptor. The most prominent co-stimulatory receptors are CD28 and CTLA-4. The specific mechanism behind TGN-1412 was to stimulate CD28 in such a vigorous way it could bypass the need for the T cell receptor. Newly quiescent Treg cells were intended to remove the brakes on the immune system and thereby invigorate the killing of tumor cells. Unfortunately, this strategy worked a bit too well, as TGN-1412 relieved many Treg brakes while simultaneously stimulating T cells throughout the body. The result of this sudden change in regulation was a vigorous cytokine storm.

A troubling outcome of the TGN-1412 trial, beyond its immediate disastrous impact on those intimately involved, was that medical scientists had not anticipated this toxicity. In retrospect, one could easily pontificate how the outcome was inevitable, but the fact no one saw it coming remained particularly troublesome. This ignorance (not intended as a derogatory term so much as a realistic one) generated considerable concern, both within the relatively small community of researchers studying monoclonal antibodies and more acutely with the population of medical researchers and physicians intent on determining if immune oncology and manipulation of Treg cells could be used to fight cancer. Indeed, early analysis of the TGN-1412 incident predicted the demise of the entire field of immune oncology even before it had been christened.

These critics would be proven wrong, but not without a fight.

### *Accomplishments Big as All Hell and Half of Texas*

The title of this section is a Texan saying and meant to provide context for the introduction of a character who would revolutionize the fields of immunology and cancer therapy. James "Jim" P. Allison was born in the sleepy southern Texan town of Alice on August 7, 1948.

It is perhaps unkind to state Alice, Texas, is only known for an abundance of cattle above and oil beneath, as it did gain national attention in 1948 with an interesting revelation about its voting patterns. It seems in the final minutes before the polls closed, the ballot boxes in Alice had suddenly been filled with 202 ballots, all for Lyndon Baines Johnson and, importantly, in alphabetical order. Now it certainly cannot be entirely eliminated that a highly organized crew of Johnson loyalists entered the polling station in alphabetic order to convey their enthusiastic support for the Democratic senate candidate, but one who maintains such a belief would be, quoting another Texan saying, "two tacos short of a number two meal."

One can assume Allison was not part of this conspiracy, given he was three months old at the time, but he gained his own notoriety when, as a sixteen-year-old high school senior, he refused to take a biology class because evolution was excluded due to objections from the surrounding religious community.[26] The feud escalated to the point where the school board intervened and eventually settled upon a compromise, allowing Allison to substitute this requirement with a correspondence course from University of Texas at Austin, an institution that would later serve as Allison's alma mater, for both his bachelor's and doctoral degrees in biology.*

Beyond a passion for the biological sciences stimulated in part by this course, Allison's maternal lineage would unexpectedly also influence his future plans. His mother had died from lymphoma when Jim was eleven, preceded by "years of radiation therapy that left her skin burned and body gaunt."[27] Preparing to go swimming one day with his friends, he was called back to the house, where he was told to go see his mother. She died soon thereafter, while Allison held her hand.[28] Over the following few years, one maternal uncle died after a similar torture during his fight with lung cancer and a second uncle refused therapy for his melanoma altogether after witnessing the anguish experienced by his two siblings. Despite this considerable family trauma, Allison was not intent on a career in cancer, as he realized the idea of tumor immunology had, up to this time, never lived up to the hype surrounding it. As one example, Allison cited a 1980 *Time* magazine cover reflecting the hysteria around the use of interferon for cancer, stating, "It was crazy because people were doing things and they didn't understand how they worked."[29]

After a postdoctoral fellowship at the Scripps Institute, Allison returned to Texas with an appointment at the Smithville Science Park, the basic science cornerstone of the prestigious M.D. Anderson. Although housed in a cancer center during a tenure lasting from 1974 until 1985, Allison pioneered fundamental scientific research to understand the immune system in general and T cells in particular. He then moved to the University of California,

---

\* Allison would return to the Texan debate on evolution in 1981, when his former eighth-grade algebra teach, who had by then moved on to become a member of the Texas legislature, invited him to speak against a bill introduced to codify the teaching of the oxymoronic "creation science" in Texas classrooms. In an impassioned speech, Allison stated, among other things, "While the theory of gravity is still controversial, apples still do indeed fall down." The bill failed. (Source: E. Benson, "The Iconoclast," *Texas Monthly*, November 2016.)

Berkeley, where he would remain until 2004, and later to the Memorial Sloan Kettering Cancer Center until 2012, and when he went back to his native Texas and M.D. Anderson.

Among Allison's science accomplishments were an elucidation of how T cells recognize foreign antigen and the structure of the T cell receptor (TCR). Allison also led efforts to understand the regulation of the TCR and the need for a co-stimulatory signal by CD28 to properly activate these vital cells (the basis of the intended efficacy of TGN-1412). Although any of the above discoveries would have secured a historical legacy for Allison, future findings would be even more monumental.

At this point, it is important to reintroduce you to some people and put them in context, so we return to the outspoken and brilliant scientist Lee Nadler. In chapter 6, we saw Nadler was the first to test monoclonal antibody drug candidates in people and was recognized for his discovery of a monoclonal antibody, which he had named B1. This antibody was later revealed to recognize CD20 (the target successfully prosecuted by rituximab and other therapies). Another of these monoclonal antibodies would point the way to an entirely new approach to treating cancer.

In October 1989, Nadler reported the identification of a molecule on the surface of B cells that he named B7.[30] An intriguing finding, to which we will soon return, was that B7 was found at high levels not only on activated B cells but in most cases of non-Hodgkin's lymphoma.

Armed with this information, we now reintroduce Peter Linsley and Jeffrey Ledbetter, who had been studying CD28 and its role as a powerful co-receptor for T cell activation. For a time, CD28 was known as an *orphan receptor* because its binding partner had not been identified. This would all change when they demonstrated Nadler's B7 was the binding partner for CD28.[31] The Seattle team at Bristol-Myers Squibb had demonstrated the binding of the B7 on the surface of antigen-presenting cells with CD28 on T cells was necessary to fully activate T cells if this signaling occurred at the same time the TCR had been stimulated.

Fortunately for science and medicine, but unfortunately for the ease of clarity, the story with B7 would not be so simple. For one thing, it turns out B7 was not a single molecule, but rather one of an ever-expanding family of proteins with at least ten family members. Two of these B7 family members (known as *B7-1* and *B7-2*) interact with CD28 and eight do not. Worse still, B7-1 and B7-2 do not interact exclusively with CD28 and instead are quite promiscuous in their choice of partners.

Allison expanded on this emerging knowledge and demonstrated B7-1 and B7-2 can also interact with another molecule on T cells, known as *CTLA-4*. Paradoxically, their binding to CTLA-4 triggers a cascade of events resulting in the exact opposite outcome of their coupling with CD28. Specifically, the binding of either B7-1 or B7-2 to CD28 promotes T cell activation, whereas their binding to CTLA-4 actively thwarts T cell activation.

Given the inherent complexity, the reader can appreciate the frustration this must have caused for some scientists, who prefer neat and clean findings. These same reductionists tend to prefer tidy hypotheses and cite pithy justifications, such as Occam's razor, to explain confounding data. The complexity of the juxtaposition between CD28 and CTLA-4 would be anathema for "hard scientists," such as physicists and chemists, who tend to measure the accuracy of their findings to the nth decimal point. This idea is reflected and parodied in the seventh season of the hit science comedy *Big Bang Theory*, when Dr. Sheldon Cooper discovers a trivial miscalculation in a formula he had crafted, conveying in disgust, "I'm worse than a fraud, I'm practically a biologist."[32] Despite the need to bear the disdain of colleagues in the physical sciences, such examples of chaos are manna for biologists, who thrive upon considering the implications of a world less tidy than originally envisioned.

Within this context, the discovery that B7 binding to CTLA-4 blocked T cell activation posed a great opportunity and challenge to Allison, who had begun collaborating with a like-minded investigator at the University of Chicago. Allison and Jeffrey A. Bluestone paired up to examine how CTLA-4 functioned to block immune cells, but their findings also laid the groundwork for understanding other similarly behaving systems. As a brief summary, their work revealed elevated levels of B7-1 or B7-2 on tumor cells could engage with CTLA-4 on T cells and thereby actively impair the ability of these T cells to recognize the tumor cells as foreign and eliminate them. This work would have implications well beyond B7, as the same themes would apply to a pair of exotic-sounding molecules known as *programmed cell death protein-1* (PD-1) and its binding partner (known as *PD-L1*), a subject to which we will soon return.

In 1996, Allison published a paper that would ensure he would be the second Nobel prize winner from sleepy Alice, Texas (the first was Robert F. Curl Jr., who received the 1996 Nobel Prize for his discovery of fullerene, a soccer-ball-shaped molecule, which provides backbone for carbon nanotubes).[33] In a manuscript published in the March 22 edition of *Science* magazine, Allison's team described a remarkable ability to fully activate T cells and direct them to kill tumor cells. This outcome was achieved following treatment with a CTLA-4 monoclonal antibody created with the intention of blocking CTLA-4 binding to its B7 ligand. In other words, Allison created a double negative by using a CTLA-4 antibody to turn off the negative regulation repressing T cells from killing tumor cells. Stated a third way, this targeting strategy could unleash the fury of the T cells to target and kill malignant cells. The approach being pioneered was later to be known as *checkpoint inhibition* based on the idea CTLA-4 (and similar effectors) represented a checkpoint to shut down auto-reactive T cells. By blocking these checkpoints, CTLA-4 antibodies might allow Treg cells to regain the ability to kill tumor cells. This was the hypothesis Allison sought to test.

The results were, to put it mildly, definitive. Tumor-bearing mice were injected with the CTLA-4 antibody and tumor survival was assessed over the following few days. According to a normally cautious Allison, "The tumors were cured. I mean it was 100% and 0%—no statistics necessary."[34]

Although such results seemed indisputable, his skeptics were hardly muted. Indeed, Allison recalled the comments of a reviewer of the paper who recommended the article be rejected since "we all know that immunotherapy's crap. It's never worked."[35]

This data containing a CTLA-4–blocking monoclonal antibody triggered a partnership with a small biotechnology company located in Princeton, New Jersey. Medarex had been founded in 1987 by a group of immunologists from the Dartmouth School of Medicine. The "secret sauce" propelling Medarex to success was the use of mice specially engineered to express human antibodies. As we have seen, mouse antibodies are inherently recognized as foreign and rejected when injected into people. This hurdle was surmounted by exchanging the genes for mice immunoglobulin with their human counterparts. The resulting "HuMAb mice" produced antibodies that appeared to be human and would therefore be accepted in patients. Using this approach, the Medarex mice were used to generate CTLA-4 antibodies to block the interaction with B7.

The resulting product, ipilimumab (trade name: Yervoy®) began clinical trials in June 2000. As is the case for all new medicines, the first and highest hurdle was to assess whether ipilimumab was safe. A total of seventeen patients, primarily suffering from prostate cancer or melanoma, were treated with the drug. Early signs were not at all promising. A few patients demonstrated the signs of inflammation and potential autoimmune disorders, and the drug was considered responsible for the deaths of some of the volunteers. These toxic outcomes had occurred five years before the fateful TGN-1412 clinical trial (had they been encountered after, it seems likely skittish regulators would have shut down the investigation). Nonetheless, the toxicity encountered with ipilimumab did recall the painful experiences with IL-2 in clinical trials, where in many cases, the toxicities from the cytokine storm triggered by treatment exceeded the severity of the disease. By this time, Bristol-Myers Squibb had joined the collaboration (they would eventually acquire Medarex in 2009) and, as a large company with the potential for reputational as well as liability risks, cancellation of the ipilimumab program seemed probable.

Compounding the problem, only three of the first seventeen patients had demonstrated any significant positive response to ipilimumab. Nonetheless, this minority of patients exposed extraordinary efficacy, reminiscent of Allison's studies in mice. One patient, Sharon Belvin, experienced a "melting away" of her tumors.

Despite this powerful display of effectiveness, the sponsors, Medarex and BMS, remained queasy. The bile rose in their throats further upon learning Pfizer, which was developing its own CTLA-4 antibody, had experienced the same toxicities. Indeed, Pfizer had become sufficiently chastened that the company elected to disgorge its own experimental CTLA-4 antibody, selling it to a rival, AstraZeneca, in 2008.

In a truly courageous decision, Medarex and BMS decided to wait out the results from an ongoing clinical trial in metastatic melanoma. The boldness of this decision is particularly clear given metastatic melanoma had long been known in the field as the "black death," not just because of its appearance on patients, but also its reputation for killing the future of all medicines developed to try and treat it. Anyone betting on a positive outcome with melanoma would have long odds and, adding the toxicities associated with ipilimumab, it seemed a good bet the drug was yet another candidate destined for the dustbin of failed experimental medicines.

On August 19, 2010, an article appeared in the *New England Journal of Medicine* titled, "Improved survival with ipilimumab in patients with metastatic melanoma."[36] In a study conducted in 125 cancer centers located in thirteen countries spread over four continents, 750 patients were randomly divided into groups and treated with ipilimumab, with or without standard therapy. By this time, prior experience with the antibody had allowed the physicians to anticipate and minimize potential side effects caused by a cytokine storm (although the drug was sadly linked to the death of fourteen patients).

Like Sharon Belvin, more patients showed remarkable tumor regressions and ipilimumab decreased the risk of cancer death by one third. Just months before, such an outcome was simply unthinkable, particularly in patients with incurable metastatic melanoma. Ipilimumab was approved by the FDA as the first "checkpoint inhibitor" on March 25, 2011. Positive results continued to arrive as the potential use of the drug was expanded to include many other cancer types since its initial approval.

Despite his initial reluctance to become a cancer researcher, Allison has remained dedicated to a science which has again come to hit a bit too close to home. In 2005, Allison was again burying a relative, this time a brother who had succumbed to prostate cancer. Later in the same year, Allison would be diagnosed with the same disease himself. In early 2016, Alison's colleagues noted a mass on his nose and suggested he needed to see a dermatologist. This was removed and Allison was informed the diagnosis was melanoma and was advised, "We want to get this out before you have to get that drug of yours."[37] Thankfully, Allison has not yet been required to take a dose of his own medicine.

Amid the excitement surrounding ipilimumab, inevitable criticism dampened enthusiasm, particularly as it pertains to safety. Invoking the dramatic outcomes of the TGN-1412 trial, concerns were vented about the likelihood the stimulation of T cells by ipilimumab would stimulate not just tumor-killing activity, but autoimmune disorders as well. A particularly scathing article appeared in the June 2012 edition of *Immunobiology*, accusing BMS of being "unmindful of the clinical trial catastrophe in London," referring to the TGN-1412 debacle.[38] Allison himself led a counterattack, leading a team of immunologists who accused their critics of "lacking in scientific rigor" and selectively using only snippets of published clinical data to support their argument (revealing some scientists are just as prone to selective filtering as many political partisans).[39] As we will see, concerns about the safety of immune oncology therapies remain prevalent and prescient.

Despite the exciting findings revealing efficacy and improved management of toxicities, such as cytokine storms, the truth nonetheless remained for many patients that ipilimumab was not effective. This fact would drive further investigation and soon ipilimumab would be joined by waves of new entrants to the rapidly burgeoning field of immune oncology.

## A Life After Programmed Death Experience

A recurring theme pervading not only the story of immune oncology, but the larger history of science, is the power of chance and epiphany. In the case of our next innovator, the beginning and end of his story were defined by antibodies. Tasuku Honjo was born on January 27, 1942, amid the tumult of the Second World War, in Kyoto, Japan. The location that would serve as a backdrop for most of Honjo's life had been the former Imperial capital of Japan for more than a millennium and had suffered many times from the ravages of war, including its sacking during the Onin civil war in the 15th century. A minor struggle for imperial succession escalated into a nationwide internecine bloodletting that would plague the nation, and repeatedly devastate Kyoto, in particular, for a century and a half. The city would eventually recover but be put to the torch again in 1864 with the Kinmon incident, a rebellion against the emperor that began with the burning of the city by the rebels. Again, Kyoto would recover and grow to become the intellectual and cultural capital of Japan, hosting at least forty colleges and universities, two thousand Buddhist and Shinto landmarks, and seventeen UNESCO World Heritage sites. All these remarkable institutions, as well as the young Tasuku Honjo, might have been but a pile of ashes but for a honeymoon trip by a man understandably reviled by many Japanese.

Three years after the Kinmon incident, Henry Stimson was born into an upper-class family a world away in Manhattan, the son of a prominent banker, surgeon, and socialite, Lewis Atterbury Stimson,[40] who had been a star among the New York elite (his patients included Ulysses S. Grant) and wrote the charter for the Cornell University Medical College, advocating for its founding in Manhattan rather than upstate Ithaca. After graduating from an elite series of schools (the Philips Academy, Yale University, and the Harvard Law School), Henry Stimson married Mabel Wellington White. This 1893 marriage would prove fateful for the people of Kyoto, as the city was chosen as the site of their honeymoon.

After a successful career as a Manhattan banker and lawyer, Stimson would later go on to serve as secretary of war under President William Howard Taft in the days immediately before the start of the First World War. He later served as the American ambassador to Nicaragua and the Philippines and, during this latter time, returned to Japan, this time to Tokyo, in 1926. Within three years, Stimson would return to the United States as secretary of state under President Herbert Hoover. He was also called to service under President Franklin Delano Roosevelt, as secretary of war, in the days immediately following the Nazi domination of France and Scandinavia as it became apparent American involvement in the burgeoning Second World War would be inevitable.

During this second stint as the nation's leading civilian figure in the Pentagon, Stimson oversaw the extraordinary buildup of forces and became the pivot point in many controversial decisions. An early fight centered upon the internment of Japanese-Americans. Although Stimson was initially opposed to this draconian measure in the days after Pearl Harbor, he spent December 1941 and the following January tending to panicked military leaders and politicians from the West Coast, eventually capitulating to demands to relocate and imprison these legal citizens of the United States. This controversy paled in comparison to a decision which would come to define the man for future generations.

Among the components of Stimson's portfolio was the Manhattan Project, tasked to design, test, and manufacture a nuclear weapon. Given the extraordinary degree of secrecy afforded to the program, its director, General Leslie Groves, reported directly to Stimson, who, as secretary of war, would not only place the program at the top of his priority list but would determine the priorities of its use. Originally conceived as a means to reverse Nazi victories, the deployment of this new wonder weapon was too late for use in Europe. To the dismay of many scientists whose energies had been invested in the program as a means to halt Hitler, Stimson and Truman were determined to use it to hasten an end to the war with Japan.[41]

The Target Committee of the Manhattan Project was charged with determining where the first bomb would be dropped. Kyoto was placed at the top of a list submitted to Stimson on May 10, 1945, followed by Hiroshima, Yokohama, Kokura Arsenal, and Niigata (Nagasaki would be added more than two months later).[42] Perhaps reflecting on his honeymoon, Stimson removed Kyoto from the list, claiming its role as an ancient capital and intellectual center. The Target Committee argued these were the exact reasons why Kyoto should be leveled. The fight was escalated to the point where Stimson personally advocated his position to President Truman and eventually won over the commander-in-chief to his preference.[43] This fateful action had doomed Nagasaki and Hiroshima but spared the life of a toddler in Kyoto who would go on to change cancer therapy.

After earning both a medical degree and a doctorate in his hometown Kyoto University, Tasuku Honjo performed research in Tokyo for a decade before returning back to Kyoto, where he has remained ever since. A year before his return to Kyoto, Honjo initiated a project to understand the extraordinary diversity allowing antibodies to recognize literally anything in nature (and even artificial molecules). Beyond the arranging of different genes (you may recall the analogy of different-colored Lego blocks) contributing to diversity, investigators had realized antibodies were subject to periods when a profound increase in the mutation rate promotes a Darwinian-like process to create antibodies with even greater affinity for their targets. Honjo built upon these theories. In 2000, he reported the characterization of a key enzyme, activated-induced cytidine deaminase (AICD), which is responsible for these brief periods of hypermutation.[44] This achievement would have been sufficient to ensure Honjo's scientific legacy for future generations but paled in comparison to a project he had begun a few years before his discovery of AICD.

In 1992, Tasuku Honjo intended to understand the basis for programmed cell death.[45] This is not an entirely new story as we have already learned about apoptosis (see chapter 1), a suicide program triggered when a cell becomes sufficiently distressed. In the early 1990s, the momentum for appreciating the importance of programmed cell death was accelerating and Honjo planned an ingenious experiment to help identify the regulators and mediators of these suicidal tendencies. What he discovered was quite unexpected indeed.

Without boring the reader with unnecessary detail, the experiment as executed used well-characterized immune cells. Cell cultures propagated in the laboratory can be quite finicky and often require the inclusion of special nutrients and chemicals necessary to prevent them from dying. Honjo's genius was to take advantage of this fact and intentionally leave out a factor to encourage them to die. He would then compare what genes were turned on (and off) to distinguish a thriving cell from its dying counterpart. An unexpected twist was that he utilized T cells and inadvertently biased the outcome for events unique to these cells.

The result of the study was the identification of PD-1 (so-named to reflects its presumed role in programmed death) as a molecule turned on in dying cells.[46] As so often occurs in science, follow-up studies revealed the higher levels of PD-1 in dying cells was a red herring and the molecule itself not directly involved in mediating apoptosis.[47] However, PD-1 did appear on the surface of immune cells following stimulation. This seemed a curious and unexpected finding.

With the proverbial bird in hand, Honjo followed his instincts and asked if this new gene might be of any interest to immunology. In the late 1990s, the field of mouse genetic engineering was at a peak and Honjo decided to make a knockout mouse lacking PD-1 and then ask if anything interesting happened in this mouse. As seen with many different knockout mice, this was a bit of a long shot, as important molecules are often compensated for by other genes. In Honjo's case, it was a mouse that changed the field of cancer.

The initial findings with the knockout mice were a bit of disappointment: Not much happened and the outcomes were all but buried in a 1998 article.[48] However, Honjo noted that these mice had been engineered using the progeny of two different strains of mice. Such genetic diversity can confound results when comparing with mice encompassing a pure lineage. Therefore, his team performed a series of what is known as *backcrossing*, to provide a pure genetic background. This seemingly minor change revealed drastic outcomes. When crossed onto a pure genetic background, the mice lacking PD-1 developed symptoms analogous to lupus and other deadly autoimmune diseases as they aged.[49] Stated another way, the presence of PD-1 in normal mice actively prevented these autoimmune indications. The question then focused on how PD-1 prevented these effects. For a molecule on the surface of T cells, such as PD-1, this meant finding its binding partner, which was likely to be found on antigen-presenting cells.

Similar to CD28, PD-1 was initially thought to be an orphan receptor but this notion was quickly dispelled with the discovery of a yet another B7 family member. In the same year the results with the PD-1 knockout mice were reported, a team at the Mayo Clinic in Rochester, Minnesota, revealed that another molecule, B7-H1, could stimulate T cells.[50] Within months, Honjo's team in Kyoto had partnered with investigators at the Dana Farber Cancer Institute to show B7-H1 was the binding partner for PD-1 (B7-H1 would later be renamed as PD-1 ligand-1 or PD-L1). At the same time, a team led by Drew Pardoll and Haruo Tsuchiya at Johns Hopkins University revealed another B7 family member, B7-Dc and demonstrated its ability to bind PD-1 and regulate T cell function.[51] In parallel, the Mayo team led by Lieping Chen countered with a landmark study in 2002, which demonstrated the presence of PD-L1 on the surface of malignant lung, ovarian, and colon, as well as melanoma, cells.[52]

With this finding, all the pieces were in place and a brief recap is crucial before moving forward. PD-1 is a receptor on the surface of T cells. Its binding partner is PD-L1, which can be found on a variety of cells and, most notably, is dramatically upregulated on tumor cells. When PD-1 on T cells binds PDL-1 on tumors cells, the T cell is functionally inactivated, rendering it unable to kill the target as normally defined by its T cell receptor. Putting it all together, the data suggested high levels of PD-L1 on cancer cells effectively inactivated (or "zombified") any T cell attempting to kill the cancer cell, creating a Treg cell in the process.

As we know from studies with BiTEs, ipilimumab, and other T cell directed therapies, these "zombified" Treg cells can be reanimated. The question then became whether PD-1 or PD-L1 blocking antibodies might provide a means to release Treg cells from their zombified state and turn them loose against cancer cells.

These ideas drove an extraordinary race forward, led by teams of academic and private sector organizations. Within months, masses of preclinical models revealed promising results. However, cynics decried the fact researchers have cured cancer in "fancy" mice thousands of times but these outcomes rarely, if ever, apply to the situation in the real world.

What was needed was a demonstration that this PD-1/PD-L1 strategy might be applicable in people.

*The Race Is on*

On May 12, 2005, Medarex, who you may recall was the purveyor of the HuMAb mice, announced a partnership with a Japanese company, Ono, to develop a monoclonal antibody intended to block PD-1. This partnership was bolstered by the participation of Honjo, who had been advising Ono. Within a remarkably short period of time, an antibody drug had been isolated and paperwork filed with the FDA to begin human trials. The resulting study of nivolumab (trade name Opdivo®) received an authorization to begin testing in people in August 2006, and the first patients began treatment two months later.

The outcomes of the first phase I clinical trial for nivolumab were promising.[53] A total of thirty-nine cancer patients volunteered to receive a single dose of the drug (in what is known as a *SAD*, or single ascending dose) trial. These brave individuals had failed all prior therapies (more accurately stated: the therapies had failed the patients) and their cancers were quite advanced (all but one had stage IV diseases, where the cancer had already spread all through the body). The primary goal of a phase I clinical trial is to ask whether an experimental drug is safe, and this definitely answered in the affirmative. Although one patient at the highest dosing level demonstrated severe colitis (inflammation of the interior lining of the colon), the malady was manageable. In a phase I clinical trial of a cancer drug, the disease in volunteers is generally so advanced it is unreasonable to expect dramatic outcomes. Nonetheless, fifteen of the thirty-nine patients showed positive responses. For the most part, the drug had served simply to stabilize the disease, preventing further progression for a time. However, three patients saw their tumors shrink. In one case, the disease disappeared altogether and remained at bay for at least twenty-one months (such an outcome is known in the medical vernacular as a "complete response," or CR). Again, recall these dramatic outcomes had occurred with only a single dose of drug.

These results inspired a study to provide multiple doses (a multiple ascending dose, or MAD trial) in a group of thirty-four patients with end-stage metastatic melanoma. Just under half (fifteen of thirty-four) of the patients showed a substantial clinical benefit. The cancer had been stopped in its tracks in seven patients and an additional eight volunteers watched as their tumors began to shrink. In two of these cases, no cancer could be detected and, remarkably, these complete responses persisted for the entire two and a half years of the study.[54]

These even more promising results inspired the advancement of studies of nivolumab in a flurry of medium-sized studies (in the range of fifty to one hundred fifty volunteers), which were overseen by Bristol-Myers Squibb (who by this time had acquired Medarex) and Ono in Japan. Many early studies focused on metastatic melanoma, a particularly bold choice as the disease had historically been obstinately resistant to new therapies. Despite dismal historical findings in melanoma with other medicines, nivolumab showed a remarkable ability to shrink tumors in roughly one third of patients and to stabilize the disease in an additional group (which ranged from 10% to more than 50% of patients, depending on the study).[55] Promising results were also emerging from additional studies of non-small cell lung cancer, renal cell carcinoma, and other cancer types. As BMS had also developed the CD28 antibody, ipilimumab, they began testing combinations of the two medicines and again were highly encouraged by positive findings.

Based on such reassuring findings, BMS expedited a phase III clinical trial to study nivolumab (with or without ipilimumab) in patients with metastatic melanoma. The study, publicized as Checkmate-037, had been designed to begin in December 2012 to evaluate 1,296 volunteers with diseases that had progressed beyond conventional therapies (including even ipilimumab). The expectation was the size of the trial and the time needed to assess patient responses would mean the trial will be completed sometime in April 2019.

Although it may not seem a big deal to many readers, a decision to move forward with a phase III clinical trial poses an extraordinary risk. In part, this risk derived from the fact a typical phase III clinical trial represents an astonishing expense, costing a minimum of hundreds of millions, and routinely exceeding billions, of dollars. Compounding these costs are the long amounts of time required to complete the trial. For example, the time spent identifying, treating, and following up with patients is expected to require six years for the Checkmate-037 trial and this does not even include the time needed to evaluate data, submit the results to the FDA, and await their analysis of the findings.

Were all of the above not sufficient to turn the stomach, the agony associated with a decision of whether to support an oncology clinical trial is worsened by the fact a positive finding in a phase II clinical trial translates into a comparable outcome in a phase III setting only 28% of the time.[56] Let's think on that a bit: If you are testing a drug with a "home run" positive outcome in a phase II clinical trial, the likelihood a positive outcome will again be achieved in a phase III trial is comparable to correctly calling the flip of a coin two times in a row. These odds seem particularly cruel given the many years and billions of dollars invested in reaching the point where one decides whether they want to try and correctly guess multiple coin flips. Needless to say, the courage to execute this decision requires cool nerves and a strong stomach.

As generally occurs in large, ambitious clinical trials, the results are analyzed at various times before study completion. These interim analyses are designed to ask whether it is beneficial for the patients (and the company) to continue a trial. This process is known as *interim* or *futility analyses* and intended to avoid unnecessary hopes and costs to patients and the sponsor, respectively, in continuing a study where early results suggest the experimental medicine is not conveying a meaningful benefit. In the case of the Checkmate-037 trial, an interim analysis would take a quick peek at the results of the first 120 patients, who had been treated with nivolumab for six months.

The results of this first interim analyses of the Checkmate-037 clinical trial were reported on September 29, 2014, at a scientific meeting in Madrid, Spain.[57] Bristol-Myers Squibb announced roughly one third of patients treated with nivolumab had demonstrated significant tumor shrinkage (as compared with 11% in patients treated with standard care). These positive responses had continued in 95% of the responding patients. These results mirrored what had been seen in the phase II studies and were deemed so striking the FDA allowed BMS to apply for an approval based on these interim data alone.

After scrutinizing the results in great detail, the FDA approved nivolumab on December 22, 2014, five years before the clinical portion of the trial had even been scheduled to conclude.[58] Within weeks, the FDA expanded the approval to include metastatic lung cancer, a decision based on an interim evaluation of another clinical trial. This trial had again revealed an improvement in overall patient survival so profound the trial had to be halted early based on ethical concerns so the drug could be offered to all participants (i.e., the patients in the control group, who had not received nivolumab). By the end of 2016, metastatic renal cancer, Hodgkin's lymphoma, head and neck cancers, urothelial carcinoma, colorectal cancer, and hepatocellular carcinoma would be added to the list of FDA-approved indications.

Although it would seem a great Hollywood ending to state nivolumab won the race to be the first PD-1 based checkpoint inhibitor approved for cancer, this was once again not to be the case, as a rival had beaten them to the punch. Whereas BMS had been responsible for the development of both ipilimumab and nivolumab, it watched its lead over the competition erode as seemingly the entire biopharmaceutical industry rushed to cash in on the demonstrated efficacy of checkpoint inhibitors. The promises and perils of this increasingly crowded space is the subject to which we will now turn as we conclude our story on immune oncology.

# 9

## *The End of the Beginning*

I pilimumab and nivolumab pioneered a new era of cancer medicine by demonstrating to the world there was promise in immune oncology. These remarkable medicines revealed metastatic melanoma, long a source of spectacular pharmaceutical failures, could be tamed, and in some patients, completely cured. Yet nivolumab would not be the first PD-1 directed immune oncology drug with a demonstrated ability to cure melanoma. Although the drug had been meticulously discovered and rigorously expedited by a superstar team and backed by Tasuku Honjo, the achievement would instead reside with the world's oldest pharmaceutical company, which, despite its age, demonstrated it could be surprisingly spry.

### *Opposites (Eventually) Attract Attention*

Gregory J. Carven was just looking for a way to remain in Boston. After graduating with a degree in chemistry from the University of Massachusetts at Amherst, he matriculated in a doctoral program at the Massachusetts Institute of Technology (MIT). His academic curiosity was drawn to the major histocompatibility complex (MHC), an arragement of two proteins, which interact with the T cell receptor to help the immune system reconnoiter the body to guard against infectious invaders.

Upon graduation in May 2004, Carven seized upon an opportunity to work in the biotechnology industry burgeoning in and around nearby Cambridge. He joined Phylogix, a start-up founded in 1998 that had raised $12 million from investors. The company focused on identifying potential therapeutics from lectins, a class of sugar-binding molecules from plants, with the potential to protect normal tissues from the lethal side effects of cancer chemotherapy (you may recall we met one lectin, ricin, in chapter 3). As often occurs in the rough and tumble world of biotechnology, Phylogix ran out of capital thirteen months after Carven's hiring, and he found himself again looking for a job in the spring of 2005.

By August, Carven's search had been successful, and he was hired by a large Dutch pharmaceutical company named Organon (a Greek name for Aristotle's teachings on logic). Although not a particularly well-known name in the United States, Organon had been founded in Oss, The Netherlands, in 1923 and by the time Carven joined, the company had twenty thousand employees, primarily in Europe. Carven had been recruited into a twenty-person outpost in Cambridge, which had just opened in the summer of 2005. The company had a long history as an innovator, being one of the first European companies to commercialize insulin, estrogens, and birth control pills. Although most Organon products were conventional small chemical-based drugs, the company had opened the Cambridge branch in part to develop monoclonal antibody products. The project assigned to Carven had begun in 2003 at Organon headquarters in Oss and was led by Andrea van Elsas, a Dutch scientist who had received a Ph.D. in immunology and oncology from the prestigious Leiden University before postdoctoral studies at the University of California, Berkeley. Their shared goal was to utilize emerging information about PD-1 to identify antibodies intended to activate PD-1. This quest was driven by the rationale these activating PD-1 antibodies would trigger a shut-down of autoreactive T cells and, as such, be utilized to alleviate certain diseases, such as rheumatoid arthritis or multiple sclerosis.

Despite strenuous efforts to identify these "agonist" molecules that stimulate PD-1, the Cambridge group was continually frustrated by the fact all their efforts had only isolated "antagonists" that blocked PD-1 activity. They were scratching their heads as to what, if anything, to do with these antagonists and considered the potential of using the antibodies to increase the efficacy of vaccines. However, the Organon scientists, like their colleagues at Medarex, Ono, and Bristol-Myers Squibb, ultimately decided to focus upon oncology.

The future of the PD-1 program seemed destined to be shelved on March 12, 2007, when the American pharmaceutical giant Schering-Plough announced it would purchase Organon for $14 billion. In a pharmaceutical world in the midst of being utterly restructured by waves of consolidation, this was a relatively minor blip for the industry, but had huge implications for the PD-1 program. The purchase of Organon was driven by Schering-Plough's need for pipeline programs close to generating revenue (in other words, relatively mature pipeline products in phase II or phase III human clinical trials). The PD-1 program had yet to enter the clinic and its most likely fate was to be binned as part of the inevitable cost-cutting measures necessary to pay off the large margins associated with mergers and acquisitions.

Fortunately for van Elsas and Carven, the PD-1 program might have been seen as too small to be placed on the chopping block. Their expenditures were sufficiently insufficient for the program to be considered in the first round of downsizing and the program remained below the radar. This delay gave them time to generate additional findings in mice. The team was beginning to put together the data needed to support an application to the FDA to begin clinical trials when again a corporate merger was announced. Almost two years to the day after Schering-Plough had devoured Organon, the company found itself the bait, consumed by an even larger predator: Merck Pharmaceuticals. On March 9, 2009, Merck announced its acquisition of the company. Again, as inevitable in such deals, this acquisition presaged yet more rounds of cuts and this time the PD-1 program was more highly visible and destined for dismantlement.

Again, van Elsas and Carven found themselves in a newly integrated company assessing its assets and planning to make substantial cuts. This version of purgatory generally takes at least a year, particularly for large mergers such as Merck and Schering-Plough (particularly since Schering-Plough had not fully digested what it had acquired from the earlier acquisition of Organon). Many projects at both firms would be abandoned altogether and a lucky few would be prepared to be sold to investors or established competitors. After experiencing the roller coaster of emotions arising from not one, but two mergers, the PD-1 team learned their program had been designated for the latter: it would be sold off.

Both van Elsas and Carven were reassigned to other projects and the business development team began to organize the PD-1 program for a sale. As they were putting together their competitive intelligence about the immune oncology marketplace (not an area of particular strength for Merck at the time), the *New England Journal of Medicine* published a paper revealing the powerful efficacy displayed by BMS's ipilimumab against metastatic melanoma. Indeed, ipilimumab would be approved by the FDA a few months later just as BMS published the first evidence of efficacy for another immune oncology drug, nivolumab, achieved during phase I clinical trial studies. The Merck executives were dutifully impressed by BMS's powerful one-two punch in the field of immune oncology and sought to determine if and how they might compete in the rapidly blossoming field.

In looking over their own assets, Merck executives suddenly realized they had their own immune oncology drug candidate, an obscure project begun at Organon. The team of van Elsas and Carven was consulted and their new bosses at Merck were impressed—they decided to bring the project back from death (or more accurately, to cancel the fire sale).

Though resigned to the fact there was no way to catch up with BMS's already approved CTLA-4 antibody and their advancing PD-1 antibody, the management at Merck performed an abrupt about-face and were adamant not only to reactivate their newly acquired PD-1 program but try to win the race against nivolumab. Pulling out all the stops, the process to file an investigative new drug application (necessary to begin testing in people) was hastily reignited. The proper paperwork was quickly filed with and approved by the FDA. Human testing in volunteers initiated in January 2011. This trial, known internally at Merck as KEYNOTE-001, would set records and precedents unlike any previous cancer trials, before or since.

The first cohort of ten volunteers in the KEYNOTE-001 trial included patients with all types of advanced solid tumors. These patients had all failed prior therapies and were treated with a single dose of the Merck PD-1 inhibitor, a monoclonal antibody named pembrolizumab (trade name: Keytruda®). The antibody was found to be generally safe and well tolerated, even at the highest doses tested. At this point, there was essentially no reason to assess the potential for efficacy as these earliest patients were intended simply to verify the safety of the experimental medicine.

As allowed by the FDA, the highest dose shown to be safe was then used to treat seven more patients. However, these patients were allowed to receive multiple doses, administered every two weeks. An additional thirteen patients were treated using an approach to escalate the dose of pembrolizumab over a three-week period. Of these first thirty patients, two demonstrated a complete response (total elimination of their tumors for at least a year), three others experienced a partial reduction in their tumor burdens, and fifteen experienced stabilization of their diseases. Altogether, two-thirds of the patients had demonstrated at least some clinical benefit: a remarkable outcome for the first experience with an experimental medicine.

Whereas such positive outcomes from the first group of patients would traditionally have been viewed as a reason to celebrate a successful conventional phase I clinical trial, Merck management was anything but conventional. Pressing forward, Merck expanded the phase I KEYNOTE-001 trial to an extreme, evolving it into a means to focus on multiple diseases (e.g., melanoma and non-small cell lung cancer), while also including patients who had received defined types of previous therapies and dosing regiments of other drugs, including nivolumab.

Essentially, the phase I trial itself metastasized into both a phase II and III study.[1] By the time the trial concluded, it had included almost 1,235 patients, an extraordinarily audacious and expensive clinical trial. However, the gamble had paid off beyond even the wildest expectations of Merck's management and scientists as unprecedented results poured in. As one example, an experienced UCLA experimental oncologist, Antoni Ribas, was quoted in a *Forbes* article as stating, "Among the first seven patients we enrolled, six patients had objective responses. I realized I was probably lucky and this high rate of response would not hold up forever."[2]

Although Ribas's experience did tend toward the extreme, the numbers put up by pembrolizumab were nonetheless jaw-dropping. Within metastatic melanoma, the drug eked out an objective response rate (a measurable reduction in tumor volume) of one in three patients. Keep in mind each of these patients had failed all prior therapies, including, in many cases, pembrolizumab or other immune oncology drugs. Amongst the responders, the beneficial effects tended to be durable, lasting for months and years. The rate of objective responses was not quite as strong for lung cancer, but still came in at an impressive 20% of patients, who were suffering from an otherwise incurable disease.[3]

Despite these impressive outcomes, Merck was still obsessed with closing the gap between the pembrolizumab development timeline and BMS's nivolumab. To complement the aggressive strategy of the KEYNOTE-001 studies, the New Jersey company utilized the even more controversial approach of deploying a linked biomarker.

As a brief aside, the idea advanced by Merck was to use a marker in the patients' cancer cells. This approach meant tumor material removed from patients would be subjected to a laboratory test requiring two weeks to process. If the test was positive, then pembrolizumab would be administered. Although scientifically sound, this action was nonetheless controversial from a business standpoint since the restrictions would limit sales and bite into profits. The challenges to this approach also were colored by the miserable experiences suffered by other biomarker-linked drugs. For example, Genentech used a biomarker test to support the early launch of Herceptin, an antibody drug for breast cancer. This biomarker test, HercepTest, proved itself to be imperfect (to be polite). Such unreliability often did not accurately identify the patients who would benefit most from the drug and very nearly scuttled the medical and commercial value Herceptin would ultimately realize.

In the case of pembrolizumab, the linked biomarker had the advantage of increasing the likelihood the clinical trial with Merck's drug would be biased toward those patients most likely to benefit from the experimental drug. By enriching for patients more likely to benefit from the drug, it was expected (and accurately so) fewer patients would be required for the clinical trials. This fact would expedite the evaluation and approval of pembrolizumab and thereby close the gap between the Merck drug and its BMS competitor.

Merck scientists selected PDL-1 as the biomarker since this is the molecule on tumor cells that binds PD-1 and forces them to become Treg cells.

This decision was based on strong scientific evidence, but again was resisted by many physicians and even some middle management at Merck, who were concerned it would preclude their ability to treat patients who might be excluded by an imperfect biomarker test.

The controversy over whether to deploy the PDL-1 biomarker eventually was so fierce it was escalated to the desk of Roger Perlmutter, the new head of Merck Research Laboratories. Perlmutter was seen as impartial, as he had just joined the organization in 2013, and this crucial decision, so early in his administration, would be closely watched. Perlmutter listened to both sides and ultimately elected to move forward with the biomarker. This decision was lambasted by many critics, including a prominent article in the March 13, 2016, edition of *The Wall Street Journal*, which also praised BMS for its own decision not to deploy a linked biomarker.[4]

In the end, the bet paid off nicely for Perlmutter and Merck as their decision to prioritize patients with high levels of PDL-1 had indeed identified those most likely to respond to the pembrolizumab. By targeting the most responsive patients, Perlmutter had also flipped the odds in the race between BMS's nivolumab and Merck's pembrolizumab. The final wild card would ultimately decide the race to determine which company would first enter the PD-1 oncology marker and was held by Merck. The company had filed for, and received, permission for pembrolizumab to be considered as a "breakthrough therapy," a designation allowing Merck to work side-by-side with its FDA regulators to expedite the final steps of the approval process.

As a consequence of this aggressive product development, pembrolizumab did indeed win the race with an FDA approval awarded to Keytruda for the treatment of metastatic melanoma on September 4, 2014. In contrast, BMS's nivolumab did not receive an approval until later that year on December 22. Keytruda continued to accrue additional uses, eventually being approved for non-small cell lung cancer, head and neck cancer, Hodgkin lymphoma, urothelial carcinoma, and gastric or gastroesophageal cancer. Furthermore, Merck broke new ground with a May 23, 2017, decision by the FDA to approve the use of pembrolizumab for any solid tumor positive for certain genetic features that predict a high occurrence of genetic defects.[5] This precedent broke with the tradition, whereby the FDA would grant approval to use a drug for a cancer in or from a particular organ. Instead, the FDA had allowed the presence of a biomarker alone to define the patients in whom the drug should be used. This action therefore precluded the need for Merck to test pembrolizumab in other cancer types. Consequently, the feared limitations of using a biomarker ironically allowed Merck to expand more efficiently the use of pembrolizumab to a much larger population of cancer patients.

The most famous patient of pembrolizumab was a former pioneer of America's nuclear submarine force, who also happened to be a former chief executive of the United States. James Earl Carter Jr. was born in the boomtown of Plains, Georgia, on October 1, 1924. Carter fulfilled a childhood dream by matriculating at the United States Naval Academy in Annapolis, Maryland, during the autumn of 1941, a few months before Pearl Harbor. With a degree granted in science, Carter began a career largely spent on submarines, and with these credentials, was personally recruited by a newly minted admiral, Hyman G. Rickover, to join an experimental program intended to create a new class of ultra-quiet submarines. These new ships were intended to render obsolete the loud, cantankerous diesel engines typical of submarines, which betrayed their presence to sonar technologies. Instead, American control of the depths would be enabled by stealth provided by the virtually inaudible power created by nuclear reactors.

Given the newness of the technology, it is unsurprising Rickover and Carter experienced unexpected setbacks, including a 1952 nuclear reactor meltdown at the Chalk River Laboratories in Canada (which had secretly partnered with the U.S Navy for the design of these small, quiet reactors). One of Carter's early leadership roles was oversight of the cleanup of the Canadian meltdown, which entailed sending men into the contaminated reactor facilities for short times to clean up the mess. This experience would serve Carter well in future years when, as president of the United States, he helped oversee federal efforts to stabilize another nuclear reactor meltdown in the spring of 1979 at the Three Mile Island complex near Harrisburg, Pennsylvania.

Although Carter's experiences at Three Mile Island were a situation of the right person being at the right place at the right time, this was the unfortunate exception rather than the rule for a presidential term marred with overwhelming challenges. Carter's term in office had begun during the sullen national morale of a nation still reeling from the dual insults

of Watergate and the Vietnam War. Where Nixon was secretive and con-
niving, Carter was transparent and guided by an ethical imperative. As
masterly described by Lawrence Wright in his 2014 book, *Thirteen Days in
September,* these characteristics allowed Carter to broker a breakthrough
in Middle East peace with the conclusion of a peace treaty between Israel
and Egypt. Despite this success, Carter's leadership approach was instead
regarded widely as naïve and ineffective by an American electorate jaded
by Watergate and prolonged economic malaise. His tenure was further burdened by domestic and international debacles, including stagflation (a lethal
combination of high inflation and economic stagnation), the Iranian Crisis
(entailing the overthrow of the shah and the later kidnapping of fifty-one
American hostages for 444 days), and the Soviet invasion of Afghanistan.
A low approval rating ensured Carter would be a one-term president.

Carter resurrected his reputation through an unprecedented series of good
works starting in the days after leaving the presidency. Rather than enriching
himself by milking the lecture circuit, he devoted his energies to popularizing
causes to help the poor (such as Habitat for Humanity) and in promoting
international diplomacy. After leaving office, his personal approval rebounded
in appreciation for these selfless efforts. The recognition of his charitable
activities earned Carter considerable recognition, including the 1998 United
Nations Human Rights Prize and the 2002 Nobel Peace Prize.

Carter has remained one of the most respected Americans well into his
nineties. Despite his advanced age, many Americans were shaken by an
August 2015 announcement that Jimmy Carter was suffering from advanced
cancer. The disease had been diagnosed on August 3, following a surgical
procedure at Emory University in Atlanta in which a mass was removed from
his liver. A week later, Carter himself announced a diagnosis of metastatic
cancer and revealed the disease had spread throughout his body. On August
20, more bad news arrived when Carter announced that the disease, later
revealed to be metastatic melanoma, had spread to his brain as well. The
prognosis seemed set in stone with the revelation the ex-president had not
one, but four separate metastatic lesions in his brain alone. In pragmatic
statements, Carter admitted he had only "a few weeks left" and was "at ease"
with his imminent demise.

The nation began to come to grips with the impending loss of a president, a relative rarity for a country with few former chief executives. Notes

of praise and admiration from public and private officials converged upon Plains, Georgia, from around the world as obituary writers updated their intended elegies for the former president amid his final struggle. As the summer of 2015 slipped into autumn, other news stories came to the fore and Carter's story faded from the headlines.

An unexpected and pleasant surprise arrived in November 2015 with an announcement Carter was improving. This announcement further indicated he would attend a Habitat for Humanity event in Memphis later in the month. Rather than being content to play a symbolic role, Carter donned a construction apron and energetically contributed to the construction of the new home. Within a month, another pleasing shock came with Carter's announcement he was cancer-free. No cancer could be detected in his brain, liver, or anywhere else in his body.

Even though he is a deeply devout man, Carter credited this remarkable outcome to a different type of miracle: pembrolizumab. The thirty-ninth president of the United States had responded well to therapy and became the poster child for immune oncology, further elevating the public's awareness of and anticipation for even more.

*Send in the Clones*

Though portrayed above as a foot race between Merck and Bristol-Myers Squibb, a wave of immune oncology drugs was building throughout the biopharmaceutical arena. Both Merck and BMS had taken an approach of blocking PD-1, whereas some competitors instead decided to target its ligand, PD-L1. Genentech, a biopharmaceutical pioneer acquired by Roche in 2009, crossed the finish line with the approval of a PD-L1 monoclonal antibody, atezolizumab (trade name: Tecentriq®), on May 18, 2016. This approval was followed a year later when FDA gave a nod to AstraZeneca's durvalumab (trade name: Imfinzi®) on May 1, 2017, and EMD Serono's avelumab (trade name: Bavencio®) eight days later.

This bolus of FDA approvals for immune oncology products, a virtually nonexistent field a few years before, was unparalleled in the history of the pharmaceutical industry. To provide some perspective, most readers are probably familiar with statins, a class of small molecule drugs, which lower cholesterol by impeding the function of a molecule known as *HMG-CoA reductase.* The development of multiple statin products within a relatively short time is frequently invoked as an example of a "fast follower drug" (these used to be called "me-too" drugs but the descriptor has been usurped rightfully by a more important movement in the past few years). The first statin (lovastatin) was approved in 1987 and a decade later, the fifth statin (atorvastatin) began to be marketed. The approval of five drugs within a decade is indeed impressive given the average time spent in clinical trials now exceeds ten years for many drugs. However, in the case of PD-1/PD-L1 drugs, five unique products had been approved between September 2014 and May 2017.

Far more PD-1 based medicines were being tested in the clinic. The pharmaceutical industry tends toward a herd mentality and the rapid-fire approvals of CTLA-4 and then PD-1/PDL-1-based therapies belied the reviewer's statement in response to one of Jim Allison's paper, which you may recall stated, "We all know that immunotherapy's crap."[6]

The herd began a stampede toward immunotherapy. According to a July 2017 report from the Pharmaceutical Research and Manufacturers of America (PhRMA), the industry was in the midst of developing more than 240 additional immuno-oncology products. This report was prefaced by a claim from the president of the American Cancer Society's Cancer Action Network: "We are at a moment of tremendous opportunity when it comes to developing therapies that can address even the most vexing cancers we see today."

By December 2017, the nonprofit Cancer Research Institute (which you may remember from chapter 5 was founded in 1953 by Helen Coley Nauts, daughter of William B. Coley) upped the count almost tenfold by announcing it was curating a database of more than two thousand different immune oncology drugs, half of which were already undergoing testing in people.[7]

These encouraging findings have eased the ability to raise investor dollars, either from venture capitalists or through an initial public offering. Beyond traditional interest in drug development, immune oncology entrepreneurship has arguably become a source of "irrational exuberance." This term accurately reflects the entry of less-experienced "dumb money" and expectations as pronounced as new investors first entering the dot-com bubble in 1999 or the housing market in early 2007. One example capturing the moment, a June 22, 2016, was a posting by the accomplished venture investor, Bruce Booth, on the LifeSciVC blog titled: "I/O: The Strategy Supernova in Cancer Today." As a brief summary in tune with this astronomical theme: Supernova provide both the source material needed for life but do so by wreaking extraordinary havoc as they explode.

Looking at the situation surrounding immune oncology from the global perspective of the pharmaceutical industry, it is important to note there are obviously finite resources available to individual companies. Consequently, every dollar invested in immune oncology necessarily is not available to invest into therapeutics for other diseases of modern society, including the growing plagues of metabolic diseases (e.g., obesity and diabetes) and neurodegeneration (e.g., Alzheimer's and Parkinson's diseases). One limitation recently capturing headlines around the world is the growing crisis of drug-resistant "superbugs." Stories of antibiotic resistant bacteria have been growing not simply due to exotic bugs, such as the stories of flesh-eating bacteria from decades past, but are also associated with far more mundane (and truly dangerous) bacteria, such as the microorganisms lining our intestines and occasionally contaminating our food (vancomycin-resistant Enterococcus), found on our skin (methicillin-resistant Staphylococcus aureus), or in our respiratory systems as deadly diseases largely forgotten in some countries, such as the United States, but persisting in the developing world and risk returning (multi-drug-resistant Mycobacterium tuberculosis). Beyond Ebola and other exotic emerging viruses, the most dangerous threats come from a recurrence of pandemic influenza viruses, and most circulating strains are already resistant to conventional antivirals (e.g., Tamiflu® and Relenza®). Consequently, the ever-increasing emphasis on the steep profits to be made from immune oncology drugs has arguably lured a disproportionate number of companies away from other public health challenges, and a halt in the pursuit of some of these other indications can be permanent.

In an extreme version, Bristol-Myers Squibb, one of the world's largest, most diverse, and storied pharmaceutical companies, has entirely bet the farm (or more accurately, pharm) on immune oncology. Throughout late 2013 and into the early days of 2014, the company announced a series of decisions to shed interests, personnel, and assets in other therapeutic areas with the goal of focusing all its efforts on immune oncology. This was quite a bold decision, as the company now seems to face a binary outcome. One possibility is BMS will win the race and dominate the immune oncology field until the patents for its landmark drugs expire and revenues from these products are hoovered up by generic competition. At this point, the company would be flat-footed in all other therapeutic areas and their continued survival would seem dubious in an industry requiring constant replenishment of its product pipeline. An alternative fate would arise if BMS does not pick the winning horses in immune oncology and sees its current lead in the field shrink, which would hasten the shuddering of the company. As the company has divested itself of all other therapeutic areas, it lacks the ability to pivot to other diseases or medical needs beyond oncology. Despite the advantages the bold decision may seem in the short term, it is challenging to understand how such trends can allow an individual company, or indeed an entire industry, to remain viable over the long term.

Although the premise of this book is fully supportive of the enthusiasm and success being realized in immune oncology by scientists, investors, and, most importantly, patients, it nonetheless bears iterating the title is *The End of the Beginning* and much work will be needed before we can progress to *The Beginning of the End* of the cancer plague. We will discuss a few of these barriers, not with the intention of discouraging enthusiasm for this coming era, but rather to manage expectations appropriately.

### *A Lawyer Walks Into a Lab . . .*

Where there is big money and expectations for making more, it is inevitable lawyers will soon join the party. In the case of immune oncology, the lines were being drawn well before the headline-making events of the past few years.

By the time the starting gun had fired in the race to gain approval for the first PD-1 inhibitors, the first salvos in the legal war had long since hit their mark. The legal actions constructed vast patent estates (collections of individual patents) as filed by virtually all the private and public sector organizations involved in the discovery or application of PD-1 and its various ligands. Major players in the fray included the academic homes of key players in our story, including the Mayo Clinic, Dana-Farber Cancer Institute, Johns Hopkins University, and myriad private sector entities with whom these organizations and others had partnered.[8] At stake were billions of dollars arising from novel therapies with the potential to cure diseases responsible for immeasurable suffering. As such, these medicines can command very high price tags from a large number of patients (and their insurers).

Rather than delving into the thicket of patent claims propelling lengthy lawsuits, some of which remain to be resolved, we will focus upon two instructive cases, both to understand the issues at hand and the possibilities for more fully realizing the potential of immune oncology in the future.

BMS's experiences in immune oncology provide one example of the roller-coaster world of pharmaceutical business. Their story began strong as the result of two acquisitions. The first was their 1985 takeover of Seattle-based Oncogen, which yielded the remarkable Seattle squad of scientists. Although the company was, in retrospect, short-sighted in terms of its decision to disband the Seattle site in 1997, the dispersal of employees to other locations facilitated the dissemination of the untapped potential surrounding immune oncology throughout other BMS sites (and at a time when the field was still largely held in contempt). These unintended outcomes nicely positioned the company to more fully realize the benefits arising from a second acquisition, that of Medarex in 2009. This Medarex purchase provided the company with two ground-breaking and commercially lucrative assets for cancer therapy: a CTLA-4 antibody (ipilimumab) and the first FDA-approved PD-1 antibody (nivolumab).

Even in losing this particular race to Merck, BMS ended up winning. This seeming paradox was resolved by the actions of its attorneys. As the rivalry grew between Merck and BMS, their patent estates began to be closely scrutinized, ultimately revealing Merck had infringed upon BMS's intellectual property assets, notably patents initiated by Medarex and Ono. In a settlement announced in January 2017, Merck agreed to pay BMS and Ono a total of $625 million plus 6.5% of Keytruda sales through 2023 (and 2.5% thereafter). Thus, even when Opdivo loses sales to Keytruda, BMS has a rather nice consolation prize.

A far more sustainable prospect for the industry, and for public health, may arise from a type of experiment initiated by the Dana-Farber Cancer Institute. The intellectual property developed by academic organizations is generally licensed to private sector companies under what is known as an *exclusive agreement*. These deals designate the corporate partner as the sole organization able to practice the inventions found in the patents they license. Most companies insist upon such terms as they do not want to compete with rivals who might outpace them much as we saw with BMS and Merck.

Although this is the standard practice, it was not the strategy practiced by Dana-Farber. Instead, it made its intellectual property surrounding PD-1 available to the private sector in a nonexclusive manner. Although each individual deal had lower financial terms, it spread the bet for Dana-Farber among multiple partners and had another even more positive outcome. The competition we have seen between Merck and BMS (both of whom licensed Dana-Farber patents) was amplified by the decisions of other partners (including Roche, Novartis, Merck Serono, and Amplimmune) to enter the race and develop their own unique PD-1 antibodies.[9] The result seems to have been a burgeoning of the breadth and depth of new cancer products predicated upon the rather Darwinian idea of the survival of the most fit. A larger number of participants in the immune oncology race increased the likelihood unique products will be developed for distinct subsets of cancer not addressed by their competitors, a subject to which we will return at the end of this story.

## If at First You Don't Succeed, Fail, Fail Again

The poster children of immune oncology, CTLA-4 and PD-1 antibodies, were developed to target regulatory T cells. However, they were not the first to do so, and indeed lagged more than a decade and a half behind. Furthermore, the forerunner leading the charge may be instructive as to the hurdles facing immune oncology in the future.

As you may recall, a key characteristic of Treg cells is the expression of a molecule known as *CD25* (a.k.a. the IL-2 receptor alpha chain). The concept of targeting Treg cells was aided by the existence of FDA-approved drugs targeting CD25 as a means to incapacitate the immune system.

In 1996, an early pioneer in the emerging field of monoclonal antibodies founded a company in Mountain View, California, to advance these new biotechnology products. As we have seen, the fact that these products had been derived from mice posed a problem since the mouse content of an antibody product would be seen as foreign and thus be rejected.

Cary Queen, a Berkeley-trained mathematician, had begun a promising academic career as a professor at Cornell University but became increasingly interested by challenges posed by biological problems. He eventually moved to the NCI in Bethesda to address questions about how mouse-derived antibodies might be made to be seen as more human by the immune system. This challenge required detailed knowledge of the structure of how antibodies interfaced with their antigens, which was right up the alley of a computational mathematician.

The company Queen cofounded in 1996 back in California was named Protein Design Labs (PDL) and its first product was a technology for a process now known as *humanization*. The word simplifies the considerable complexity required for swapping out mouse portions of an antibody and replacing them with equivalent human portions. This may seem like simply replacing a red Lego block with a blue one, but the complexity arises when one considers such a swap can cause a rather dramatic change in the shape of the entire structure. Rather than Legos, this approach is more akin to another childhood game, Jenga, where subtle changes to the blocks can cause the tower to plummet. PDL had mastered the approaches needed for humanization and licensed this knowledge to many early biotechnology companies, including Genentech, Roche, and MedImmune.

In parallel, PDL was developing its own monoclonal antibody product, which gained an FDA approval within a year after the formation of PDL. This product, daclizumab (trade name: Zenapax®), was a monoclonal antibody targeting CD25 and its FDA-approved use in 1997 was to prevent tissue rejection following organ transplant. Given the prominence IL-2 plays in governing the immune response, the drug was essentially meant to be a sledgehammer to prevent the body from rejecting a transplanted liver. This might seem a bit extreme until one considers the drug had been intended to replace muromonab-CD3, a mouse antibody designed to seek out and destroy all T cells in the body.

By the time of its approval, PDL had licensed Zenapax to Roche Pharmaceuticals and the drug had been anticipated to generate something around a quarter billion dollars in annual sales for transplantation use alone. However, this was intended to be the tip of the iceberg as PDL and Roche began exploring the use of Zenapax for asthma and other inflammatory diseases of the lungs. Another biotechnology pioneer, Biogen-IDEC, also initiated a partnership with PDL in 2005 to expand the use further, quite possibly to include other autoimmune diseases, the most prominent of which was multiple sclerosis, an otherwise challenging disease (as well as a great market opportunity) where clinical trials of Zenapax showed particular promise. A 2008 announcement revealed PDL would spin out daclizumab, along with a few other antibody products, into a new venture called Facet Biotech Corporation, which was interpreted as an indication of additional enthusiasm for the product but now might be viewed a bit differently.

Unexpectedly, the bubble of interest in Zenapax suddenly burst in 2008 when Roche announced it was ending it partnership with PDL. A year later, a second surprise shook the biotechnology world when Zenapax was unexpectedly pulled off the market in 2009. The reason cited for this action was "diminishing market demand." Why the sudden changes?

Market demand may have been a consideration but another persistent concern plaguing Zenapax centered upon toxicity. The targeting of CD25 was a blunt object as the molecule was on the surface of both cytotoxic (killer) T cells as well as many helper T cells. The projection was that daclizumab was predicted to cause severe immune suppression. The reality was both expected and yet surprising.

The primary toxicities associated with Zenapax included risks of infection, which had been anticipated as the mechanism of the drug was based upon suppressing the immune system. A 2014 review of daclizumab efficacy and safety stated, "Common infections including viral meningitis, lymphadenopathy, [and] allergic reactions."[10] Another patient was reported to have developed psoriasis. Evaluated in retrospect, lymphadenopathy, allergic reactions, and psoriasis are all widely understood to be autoimmune or inflammatory indications, which can result from infection but often do not. However, reflecting on the assumption the molecule would be wildly immunosuppressive, most experts dismissed these symptoms as indications of infection by various pathogens newly freed from constraints placed upon them by a fully functioning immune system.

After the withdrawal of Zenapax from the market, these side effects were largely forgotten. Behind the scenes, though, business development activities, including the purchase of Facet Biotech by Abbott, meant the team behind Zenapax (Roche and PDL) would soon be replaced by one consisting of Biogen and AbbVie (an offshoot of Abbott Pharmaceuticals). The target of this newfound interest in daclizumab was multiple sclerosis.

Multiple sclerosis is a debilitating and life-threatening autoimmune disease suffered by at least 400,000 Americans. The disease generally strikes women at a rate three times higher than men and its prevalence tends to peak in patients between the ages of forty-five and forty-nine.[11] The disease has other demographic and geographic oddities including a higher prevalence in the Northeastern and Midwestern United States as compared with either the American South or West, perhaps suggesting an environmental contribution. Beyond the devastation wrought by the disease, multiple sclerosis tends to prevail in relatively prosperous individuals who usually have health insurance and thus are particularly attractive to the pharmaceutical industry.

A new name, Zinbryta®, was given to daclizumab and subsequent clinical trial data from phase II and phase III studies revealed considerable promise for the product in multiple sclerosis. The results of a phase II trial revealed Zinbryta was superior to the existing therapy for it slowed the relapse rate and number of lesions for multiple sclerosis by 45%, a stunning outcome for a disease which has proven itself to be largely unresponsive to therapy.[12] Although hailed by patient advocacy groups, many regulators were less cheered, because the top-level headlines touting the phase III trial data gave less attention to the drug's side effects. For example, an appraisal by United Kingdom's National Institute for Health and Care Excellence (NICE) cited a high prevalence of infectious diseases as well as inflammatory reactions in the liver and the skin. Such reactions were met with scorn as underscored by an October 3, 2016, statement from Amy Bowen, a director of the MS Trust, which related, "it is very frustrating that, yet again, access to an effective new treatment will be further delayed by the NICE appraisal system."[13] Indeed, this statement was released five months after the U.S. FDA had approved Zinbryta for the treatment of multiple sclerosis. Bowing to pressure from the MS Trust, NICE eventually relented, approving the use of Zinbryta in England and Wales on March 15, 2017 (Scotland approved its use a month later).

Sadly, this success would prove to be short-lived, as in March 2018, Biogen and AbbVie announced the voluntary withdrawal of Zinbryta worldwide. The companies were not able to cite a lack of market demand and the reason for this second withdrawal was attributed to massive inflammation in the brain, which had triggered deadly encephalitis and other autoimmune and inflammatory effects.

The mechanism of this toxicity harkens back to Treg cells. The presence of the CD25 molecule, the target for daclizumab, was a hallmark of Treg cells. As such, Zenapax/Zinbryta had released the brakes holding back unwanted inflammatory and autoimmune damage. Such an outcome should not have been unexpected, particularly given the lessons learned by TGN-1412. Indeed, the idea that daclizumab would target Treg cells had been demonstrated during a 2009 study, which showed daclizumab would block Treg cells to amplify antitumor immunity with breast cancer vaccines.[14] Indeed, the yin of efficacy versus the yang of toxicity are the sides to a balancing act that closes out the beginning of the immune-based war on cancer.

### Careful What You Wish For

For the first generation of immune therapies developed over the past decade, it seems virtually inevitable expectations must be tempered by reality. The first cautionary note is that not every cancer will be amenable to immune-based therapies. Even within melanoma, one of the more responsive diseases to these new therapies, approximately one-third of patients are helped by immune therapies. For these lucky few, the responses appear largely durable, lasting for years and perhaps even providing the rare opportunity to use the word *cure*.

Nonetheless, the majority of patients do not yet respond to these therapies and this creates its own set of problems. Much attention is rightfully being placed upon identifying those patients who will respond to therapy and expediting their treatment with immune therapies. Indeed, regulators and biopharmaceutical companies have emphasized the need for innovative new approaches as evidenced by the first-ever approval of a cancer drug, Keytruda, for a genetically defined set of cancers. In parallel, investigation can and should continue to determine if different therapies might be developed for those patients who do not respond to current immune-based therapies. As more knowledge about Treg cells and their role in cancer comes to light, new opportunities open up for even greater improvements to immune therapies.

Moreover, patients and physicians alike should recognize an inevitable outcome of immune therapy is an increased risk of inflammatory and autoimmune disease. Word choice is crucial here because while *inevitable* does not apply to each individual, it will undoubtedly apply to each new immune therapy. Much as was seen with daclizumab, some patients will respond negatively, and much emphasis will be needed to avoid treating individuals at risk for toxicity, and in parallel to treat those likely to respond productively and without (or with manageable) toxicities.

One can look at daclizumab as an example of failing to act upon these concerns. The drug had demonstrated unprecedented abilities to treat multiple sclerosis but ultimately was abandoned due to an inability to distinguish those patients in whom therapy would be more beneficial than harmful. Although it seems highly unlikely daclizumab will be resurrected yet again, the experiences gained from the experience could still be put to good use to avoid future repetitions of throwing out the proverbial baby with the bathwater for other medicines if the risk-to-benefit ratio can be minimized.

Along these same lines, we will come full circle back to the question of when and whether treatment should take place. At the beginning of the book, I related my shock in learning of the prevalence, indeed inevitability, of metastatic prostate cancer. The key point was, absent improvements in our ability to detect the disease, many men with the disease would have expired due to natural causes utterly unrelated to the metastatic disease within. Although chemotherapeutic regimens have always entailed risk, they have generally tended to be relatively acute (hair loss, gastrointestinal distress, and immune depletion). In contrast, new immune-based therapies differ due to their durability, both in terms of efficacy and toxicity, which in both cases may last decades.

### *The Beginning of the End*

Harkening back to Winston Churchill's 1942 speech celebrating victory in the Second Battle of El Alamein, it seems likely we are now preparing to transition to a period that might be considered the Beginning of the End. Second Alamein was just the first step toward ejecting Rommel's forces from North Africa and many struggles and setbacks remained until the final victory. Likewise, the war on cancer will entail far too many fatalities and setbacks. However, the momentum seems to be moving inevitably forward.

Much as was the case in the Second World War, the battle will take place in two major theaters. The first is the battle against cancer itself, while a second front will need to be expanded to counter some of the more detrimental outcomes of immune therapy. Although we will focus most of our remaining time on the former, it nonetheless is worth taking a moment or two to address steadily rising concerns about induced autoimmunity. It is inevitable that increasing emphasis on immune-based oncology products will increase the incidence and severity of inflammatory and autoimmune diseases. These detrimental effects may be somewhat self-correcting as it is likely greater emphasis will be placed upon the means to manage autoimmune reactions. This is likely to take two approaches. In one case, such outcomes would give rise to blunt instruments meant to battle autoimmune diseases. The current blunt objects include steroids or therapies, such as CD20 or cytokine antibodies, meant to block key components of inflammatory/autoimmune damage. Given the likelihood the incidence of such diseases will increase, pressures will comparably escalate to create more targeted drugs, which do not wholly immobilize the body's defenses but are directed to block only the subset of autoreactive cells responsible for the damage. As knowledge increases about the identity and interactions among these cells, one can anticipate the creation of more "designer" medicines meant to inactivate, perhaps via induction of a Treg behavior, only those cells doing harm. In a similar manner, future medicines are likely to de-regulate those Treg cells responsible for curtailing attacks against tumor cells (rather than the current sledgehammers to de-activate all Treg cells).

Another case indicates further improvements will follow upon the discovery of novel neoantigens, as advanced by Robert Schreiber, to be exploited to give rise to new cancer vaccines and/or targets for new generations of highly specific monoclonal antibody–based therapies. As the accumulation of this information continues to expand at an exponential basis, it will provide an ever-increasing array of opportunities for new therapies.

The technologies used to combat cancer will continue to improve. Just over a quarter century ago, monoclonal antibody therapies were widely considered to be far too speculative and expensive to be practical. Likewise, the feasibility of cell-based therapies continues to be dismissed by many today. Nonetheless, these two approaches are now being constantly refined through biomedical and engineering improvements that have steadily increased their efficacy and ability to be deployed (e.g., by reducing the cost of manufacturing by many magnitudes).

At its most fundamental level, cancer is a disease of mutation. In this way, the treatment of cancer is reminiscent of many infectious diseases. As is widely known, humanity has been at war with bacteria and viruses from the birth of our species and the battles only escalated with the advent of antibacterial and antiviral medicines starting in the early to mid-20th century. Although these technological improvements gave humans the upper hand for a time, a combination of evolution and a high mutation and proliferation rate among our microbial adversaries soon leveled the playing field, abrogating the efficacy of therapies developed only years before. A representative example is found in the struggle against HIV/AIDS in the 1990s and early 2000s. When challenged with individual drugs, the virus was placed under a classical Darwinian pressure to select for mutants able to escape the drug. This outcome is indeed what occurred. The real breakthrough was the combination of medicines, each targeting a different weakness in the virus, which put such overwhelming pressure on the virus that it was unable to deploy its mutational advantage to escape. A similar strategy can be used against cancer.

While therapies with cocktails of conventional cancer agents have been used for the past few decades, the same is now being done with immune therapies. For example, multiple tweaks against different immune mechanisms (e.g., CD28, CTLA-4, PD-1, and PD-L1) might improve the breadth or depth of immune responses against tumors. Such an approach might be strengthened further if combined with CAR-T cells and/or vaccines targeting neo-antigens. Such approaches are still in their infancy, due in part because most of these therapies are still quite new. However, the cost of such combinations will undoubtedly convey a practical hurdle impossible to overcome. The expense of cell-based therapies now routinely exceeds $500,000 and combinations may be prohibitively expensive to test, even on an experimental basis. Unlike conventional small molecule medicines, which eventually become more affordable as key patents expire, the intellectual property minefields to protect antibody- and cell-based therapies from being cannibalized by generic competitors are far more complex. This fact may curtail the deployment of exotic combinations of immune oncology medicines. Such an outcome may seem to be bad news but likely represents a mere speed bump as these technologies will soon enough find themselves utterly disrupted by a new wave of biomedical products.

By the end of the next decade, antibody- and cell-based immune oncology drugs will likely be viewed to be as quaint, unsophisticated and dated as a 2018 Tesla Model-X owner would view a 1908 Ford Model-T. Although incremental improvements to conventional antibody- and cell-based technologies will continue for a time, disruptive technologies will reshape immune therapies. The first of these technologies, genome editing, facilitates a facile modification of the fundamental DNA code. This could make it possible not only to identify and fix a disease-causing defect (be it in a cancer cell or in an autoimmune cell), but to prevent the disease or symptoms from arising before they are even felt.

The most hyped of these first-generation genomic engineering techniques is known as *CRISPR/Cas9* and is already being tested in people. Without boring the reader with detailed explanations of how the DNA and genetic code can now be readily manipulated, it suffices to state this technology is one offshoot of DNA sequencing technology, which itself arose from the Human Genome Project of the 1990s. As our understanding of the composition of DNA in humans (and other species) increased throughout the final quarter of the 20th century, parallel advancements were unfolding in our ability to modify DNA, first at the most fundamental level (known as an *individual nucleotide*) and progressively through the large-scale level of chromosomes, which can be comprised of hundreds of millions of nucleotide pairs.

These new genome-editing technologies will truly reflect a buzzword among medical researchers: "personalized therapy." DNA sequencing in the 1980s required intensive and expensive efforts in which a few hundred DNA nucleotides might be sequenced by a laboratory in a week or two. Now, the newest DNA sequencers can sequence entire genomes (three billion bases) within hours, and one machine, the MinION by Nanopore Technologies, is roughly the size of a smartphone. Likewise, the ability not only to identify DNA mutations, but to correct them, has been improving with comparable efficiency.

Beyond the extraordinary potential for correcting defects to prevent or treat disease, this technology differs fairly dramatically from antibody- or cell-based therapies since genome editing might actually be less expensive to put in place than even conventional antibody- or cell-based therapies. Were these improvements to be realized, it is conceivable cancer will soon be rendered to be a historical footnote for future generations (much as smallpox, once the scourge of the planet, is regarded today).

# *Epilogue*

The coming years will witness a continued acceleration in the rate and breadth of cancers able to be cured with immune-based therapies. Beyond the recent renaissance in therapy for melanoma, which has resulted in cures for a disease that had utterly defeated most conventional medicines, other solid and liquid tumors are beginning to fall to drugs, such as CTLA-4, PD-1, and PD-L1 inhibitors. Moreover, there are hundreds, if not thousands, of new drugs under investigation. There is no reason to believe the three targets mentioned above will ultimately prove to be the only, or even the best, targets for immune-based oncology.

Particular advantages will undoubtedly be obtained by combining different immune oncology drugs. Taking a cue from successes in the war against HIV/AIDS, it can be argued the major breakthrough arose not in the form of a new miracle drug, but from combinations of drugs, which synergized in combination. These groupings decrease the likelihood that mutant, drug-resistant viruses will emerge and render current therapies useless. A milestone indicative of this success arose in the early years of the 20th century when life insurance companies began issuing policies to individuals with an HIV-positive status (under the proviso they continue to faithfully adhere to therapy). It is quite conceivable a similar approach of combining immune oncology drugs could yield comparable outcomes for cancer.

Combination therapy comes at a price—literally. A key problem moving forward will reflect the fact immune oncology drugs will require a high price tag. For example, a year's worth of treatment with ipilimumab (Yervoy®) comes in at $120,000 and nivolumab (Keytruda®) has been priced at $150,000 per year. A combination of these medicines (and more) could therefore easily exceed $500,000 per year. Furthermore, monoclonal antibody therapies, such as Yervoy and Keytruda, tend to be less susceptible to generic competition, particularly in the United States, where a debate about "biosimilars" has been raging for decades. Therefore, one should not expect the extraordinary costs of these remarkable medicines are likely to retreat any time soon.

Another important factor to consider is the early experience with immune oncology drugs, which conveys a benefit to roughly a quarter to a third of all patients. Those responding tend to have dramatic outcomes, with a sustained loss of tumors and something akin to a cure. However, the remaining patients either do not respond at all or have a limited duration of response. It may be these patients have not yet been matched with the best drug for them. This optimistic view suggests it is only a matter of time (or perhaps genetics) until personalized treatment regimens can be identified for each and every person with cancer (who can afford to do so).

Were time to grant this outcome, it is entirely conceivable cancer could be relegated to the dustbin of diseases, alongside other serial killers like smallpox and scurvy. The promising results with HPV, EBV, and HBV vaccines may portend a future in which many cancers might be prevented before they occur (or at least, before any symptoms are felt). As the saying goes, an ounce of prevention is worth a pound of cure. Given the fractional costs of vaccines as contrasted with, for example, immune therapy drugs, increased investment in understanding the causes and ability to prevent the rise of cancer in the first place should be explored as a more efficient means than continued reliance upon therapeutic strategies. The primary issue with vaccines, as identified in my second book, *Between Hope and Fear*, is that the business case for vaccines developers and manufacturers seems to be in rather steep decline, which could preclude future advances.

Were we to succeed in achieving an unconditional surrender in our war against cancer, which is now at an early stage but potentially realistic, a predictable outcome will be a coincident increase in autoimmune diseases. Many have argued this is a price worth paying but rather than simply resigning ourselves to such an inevitability, a more constructive, and lucrative, decision could be to increase our investment in treatments for those diseases. Much of the same knowledge about Treg cells, which helped usher in a new era of immune oncology, could be used to tweak these cells toward a favorable balance between blocking cancer while preventing autoimmune damage.

We may soon look back on the latest generation of immune oncology drugs, such as those targeting CTLA-4 and PD-1, and conclude these were sledgehammers much in the same way we now look back upon arsenic and mercury as treatments for syphilis or at nitrogen mustards and antimetabolite drugs for cancer. Therefore, advice for potential investors and regulators would be to seek out and incentivize opportunities to create more nuanced immune oncology treatment regimens designed to maximize the ratio of benefit to toxicity.

Overall, the opportunities arising from the ongoing revolution in immune oncology would seem to far exceed the costs and risks. The next few years will witness waves of improvements in immune oncology as the miraculous cures witnessed over the past few years will undoubtedly be refined and improved, likely yielding a time in the near future when an increasing frequency of cures will transition from the end of the beginning to the beginning of the end of cancer.

# Acknowledgments

There are many people without whom this book could not have been
completed. Always the first to receive my humble thanks and love is my
family. As indicated in the text, the health and happiness of my family
has consistently underpinned the many choices faced throughout my life,
from a decision to pursue to cancer research to choices that ultimately led
my wife and me to leave academia and move around the country, dragging
our family from North Carolina to Indiana to Maryland to Connecticut and
finally (hopefully) to Missouri. As related in the introduction to this book,
my mother, Sue Kinch, had to endure and witness firsthand the trauma of
cancer, including, but not limited to, the loss of her father and her brother,
who were taken from this world by cancer at too young an age. The loss
of Harold Noe, Thomas Noe, and William Zellner to cancer irreversibly
affected the lives of my sister, Beth Anne Vasilakos, and me and in ways
inexpressible in words alone.

My wife, Dr. Kelly Carles-Kinch, and our children, Sarah and Grant,
have provided continual inspiration and deserve all the credit for tolerating

the time and focus necessary to sustain the efforts required to research and write this manuscript.

I would also like to thank my extended work family, especially my professional inspiration, Dr. Holden Thorp, who encouraged and helped expand my horizons, for supporting our work at the Center for Research Innovation in Biotechnology (CRIB) at Washington University in St Louis, which provided the foundation for this book. Our CRIB team of Rebekah Griesenauer, Constantino Schillebeeckx, and David Maness has been exceptionally understanding given the many distractions this work had caused.

My deepest thanks are also given to the many people who have helped in the preparation needed to publish this book. In particular, I would like to single out my literary agent, Don Fehr at Trident Media Group, for helping to seal a partnership with Pegasus Books, which allowed for the publication of *Between Hope and Fear* and the current manuscript. The folks at Pegasus Books, and in particular Jessica Case, have provided extraordinary help to mask my extraordinary incompetence in preparing a trade book and have somehow managed not to laugh out loud at my naïveté.

I would like to thank the many scientists and physicians who have dedicated their lives to the eradication of cancer. The stories found herein are small snippets of a larger story, far too large to convey or even for anyone to digest, and by no means comprise a comprehensive review of all the brilliant minds and tireless hours of multitudes of cancer researchers around the world. Many names have been lost to time or insufficiently recalled. Any forgotten individuals are the result of my notoriously awful memory and I ask for their forgiveness.

Most importantly, the greatest thanks go to the unsung heroes of this book: the nameless patients, who volunteered for countless clinical trials and, despite being afflicted with deadly diseases, never hesitated to endure experimental treatment to try and use their remaining years, months, or days to help advance medical research. Their efforts were not in vain and the dividends are now finally being realized by a grateful generation. Their stories must never be forgotten.

# Endnotes

## 1: A GROWING CONCERN

1   D. Waters, D. Bostwick, and G. Murphy, "First international workshop on animal models of prostate cancer," *Prostate* 36 (1998): 45–67.

2   W. Sakr, et al., "The frequency of carcinoma and intraepithelial neoplasia of the prostate in young male patients," *The Journal of Urology* 150, no. 2 (1993): 379–85.

3   I. J. Powell, et al., "Prostate cancer biochemical recurrence stage for stage is more frequent among African-American than white men with locally advanced but not organ-confined disease," *Urology* 55, no. 2 (2000): 246–51.

4   A. R. Rich, "On the frequency of occurrence of occult carcinoma of the prostate," *CA: A Cancer Journal for Clinicians* 29, no. 2 (1979): 115–9.

5   J. M. Gulleyardo, et al., "Prevalence of latent prostate carcinoma in two US populations," *Journal of the National Cancer Institute* 65, no. 2 (1980): 311–6.

6   I. M. Thompson, M.S. Lucia, and C.M. Tangen, "Commentary: The ubiquity of prostate cancer: echoes of the past, implications for the present," *International Journal of Epidemiology* 36, no. 2 (2007): 287–9.

7   E. Bianconi, et al., "An estimation of the number of cells in the human body," *Annals of Human Biology* 40, no. 6 (2013): 463–71.

8   C. Sagan, *Cosmos* (New York, NY: Random House, 1980).

9   A. Derkachov and D. Jakubczyk, *Nanomedicine and Tissue Engineering State of the Art and Recent Trends* (Oakville, Ontario: Apple Academic Press, 2015).

10   J. Kerr, "A histochemical study of hypertrophy and ischaemic injury of rat liver with special reference to changes in lysosomes," *The Journal of Pathology and Bacteriology* 90, no. 2 (1965): 419–35.

11   J. E. Duque-Parra, "Note on the origin and history of the term 'apoptosis,'" *The New Anatomist* 283, no. 1 (2005): 2–4.

12   H. R. Horvitz, "Worms, life, and death (Nobel lecture)," *ChemBioChem* 4, no. 8 (2003): 697–711.

13   S. Brenner, "Nobel lecture: nature's gift to science," *Bioscience Reports* 23, no. 5 (2003): 225–37.

14   S. M. Frisch and H. Francis, "Disruption of epithelial cell-matrix interactions induces apoptosis," *Journal of Cell Biology* 124, no. 4 (1994): 619.

15    D. Oken, "What to tell cancer patients: a study of medical attitudes," *Journal of the American Medical Association* 175, no. 13 (1961): 1120–8.

16    C. Neal, et al., *Cancer Stigma and Silence Around the World: A Livestrong Report* (Austin, TX: Livestrong Foundation, 2007).

17    L. A.V. Marlow, J. Waller, and J. Wardle, "Variation in Blame Attributions across Different Cancer Types," *Cancer Epidemiology Biomarkers & Prevention* 19, no. 7 (2010): 1799–805.

18    M. J. Lerner and S. Clayton, *Justice and Self-Interest: Two Fundamental Motives* (Cambridge, United Kingdom: Cambridge University Press, 2011).

19    Neal, *Cancer Stigma and Silence Around the World.*

20    J. W. Johnsson and K. Dehlholm, *Den danske Laegestand 1901–1907* (Copenhagen, Denmark: Jacob Lunds Forlag, 1907).

21    V. Ellerman, "A new strain of transmissible leucemia in fowls (strain H)," *Journal of Experimental Medicine* 33, no. 4 (1921): 539–52.

22    O. Thomsen and V. Jensen, "Shaving brushes infected with anthrax spores," *Acta Pathologica Microbiologica Scandinavica* 1, no. 2 (1924): 114–31.

23    C. M. Szablewski, et al., "Anthrax Cases Associated with Animal-Hair Shaving Brushes," *Emerging Infectious Diseases* 23, no. 5 (2017): 806.

24    "British Medical Journal," *Br Med J* 1, no. 3349 (1925): 467–73.

25    Szablewski, "Anthrax Cases Associated with Animal-Hair Shaving Brushes," 806.

26    T. Christofferson, *Tripping over the Truth: How the Metabolic Theory of Cancer Is Overturning One of Medicine's Most Entrenched Paradigms* (Hartford, VT: Chelsea Green Publishing, 2017).

27    "Peyton Rous—Biographical," in Nobel Lectures, *Physiology or Medicine 1963–1970* (Amsterdam: Elsevier Publishing Company, 1972). Found online, accessed April 3, 2018, https://www.nobelprize.org/nobel_prizes/medicine/laureates/1966/rous-bio.

28    Ibid.

29    J. T. Flexner, *An American Saga: The Story of Helen Thomas and Simon Flexner* (New York: Fordham University Press, 1993).

30    P. Rous, "A transmissible avian neoplasm," *Journal of Experimental Medicine* 12, no. 5 (1910): 696.

31    P. Rous, "A sarcoma of the fowl transmissible by an agent separable from the tumor cells," *Journal of Experimental Medicine* 13, no. 4 (1911): 397–411.

32    Rous, "A sarcoma of the fowl transmissible by an agent separable from the tumor cells," 397–411.

33    R. E. Shope and E.W. Hurst, "Infectious papillomatosis of rabbits: with a note on the histopathology," *Journal of Experimental Medicine* 58, no. 5 (1933): 607.

34    E. J. Odes, et al., "Earliest hominin cancer: 1.7-million-year-old osteosarcoma from Swartkrans Cave, South Africa," *South African Journal of Science* 112, no. 7–8 (2016): 1–5.

35    G. K. Ostrander, et al., "Shark cartilage, cancer and the growing threat of pseudoscience," *Cancer Research* 64, no. 23 (2004): 8485–91.

36    J. Graham, "Cancer and evolution: synthesis," *Journal of Theoretical Biology* 101, no. 4 (1983): 657–9.

37    J. Graham, *Cancer selection: The New Theory of Evolution* (Lexington, VA: Aculeus Pr, 1992).

38    A. M. Leroi, V. Koufopanou, and A. Burt, "Cancer selection," *Nature Reviews Cancer* 3, no. 3 (2003): 226–31.

39    L. M. Merlo, et al., "Cancer as an evolutionary and ecological process," *Nature Reviews Cancer* 6, no. 12 (2006): 924–35.

40    E. Littré, *Oeuvres Complètes d'Hippocrate,* vol. 10 (Paris, France: JB Baillière, 1861).

41    S. Gibaud and G. Jaouen, *Medicinal Organometallic Chemistry* (New York: Springer, 2010), 1–20.

42 F. Bosch and L. Rosich, "The contributions of Paul Ehrlich to pharmacology: a tribute on the occasion of the centenary of his Nobel Prize," *Pharmacology* 82, no. 3 (2008): 171–9.

43 W. S. Halsted, "I. The results of operations for the cure of cancer of the breast performed at the Johns Hopkins Hospital from June, 1889, to January, 1894," *Annals of Surgery* 20, no. 5 (1894): 497.

44 J. Toland, *Adolf Hitler* (Garden City, NY: Doubleday, 1976).

45 M. S. Kinch, *A Prescription For Change: The Looming Crisis in Drug Discovery* (Chapel Hill, NC: UNC Press, 2016).

46 E. C. Miller and J.A. Miller, "Charles Heidelberger: December 23, 1920-January 18, 1983," *Biographical Memoirs. National Academy of Sciences (US)* 58 (1989): 259.

## 2: SURVEILLANCE STATE

1 G. Weissmann, *Lewis Thomas*, in *Biographical Memoirs*, vol. 85 (Washington, D.C.: The National Academies Press, 2004), 315–35.

2 Ibid.

3 G. Weissmann, "Arts and Science: Lewis Thomas and F. Scott Fitzgerald," *FASEB Journal* 25, no. 3 (2011): 809–12.

4 Ibid.

5 H. Zinsser, *Rats, Lice and History* (Boston, MA: Little Brown, 1935).

6 W. C. Summers, "Hans Zinsser: a tale of two cultures," *The Yale Journal of Biology and Medicine* 72 no. 5 (1999): 341.

7 Weissmann, *Lewis Thomas*, 315–35.

8 H. S. Lawrence, *Cellular and Humoral Aspects of the Hypersensitive States: A Symposium Held at the New York Academy of Medicine* (New York: PB Hoeber, 1959).

9 Ibid.

10 P. R. Ehrlich and F. Himmelweit, *The Collected Papers of Paul Ehrlich*, vol. 1 (Oxford, UK: Pergamon, 1956).

11 M. S. Kinch, *Between Hope & Fear: A History of Vaccines and Human Immunity* (New York: Pegasus Books, 2018), 360.

12 M. S. Kinch, *A Prescription for Change* (Chapel Hill, NC: UNC Press, 2016).

13 "Geschichte des Paul-Ehrlich-Instituts," Paul-Ehrlich-Institute, accessed April 5, 2018, https://www.pei.de/DE/institut/geschichte/geschichte-node.html.

14 Ibid.

15 H. Pakula, *An Uncommon Woman: The Empress Frederick, Daughter of Queen Victoria, Wife of the Crown Prince of Prussia, Mother of the Kaiser Willheim* (New York: Simon and Schuster, 1997).

16 M. Fulbrook, *A Concise History of Germany* (Cambridge, United Kingdom: Cambridge University Press, 2004).

17 Pakula, *An Uncommon Woman*.

18 G. MacDonogh, *The Last Kaiser: William the Impetuous* (London: Weidenfeld & Nicolson, 2000).

19 J. C. Röhl, *Young Wilhelm: The Kaiser's Early Life, 1859–1888* (Cambridge, United Kingdom: Cambridge University Press, 1998).

20 R. K. Massie, *Dreadnought: Britain, Germany, and the Coming of the Great War* (New York: Random House, 2007).

21 MacDonogh, *The Last Kaiser*.

22 Röhl, *Young Wilhelm*.

23 Pakula, *An Uncommon Woman*.

24 Ibid.

25 "Geschichte des Paul-Ehrlich-Instituts."

26    Ehrlich and Himmelweit, *The Collected Papers of Paul Ehrlich.*

27    A. Gelpi, A. Gilbertson, and J.D. Tucker, "Magic bullet: Paul Ehrlich, Salvarsan and the birth of venereology," *Sexually Transmitted Infections* 91, no. 1 (2015): 68–9.

28    H. O., Schembs, G. Speyer, and F. Speyer, *Georg und Franziska Speyer-Stifter und Mäzene für Frankfurt am Main* (Frankfurt am Main, Germany: Waldemar Kramer, 2001).

29    F. Heynick, *Jews and Medicine: An Epic Saga* (Brooklyn, NY: KTAV Publishing House, Inc., 2002).

30    M. Burnet, "Cancer—a biological approach: I. The processes of control. II. The significance of somatic mutation," *British Medical Journal* 1, no. 5022 (1957): 779.

31    R. A. Kyle and M.A. Shampo, "Peter Medawar—Discoverer of Immunologic Tolerance," *Mayo Clinic Proceedings* 78, no. 4 (2003): 401–3.

32    Ibid.

33    R. E. Billingham, L. Brent, and P. B. Medawar, "Quantitative studies on tissue transplantation immunity. III. Actively acquired tolerance," *Philosophical Transactions of the Royal Society of London* 239, no. 666 (1956): 357–414.

34    D. Grimm, "Dawn of the dog," *Science* 348, no. 6,232 (2015): 274–9.

35    L. R. Botigué, et al., "Ancient European dog genomes reveal continuity since the Early Neolithic," *Nature Communications* 8 (2017).

36    D. Palmer, "Obituary: Norman Roy Grist (1918–2010)," *The Glasgow Naturalist* 25 (2012), https://www.glasgownaturalhistory.org.uk/gn25_4/obit_norman_grist.pdf.

37    "Laboratory Animals: Origin of nude mouse," *Nature* 224 (1969): 114–5.

38    M. Nehls, et al., "Two Genetically Separable Steps in the Differentiation of Thymic Epithelium," *Science* 272, no. 5263 (1996): 886–9.

39    A. J. Laster, et al., "The human thymic microenvironment: thymic epithelium contains specific keratins associated with early and late stages of epidermal keratinocyte maturation," *Differentiation* 31, no. 1 (1986): 67–77.

40    M. Nishino, et al., "The thymus: a comprehensive review," *Radiographics* 26, no. 2: 335–48.

41    Laster, "The human thymic microenvironment," 67–77.

42    A. Liston, "The development of T-cell immunity:, no," *Progress in Molecular Biology and Translational Science* 92 1–3.

43    J. F. Miller, "A scientific odyssey: unravelling the secrets of the thymus" *Medical Journal of Australia* 183, no. 11–12: 582–4.

44    J. F. Miller, (1999): "Immunological function of the thymus," *The Lancet* 278, no. 7205: 748–9.

45    Ibid.

46    J. F. Miller, "Discovering the origins of immunological competence," *Annual Review of Immunology* 17 (2005), no. 1–17.

47    A. Luch, "Nature and nurture-lessons from chemical carcinogenesis," *Nature Reviews: Cancer* 5, no. 2 (2005): 113.

48    J. R. Brown and J.L. Thornton, "Percivall Pott (1714–1788) and chimney sweepers' cancer of the scrotumt zu Tokyo," *British Journal of Industrial Medicine* 1 (1915): 68.

49    K. Yamagiwa and K. Ichikawa, *Experimentelle Studie über die Pathogenese der Epithelialgeschwülste* no. 24, (1974): (Tokyo, Japan: Medizinische Facultat der Kaiserlichen Universit) 295–344.

50    O. Stutman, "Tumor development after 3-methylcholanthrene in immunologically deficient athymic-nude mice." *Science* 183(4124): (1974): 534–6.

51    V. Vetvicka, et al., "Macrophages of athymic nude mice: Fc receptors, C receptors, phagocytic and pinocytic activities" *European Journal of Cell Biology* 35(1): (1984): 35–40.

52    I. S. Pogany, *Righting Wrongs in Eastern Europe* (Manchester, United Kingdom: Manchester University Press, 1997).

53    D. S. Cornelius, *Hungary in World War II: Caught in the Cauldron* (New York: Fordham University Press, 2011).

54    Ibid.

55    T. Sakmyster, "From Habsburg Admiral to Hungarian Regent: The Political Metamorphosis of Miklós Horthy, 1918–1921," *East European Quarterly* 17, no. 2 (1983): 129.

56    J. Bierman, *Righteous Gentile: The Story of Raoul Wallenberg, Missing Hero of the Holocaust* (London: Penguin UK, 1995).

57    G. Klein and E. Klein, "How one thing has led to another," *Annual Review of Immunology* 7, no. 1 (1989): 1–34.

58    K. Rajewsky, "George Klein: 1925–2016," *Proceedings of the National Academy of Sciences* 114, no. 13 (2017): 3275–7.

59    E. Klein, et al., "Surface IgM-kappa specificity on a Burkitt lymphoma cell in vivo and in derived culture lines," *Cancer Research* 28, no. 7 (1968): 1300–10.

60    R. Kiessling, E. Klein, and H. Wigzell, "'Natural' killer cells in the mouse. I. Cytotoxic cells with specificity for mouse Moloney leukemia cells. Specificity and distribution according to genotype," *European Journal of Immunology* 5, no. 2 (1975): 112–7.

61    R. Kiessling, et al., "'Natural' killer cells in the mouse. II. Cytotoxic cells with specificity for mouse Moloney leukemia cells. Characteristics of the killer cell," *European Journal of Immunology* 5, no. 2 (1975): 117–21.

62    H.F. Pross and M. Jondal, "Cytotoxic lymphocytes from normal donors. A functional marker of human non-T lymphocytes," *Clinical and Experimental Immunology* 21, no. 2 (1975): 226–35.

63    W. Budzynski and C. Radzikowski, "Cytotoxic cells in immunodeficient athymic mice," *Immunopharmacology and Immunotoxicology* 16, no. 3 (1994): 319–46.

64    M. Kaposi, "Idiopathisches multiples pigmentsarkom der haut," *Archives of the Dermatology and Syphilology* 4 (1872): 265–73.

65    M. Schalling, et al., "A role for a new herpes virus (KSHV) in different forms of Kaposi's sarcoma," *Nature Medicine* 1, no. 7 (1995): 707–8.

66    M. Hutt, "The Epidemiology of Kaposi's Sarcoma," in *Kaposi's Sarcoma* (Basel, Switzerland: Karger Publishers, 1981): 3–8.

67    R. Shiels, "A history of Kaposi's sarcoma," *Journal of the Royal Society of Medicine* 79, no. 9 (1986): 532–4.

68    G. Sternbach and J. Varon, "Moritz Kaposi: idiopathic pigmented sarcoma of the skin," *The Journal of Emergency Medicine* 13, no. 5 (1995): 671–4.

69    A. Friedman-Kien, et al., "Kaposis sarcoma and Pneumocystis pneumonia among homosexual men—New York City and California," *MMWR: Morbidity and Mortality Weekly Report* 30, no. 25 (1981): 305–8.

## 3: THAT WHICH DOESN'T KILL YOU . . .

1    A. A. Sall, et al., "Yellow Fever Virus Exhibits Slower Evolutionary Dynamics than Dengue Virus," *Journal of Virology* 84, no. 2 (2010): 765–72.

2    W. S. Middleton, "The Yellow Fever Epidemic of 1793 in Philadelphia," *Annals of Medical History* 10, no. 4 (1928).

3    M. S. Kinch, *Between Hope & Fear: A History of Vaccines and Human Immunity* (New York: Pegasus, 2018).

4    W. Dunn, "Adrian Stokes, D.S.O., O.B.E., M.D.Dubl., F.R.C.S.I., M.R.C.P.Lond., Sir William Dumn Professor Of Pathology At Guy's Hospital, London University," *The British Medical Journal* 2, no. 3,482 (1927): 615–8.

5    Ibid.

6    N. P. Hudson, "Adrian Stokes and yellow fever research: a tribute," *Transactions of the Royal Society of Tropical Medicine and Hygiene* 60, no. 2 (1966): 170–4.

7    G. W. Corner, *A History of the Rockefeller Institute, 1901–1953: Origins and Growth* (New York: Rockefeller University Press, 1965).

8    Dunn, "Adrian Stokes," 615–8.

9    A. Stokes, J.H. Bauer, and N.P. Hudson, "Experimental Transmission of Yellow Fever to Laboratory Animals 1," *The American Journal of Tropical Medicine and Hygiene* 1, no. 2 (1928): 103–64.

10   Corner, *A History of the Rockefeller Institute, 1901–1953*.

11   Stokes, Bauer, and Hudson, "Experimental Transmission of Yellow Fever to Laboratory Animals," *The American Journal of Tropical Medicine and Hygiene* 8, no. 2 (1928): 103–64.

12   A. W. Sellards, "The behavior of the virus of yellow fever in monkeys and mice," *Proceedings of the National Academy of Sciences* 17, no. 6 (1931): 339–43.

13   N. C. Davis, W. Lloyd, and M. Frobisher Jr., "The transmission of neurotropic yellow fever virus by Stegomyia mosquitoes," *Journal of Experimental Medicine* 56, no. 6 (1932): 853.

14   N. R. Grist, "Frederick Ogden MacCallum," *Bulletin of the Royal College of Pathology* 90 (1995): 6–7.

15   G. Findlay and F. MacCallum, "An interference phenomenon in relation to yellow fever and other viruses," *The Journal of Pathology* 44, no. 2 (1937): 405–24.

16   N. R. Grist, "Frederick Ogden MacCallum," *Bulletin of the Royal College of Pathology* 90, no. 10 (1995): 6–7.

17   L. C. Norkin, *Virology: Molecular Biology and Pathogenesis* (Sterling, VA: American Society for Microbiology Press, 2010).

18   J. K. Taubenberger and D.M. Morens, "1918 Influenza: the Mother of All Pandemics," *Emerging Infectious Diseases* 12, no. 1 (2006): 15–22.

19   M. S. Kinch, *A Prescription For Change: The Looming Crisis in Drug Discovery* (Chapel Hill, NC: UNC Press, 2016).

20   C. H. Andrewes, "Alick Isaacs. 1921–1967," *Biographical Memoirs of Fellows of the Royal Society* 13 (1967): 205–21.

21   A. Isaacs and M. Edney, "Interference between inactive and active influenza viruses in the chick embryo: I. Quantitative aspects of interference," *Australian Journal of Experimental Biology & Medical Science* 28, no. 2 (1950).

22   A. Isaacs and M. Edney, "Interference between inactive and active influenza viruses in the chick embryo: II. The site of interference," *Australian Journal of Experimental Biology & Medical Science* 28, no. 2 (1950).

23   C. H. Andrewes, "Alick Isaacs, 1921–1967," *Biographical Memoirs of Fellows of the Royal Society* 13: (1967): 204–21.

24   A. Isaacs and J. Lindenmann, "Virus interference. I. The interferon," *Proceedings of the Royal Society of London* 147, no. 927 (1957): 258–67.

25   A. Isaacs, J. Lindenmann, and R.C. Valentine, "Virus interference. II. Some properties of interferon," *Proceedings of the Royal Society of London* 147, no. 927 (1957): 268–73.

26   J. Lindenmann, D. Burke, and A. Isaacs, "Studies on the production, mode of action and properties of interferon," *British Journal of Experimental Pathology* 38, no. 5 (1957): 551.

27   D. Burke, "The purification of interferon," *Biochemical Journal* 78, no. 3 (1961): 556.

28   I. Gresser and C. Bourali, "Antitumor effects of interferon preparations in mice," *Journal of the National Cancer Institute* 45, no. 2 (1970): 365–76.

29   E. Landhuis and M. Jones, "Mathilde Krim's Life of Causes," LSF Magazine, accessed April 24, 2018, https://medium.com/lsf-magazine/mathilde-krim-a707d55e7bef.

30   E. Pace, "Arthur B. Krim, 89, ex-chief of movie studios," *The New York Times*, September 22, 1994, http://query.nytimes.com/gst/fullpage.html?res=9C01EED6163AF931A1575 AC0A962958260.

31    D. E. Lipstadt, "The Third Reich in the Ivory Tower: Complicity and Conflict on Amer-
      ican Campuses," *American Jewish History* 95, no. 3 (2009): 313–5.

32    Pace, "Arthur B. Krim, 89, ex-chief of movie studios."

33    Landhuis and Jones, "Mathilde Krim's Life of Causes."

34    G. Johnson, "Dr. Krim's Crusade," *The New York Times Magazine*, February 14, 1988.

35    Landhuis and Jones, "Mathilde Krim's Life of Causes."

36    J. Klemesrud, "Dr. Mathilde Krim: Focusing attention on AIDS research," *The New York
      Times*, November 3, 1984, http://www.nytimes.com/1984/11/03/style
      /dr-mathilde-krim-focusing-attention-on-aids-research.html.

37    Johnson, "Dr. Krim's Crusade."

38    D. Goldstein and J. Laszlo, "The role of interferon in cancer therapy: a current perspective,"
      *CA Cancer Journal for Clinicians* 38, no. 5 (1988): 258–77.

39    S. D. Fossa, "Interferon in metastatic renal cell carcinoma," *Seminars in Oncology* 27, no. 2
      (2000): 187–93.

40    R. Lancour, "Beaver Castor," North American Fur Auctions, accessed April 19, 2018,
      http://www.nafa.ca/wp-content/uploads/Beaver-Castor.pdf.

41    S. Lohman, "A Brief History of Castoreum, the Beaver Butt Secretion Used as
      Flavoring," Mental Floss, June 13, 2017, http://mentalfloss.com/article/501813/
      brief-history-castoreum-beaver-butt-secretion-used-as-flavoring.

42    A. M. Carlos and F. D. Lewis, "The Economic History of the Fur Trade: 1670 to 1870,"
      EH.net, March, 16, 2008, https://eh.net/encyclopedia/the-economic
      -history-of-the-fur-trade-1670-to-1870/. *EH. Net Encyclopedia*.

43    H. Mutlu and M. A. Meier, "Castor oil as a renewable resource for the chemical industry,"
      *European Journal of Lipid Science and Technology* 112, no. 1 (2010): 10–30.

44    T. Anderson, *Monkeys, Myths, and Molecules: Separating Fact from Fiction in the Science of
      Everyday Life* (New York: Reed Business Information, 2015).

45    Kinch, *Between Hope & Fear.*

46    D. R. Franz and N.K. Jaax, "Ricin toxin," *Medical Aspects of Chemical and Biological War-
      fare* (1997): 631–42.

47    D. B. Roth, "Peter C. Nowell, MD, 1928–2016," *American Journal of Pathology* 187, no. 4
      (2017): 696.

48    E. Benton, *US Naval Radiological Defense Laboratory* (1968), *San Francisco Report*
      NRDL-TR-68-14.

49    P. C. Nowell and D. A. Hungerford, "Chromosome studies on normal and leukemic human
      leukocytes," *Journal of the National Cancer Institute* 25, no. 1 (1960): 85–109.

50    P. C. Nowell, "Discovery of the Philadelphia chromosome: a personal perspective," *Journal
      of Clinical Investigation* 117, no. 8 (2007): 2033.

51    J. D. Rowley, "A new consistent chromosomal abnormality in chronic myelogenous leu-
      kaemia identified by quinacrine fluorescence and Giemsa staining," *Nature* 243, no. 5,405
      (1973): 290–3.

52    R. Capdeville, et al., "Glivec (STI571, imatinib), a rationally developed, targeted anticancer
      drug," *Nature Reviews in Drug Discovery* 1, no. 7 (2002): 493–502.

53    P. C. Nowell, "Phytohemagglutinin: an initiator of mitosis in cultures of normal human
      leukocytes," *Cancer Research* 20, no. 4 (1960): 462–6.

54    S. A. Rosenberg, "IL-2: the first effective immunotherapy for human cancer," *The Journal of
      Immunology* 192, no. 12 (2014): 5451–8.

55    N. R. Faria, et al., "The early spread and epidemic ignition of HIV-1 in human popula-
      tions." *Science* 346, no. 6,205 (2014): 56–61.

56    S. Kasakura and L. Lowenstein, "A factor stimulating DNA synthesis derived from the
      medium of leucocyte cultures," *Nature* 208, no. 5,012 (1965): 794–5.

57    J. Gordon and L. MacLean, "A lymphocyte-stimulating factor produced in vitro," *Nature* 208, no. 5,012 (1965): 795–6.

58    K. A. Smith and C.E. Mengel, "Association of iron-dextran-induced hemolysis and lipid peroxidation in mice," *The Journal of Laboratory and Clinical Medicine* 72, no. 3: (1968) 505–10.

59    K. A. Smith, "The discovery of the interleukin 2 molecule," Dr. Kendall Smith's Immunology resource site, accessed April 19, 2018, http://www.kendallasmith.com/molecule.html.

60    Ibid.

61    R. C. Gallo and L. Montagnier, "The discovery of HIV as the cause of AIDS," *New England Journal of Medicine* 349, no. 24 (2003): 2283–5.

62    L. Montagnier, "A history of HIV discovery," *Science* 298, no. 5,599 (2002): 1727–8.

63    J. W. Mier and R. C. Gallo, "Purification and some characteristics of human T-cell growth factor from phytohemagglutinin-stimulated lymphocyte-conditioned media," *Proceedings of the National Academy of Sciences* 77, no. 10 (1980): 6134–8.

64    D. A. Morgan, F. W. Ruscetti, and R. Gallo, "Selective in vitro growth of T lymphocytes from normal human bone marrows," *Science* 193, no. 4,257 (1976): 1007–8.

65    Smith, "The discovery of the interleukin 2 molecule."

66    R. J. Robb, A. Munck, and K. A. Smith, "T cell growth factor receptors. Quantitation, specificity, and biological relevance," *Journal of Experimental Medicine* 154, no. 5 (1981): 1455–74.

67    K. A. Smith, M. F. Favata, and S. Oroszlan, "Production and characterization of monoclonal antibodies to human interleukin 2: strategy and tactics," *The Journal of Immunology* 131, no. 4 (1983): 1808–15.

68    A. Pope, *Pope's Rape of the Lock* (London: Blackie & Son, 1899).

69    H. Harrer, *Seven Years in Tibet* (London: Penguin UK, 2009).

70    J.-b. Wang and L. Wang, "A Study of P. 3492v: A Fragment of Tang Dynasty's Divination Book for Moles," *Dunhuang Research* 1 (2005): 3.

71    F. Rochberg, *The Heavenly Writing: Divination, Horoscopy, and Astronomy in Mesopotamian Culture* (Cambridge, United Kingdom: Cambridge University Press, 2004).

72    B. Urteaga and G.T. Pack, "On the antiquity of melanoma," *Cancer* 19, no. 5 (1966): 607–10.

73    A. Jemal, et al., "Recent trends in cutaneous melanoma incidence among whites in the United States," *Journal of the National Cancer Institute* 93, no. 9 (2001), 678–83.

74    D. Albreski and S.B. Sloan, "Melanoma of the feet: misdiagnosed and misunderstood," *Clinics in Dermatology* 27, no. 6 (2009): 556–63.

75    S. A. Rosenberg and J.M. Barry, *The Transformed Cell: Unlocking the Mysteries of Cancer* (New York: Putnam, 1992).

76    Rosenberg, "IL-2: the first effective immunotherapy for human cancer," 5451–8.

77    A. Pollack, "Setting the Body's 'Serial Killers' Loose on Cancer," *The New York Times*, August 1, 2016, https://www.nytimes.com/2016/08/02/health/cancer-cell-therapy-immune-system.html.

78    R. McManus, "NIH science permits 'command performance,'" *NIH Record* 66, no. 2 (2014): 1.

79    Ibid.

## 4: DEADLY SINS

1    H. Wallop, "The day I tried to match Churchill drink for drink," *The Telegraph*, January 28, 2015, http://www.telegraph.co.uk/food-and-drink/drinks/the-day-i-tried-to-match-churchill-drink-for-drink/.

2    D. B. Goldstein, "Effect of alcohol on cellular membranes," *Annals of Emergency Medicine* 15, no. 9 (1986): 1013–8.

3    E. Cockayne, "Catarrhal jaundice, sporadic and epidemic, and its relation to acute yellow atrophy of the liver," *QJM: An International Journal of Medicine* no. 1 (1912): 1–29.

4    G. Findlay and F. MacCallum, "Note on acute hepatitis and yellow fever immunization," *Transactions of the Royal Society of Tropical Medicine and Hygiene* 31, no. 3 (1937): 297–308.

5    A. Lürman, "Eine icterusepidemie," *Berlin Klinische Wochenschrift* 22 (1885): 20–3.

6    J. R. Paul, et al., "Transmission experiments in serum jaundice and infectious hepatitis," *Journal of the American Medical Association* 128, no. 13 (1945): 911–5.

7    J. A. Cuthbert, "Hepatitis A: old and new," *Clinical Microbiology Reviews* 14, no. 1 (2001): 38–58.

8    S. M. Feinstone, A.Z. Kapikian, and R.H. Purcell, "Hepatitis A: detection by immune electron microscopy of a virus-like antigen associated with acute illness," *Science* 182, no. 4,116 (1973): 1026–8.

9    E. K. Thelin, *Unforgettable* (Berkeley, CA: M&P Publishers, 2017).

10   B. S. Blumberg, *Hepatitis B: The Hunt for a Killer Virus* (Princeton, NJ: Princeton University Press, 2002).

11   C. Darwin, F. Burkhardt, and S. Smith, *The Correspondence of Charles Darwin: 1856–1857,* vol. 6. (Cambridge, United Kingdom: Cambridge University Press, 1985).

12   J. Huxley, *New systematics* (Oxford, United Kingdom: Oxford University Press, 1940).

13   M. Hasan and P. R. de Olano, *The House of Wisdom: How Arabic Science Saved Ancient Knowledge and Gave Us the Renaissance* (College Park, MD: American Association of Physics Teachers, 2012).

14   M. Qari, "Abul Qasim Khalaf ibn al-Abbas al-Zahrawi (Abulcasis)," *Journal of Applied Hematology* 1, no. 1 (2010): 66.

15   V. A. McKusick, "The royal hemophilia," *Scientific American* 213, no. 2 (1965): 88–95.

16   S. S. Montefiore, *The Romanovs: 1613-1918* (New York: Vintage, 2017).

17   M. E. Reid, C. Lomas-Francis, and M.L. Olsson, *The Blood Group Antigen Factsbook* (Ontario, Canada: Academic Press, 2012).

18   C. J. Chen, L. Y. Wang, and M. W. Yu, "Epidemiology of hepatitis B virus infection in the Asia–Pacific region," *Journal of Gastroenterology and Hepatology* 15, no. s2 (2000).

19   D. Dane, C. Cameron, and M. Briggs, "Virus-like particles in serum of patients with Australia-antigen-associated hepatitis," *The Lancet* 295, no. 7,649 (1970): 695–8.

20   M. Patlak et al., *The Hepatitis B Story. Beyond Discovery: The Path from Research to Human Benefit* (Washington, D.C.: National Academy of Science, 2000).

21   L. C. Norkin, *Virology: Molecular Biology and Pathogenesis* (Sterling, VA: American Society for Microbiology Press, 2010).

22   P. A. Offit, *Vaccinated: One Man's Quest to Defeat the World's Deadliest Diseases* (New York: Harper Collins, 2007).

23   Ibid.

24   M. S. Kinch, *Between Hope & Fear: A History of Vaccines and Human Immunity* (New York: Pegasus, 2018), 360.

25   E. B. Buynak, et al., "Vaccine against human hepatitis B," *Journal of the American Medical Association* 235, no. 26 (1976): 2832–4.

26   M. S. Kinch, *Between Hope & Fear: A History of Vaccines and Human Immunity* (New York: Pegasus, 2018).

27   L. G. Horowitz, "About Dr Len Horowitz," accessed March 23, 2018, http://drlenhorowitz.com/about 2017.

28   G. O'Connor, *Alec Guinness: The Unknown* (London: Pan, 2003).

29   P. P. Read, *Alec Guinness: The Authorised Biography* (New York: Simon and Schuster, 2003).

30   H. Tang, et al., "Molecular functions and biological roles of hepatitis B virus x protein," *Cancer Science* 97, no. 10 (2006): 977–83.

31    S. Katyal, et al., "Extrahepatic metastases of hepatocellular carcinoma," *Radiology* 216, no. 3 (2000): 698–703.

32    P. A. Offit, *Deadly Choices: How the Anti-vaccine Movement Threatens Us All* (New York: Basic Books, 2015).

33    A. Sayeed, *Women and the Transmission of Religious Knowledge in Islam* (Cambridge, United Kingdom: Cambridge University Press, 2013).

34    B. Moor and E. Rezvan, "Al-Qazwīnī's' Ajā'ib Al-MakhlŪqāt wa Gharā'ib Al-MawjŪdāt: Manuscript D 370," *Manuscripta Orientalia* 8, no. 4 (2002): 38–68.

35    J. Bonar, *Pride, Power, Progress: Wyoming's First 100 Years* (Laramie, WY: Wyoming Historical Press, 1987).

36    L. Hancock, "Wyoming Lawmakers Consider Declaring Jackalope State's Official Mythical Creature," January 12, 2013, https://trib.com/news/state-and-regional /govt-and-politics/wyoming-lawmakers-consider-declaring-jackalope-state-s -official-mythical-creature/article_3c49017f-1bfd-5c07-a9cd-c7fb707b210e.html.

37    L. P. Gross, J.S. Katz, and J. Ruby, *Image Ethics in the Digital Age* (Minneapolis, MN: University of Minnesota Press, 2003).

38    A. Erkoreka, "Origins of the Spanish Influenza pandemic (1918–1920) and its relation to the First World War," *Journal of Molecular and Genetic Medicine* 3, no. 2 (2009): 190–4.

39    W. Smith, C. Andrewes, and P. Laidlaw, "A virus obtained from influenza patients," *The Lancet* 222, no. 5,732 (1933): 66–8.

40    R. E. Shope, "A transmissible tumor-like condition in rabbits," *Journal of Experimental Medicine* 56, no. 6 (1932): 793–802.

41    R. E. Shope and E.W. Hurst, "Infectious papillomatosis of rabbits: with a note on the histopathology," *Journal of Experimental Medicine* 58, no. 5 (1933): 607.

42    D. Burns, "'Warts and all'-the history and folklore of warts: a review," *Journal of the Royal Society of Medicine* 85, no. 1 (1992): 37.

43    D. Chouhy, et al., "Analysis of the genetic diversity and phylogenetic relationships of putative human papillomavirus types," *Journal of General Virology* 94, no. 11 (2013): 2480–8.

44    S. Jablonska, J. Dabrowski, and K. Jakubowicz, "Epidermodysplasia verruciformis as a model in studies on the role of papovaviruses in oncogenesis," *Cancer Research* 32, no. 3 (1972): 583–9.

45    N. Ramoz, et al., "Mutations in two adjacent novel genes are associated with epidermodysplasia verruciformi,." *Nature Genetics* 32, no. 4 (2002): 579–81.

46    D. P. Burkitt, "Charles S. Mott Award. The discovery of Burkitt's lymphoma," *Cancer* 51, no. 10 (1983): 1777–86.

47    Ibid.

48    D. Chen and B. Yen-Lieberman, "Epstein-Barr Virus," in *Clinical Virology Manual, Fifth Edition* (Washington, D.C.: American Society of Microbiology, 2010).

49    D. Esau, "Viral Causes of Lymphoma: The History of Epstein-Barr Virus and Human T-Lymphotropic Virus 1," *Virology: Research and Treatment* 8 (2017).

50    D. Holmes, "The cancer-virus cures," *Nature Medicine* 20 (2014): 571–4.

51    W. Henle, et al., "Herpes-type virus and chromosome marker in normal leukocytes after growth with irradiated Burkitt cells," *Science* 157, no. 3,792 (1967): 1064–5.

52    J. I. Cohen, et al., "Epstein-Barr virus: an important vaccine target for cancer prevention," *Science Translational Medicine* 3, no. 107 (2011): 107fs7-fs7.

53    "Harald zur Hausen—Biographical," NobelPrize.org, November 2, 2018, https://www .nobelprize.org/nobel_prizes/medicine/laureates/2008/hausen-bio.html.

54    R. Skloot, *The Immortal Life of Henrietta Lacks* (New York: Crown, 2010).

55    I. Petrea, "Aurel A. Babes (1886-1961)," *Neoplasma* 9 (1961): 445–6.

56    B. Naylor, et al., "In Romania it's the Méthode Babeş-Papanicolaou," *ACTA Cytologica* 46, no. 1 (2002): 1–12.

57    C. Daniel, "Babes A. Posibilitatea diagnosticului cancerului cu ajutorul frotiului," *Proceedings of the Bucharest Gynecology Society* 55 (1927).

58    B. Naylor, "The century for cytopathology," *ACTA cytologica* 44, no. 5 (2000): 709–25.

59    P. A. Elgert and G. W. Gill, "George N. Papanicolaou, MD, PhDCytopathology," *Laboratory Medicine* 40, no. 4 (2009): 245–6.

60    I. N. Mammas and D. A. Spandidos, "George N. Papanicolaou (1883–1962), an exceptional human, scientist and academic teacher: An interview with Dr Neda Voutsa-Perdiki," *Experimental and Therapeutic Medicine* 14, no. 4 (2017): 3346–9.

61    S. Y. Tan and Y. Tatsumura, "George Papanicolaou (1883–1962): Discoverer of the Pap smear," *Singapore Medical Journal* 56, no. 10 (2015): 586–7.

62    G. N. Papanicolaou and H. F. Traut, "The diagnostic value of vaginal smears in carcinoma of the uterus," *American Journal of Obstetrics and Gynecology* 42, no. 2 (1941): 193–206.

63    S. McGuire, "World cancer report 2014. Geneva, Switzerland: World Health Organization, international agency for research on cancer, WHO Press, 2015," *Advances in Nutrition: An International Review Journal* 7, no. 2 (2016): 418–9.

64    I. Frazer and R. Williams, "Professor Ian Frazer, immunologist," Australian Academy of Science, 2008, https://www.science.org.au/learning/general-audience/history/interviews -australian-scientists/professor-ian-frazer-immunologist.

65    Ibid.

66    R. E., Billingham, L. Brent, and P. B. Medawar, "Quantitative studies on tissue transplantation immunity. III. Actively acquired tolerance," *Philosophical Transactions of the Royal Society of London* 239, no. 666 (1956): 357–414.

67    J. T. Bryan, et al., "Prevention of cervical cancer: journey to develop the first human papillomavirus virus-like particle vaccine and the next generation vaccine," *Current Opinions in Chemical Biology* 32 (2016): 34–47.

68    K. N. Zhao, L. Zhang, and J. Qu, "Dr. Jian Zhou: The great inventor of cervical cancer vaccine," *Protein & Cell* 8, no. 2 (2017): 79–82.

69    J. Zhou, et al., "Expression of vaccinia recombinant HPV 16 L1 and L2 ORF proteins in epithelial cells is sufficient for assembly of HPV virion-like particles," *Virology* 185, no. 1 (1991): 251–7.

70    Frazer and Williams, "Professor Ian Frazer, immunologist."

71    S. Inglis, A. Shaw, and S. Koenig, "HPV vaccines: commercial research & development," *Vaccine* 24 (2006): S99-S105.

72    J. L. Grimes, "HPV vaccine development: a case study of prevention and politics," *Biochemistry and Molecular Biology Education* 34, no. 2 (2006): 148–54.

73    J. Walker, "Tribute to vaccine's forgotten man," *The Australian*, May 3, 2008, http://www .theaustralian.com.au/archive/news/tribute-to-vaccines-forgotten-man /news-story/d9a9c9f41d2c3668048cc8e61a57c9b8.

74    A. Forster, et al., "Passport to promiscuity or lifesaver: press coverage of HPV vaccination and risky sexual behavior," *Journal of Health Communication* 15, no. 2 (2010): 205–17.

75    A. Gillen and R. Gibbs, "Serratia marcescens: The Miracle Bacillus," Answers in Genesis, July 20, 2011, https://answersingenesis.org/biology/microbiology/serratia -marcescens-the-miracle-bacillus/.

76    N. Gibbs, "Defusing the war over the 'promiscuity' vaccine," *Time Magazine Online,* June 21, 2006, http://content.time.com/time/nation/article/0,8599,1206813,00.html.

77    S. L. Small, "Warts and All: HPV Vaccine Uptake" (PhD diss., University of Michigan, 2011), https://deepblue.lib.umich.edu/bitstream/handle/2027.42/89781/stesmall_1.pdf ?sequence=1.

78    J. S. Lawson, et al., "Human Papilloma Viruses and Breast Cancer," *Frontiers in Oncology* 5 (2015): 277.

79    M. Pascale, et al., "Is Human Papillomavirus Associated with Prostate Cancer Survival?," *Disease Markers* 35, no. 6 (2013): 607–13.

## 5: AN OLD STORY

1    R. Chernow, *Titan: The Life of John D. Rockefeller, Sr.* (New York: Random House, 1998).

2    J. Corbett, "Meet William Rockefeller, Snake Oil Salesman," The Corbett Report, June 22, 2011, https://www.corbettreport.com/meet-william-rockefeller-snake-oil-salesman/.

3    P. B. Doran, *Breaking Rockefeller: The Incredible Story of the Ambitious Rivals Who Toppled an Oil Empire* (New York: Viking, 2016).

4    G. S. Kienle, "Fever in Cancer Treatment: Coley's Therapy and Epidemiologic Observations," *Global Advances in Health and Medicine* 1, no. 1 (2012): 92–100.

5    C. Engelking, "Germ of an Idea: William Coley's Cancer-Killing Toxins," *Discover Magazine*, April 21, 2016.

6    S. S. Hall, *A Commotion in the Blood* (New York: Henry Holt, 1997).

7    A. F. Schenkel, *The Rich Man and the Kingdom: John D. Rockefeller, Jr., and the Protestant Establishment* (Minneapolis, MN: Augsburg Fortress Publishers, 1996).

8    E. Shorter, *The Health Century* (New York: Doubleday, 1987).

9    W. Busch, "Aus Der Sitzung Der Medicinischen Section Vom 13. November 1867," *Berliner Klinische Wochenschrift* 5 (1868): 137.

10    P. Bruns, "Die Heilwirkung Des Erysipels Auf Geschwulste," *Beitrage fur Klinische Chirugie* 3, no. 3 (1887): 443–66.

11    F. Fehleisen, "Ueber Die Züchtung Der Erysipelkokken Auf Künstlichem Nährboden Und Ihre Übertragbarkeit Auf Den Menschen," *Deutsche Medizinische Wochenschrift* 8 (1882): 553–54.

12    W. F. Morano et al., "Intraperitoneal Immunotherapy: Historical Perspectives and Modern Therapy," *Cancer Gene Therapy* 23, no. 11 (2016): 373.

13    B. Wiemann and C. O. Starnes, "Coley's Toxins, Tumor Necrosis Factor and Cancer Research: A Historical Perspective," *Pharmacology & Therapeutics* 64, no. 3 (1994): 529–64.

14    H. C. Nauts, W. E. Swift, and B. L. Coley, "The Treatment of Malignant Tumors by Bacterial Toxins as Developed by the Late William B. Coley, MD, Reviewed in the Light of Modern Research," *Cancer Research* 6, no. 4 (1946): 205–16.

15    D. B. Levine, "The Hospital for the Ruptured and Crippled: William Bradley Coley, Third Surgeon-in-Chief 1925–1933," *Hospital for Special Surgery Journal* 4, no. 1 (2008): 1–9.

16    E. Nagourney, "Helen C. Nauts, 93, Champion of Her Father's Cancer Work," *The New York Times*, January 9, 2001.

17    M. Tontonoz, "Beyond Magic Bullets: Helen Coley Nauts and the Battle for Immunotherapy," Cancer Research Institute, April 1, 2015, https://cancerresearch.org/blog/april-2015/helen-coley-nauts-and-the-battle-for-immunotherapy.

18    B. Benacerraf, *From Caracas to Stockholm: A Life in Medical Science* (New York: Prometheus Books, 1998).

19    H. S. Jennings, "Biographical Memoir of Raymond Pearl," in *Biographical Memoirs* (Washington, D.C.: National Academy of Sciences, 1942): 293–347.

20    M. S. Kinch, *A Prescription for Change* (Chapel Hill, NC: UNC Press, 2016).

21    R. Pearl, "Cancer and Tuberculosis," *American Journal of Epidemiology* 9, no. 1 (1929): 97–159.

22    E. A. Boyse, and Old, L.J. "Some Aspects of Normal and Abnormal Cell Surface Genetics," *Annual Review of Genetics* 3, no. 1 (1969): 269–90.

23    A. Govaerts, "Cellular Antibodies in Kidney Homotransplantation," *The Journal of Immunology* 85, no. 5 (1960): 516–22.

24    Y. Nishizuka and T. Sakakura, "Thymus and Reproduction: Sex-Linked Dysgenesis of the Gonad after Neonatal Thymectomy in Mice," *Science* 166, no. 3,906 (1969): 753–55.

25    M. E. Dorf, and B. Benacerraf, "I-J as a Restriction Element in the Suppressor T Cell System," *Immunology Reviews* 83 (April 1985): 23–40.

26    iayork, "How to Embarass an Immunologist: The I-J Story," Mystery Rays from Outer Space., accessed April 27, 2018, http://www.iayork.com/MysteryRays/2007/11/02/how-to -embarass-an-immunologist-the-i-j-story/.

## 6: SMART BOMBS AND PAYLOADS

1    L. M. Nadler, et. al., "Serotherapy of a Patient with a Monoclonal Antibody Directed against a Human Lymphoma-Associated Antigen," *Cancer Research* 40, no. 9 (1980): 3147–54.

2    S. Mukherjee, *The Emperor of All Maladies: A Biography of Cancer* (New York: Simon and Schuster, 2010).

3    D. R. Miller, "A Tribute to Sidney Farber—the Father of Modern Chemotherapy," *British Journal of Haematology* 134, no. 1 (2006): 20–26.

4    G. MarieKrueger, "'For Jimmy and the Boys and Girls of America': Publicizing Child-hood Cancers in Twentieth-Century America," *Bulletin of the History of Medicine* 81, no. 1 (2007): 70–93.

5    D. Martin, "Einar Gustafson, 65, 'Jimmy' of Child Cancer Fund, Dies," *The New York Times*, January 24, 2001.

6    Miller, "A Tribute to Sidney Farber—the Father of Modern Chemotherapy," 20–26.

7    S. Farber, et. al., "Temporary Remissions in Acute Leukemia in Children Produced by Folic Acid Antagonist, 4-Aminopteroyl-Glutamic Acid (Aminopterin)," *New England Journal of Medicine* 238, no. 23 (1948): 787–93.

8    L. M. Nadler and W. C. Roberts, "Lee Marshall Nadler, MD: A Conversation with the Editor," *Baylor University Medical Center Proceedings* 20, no. 4 (2007): 381–89.

9    J. Toobin, *The Nine: Inside the Secret World of the Supreme Court* (New York: Anchor, 2008).

10    M. Bailey, "How a Former 'Street Kid' Scooped up NIH Grants and Shook up Medical Research," STAT News, December 3, 2015, https://www.statnews.com/2015/12/03/lee -nadler-harvard/.

11    Nadler and Roberts, "Lee Marshall Nadler, MD: A Conversation with the Editor," 381–89.

12    Ibid.

13    M. S. Kinch, *A Prescription for Change* (Chapel Hill, NC: UNC Press, 2016).

14    M. S. Kinch, *Between Hope & Fear: A History of Vaccines and Human Immunity* (New York: Pegasus Books, 2018).

15    L. M. Nadler, P. Stashenko, R. Hardy, and S.F. Schlossman, "A monoclonal antibody defining a lymphoma-associated antigen in man," *The Journal of Immunology* 125, no. 2 (1980): 570–77.

16    Ibid.

17    Nadler, et. al., "Serotherapy of a Patient with a Monoclonal Antibody Directed against a Human Lymphoma-Associated Antigen," 3147–54.

18    Ibid.

19    Nadler, Stashenko, Hardy, and Schlossman, "A monoclonal antibody defining a lymphoma-associated antigen in man," 570–77.

20    H. C. Oettgen, et.al., "Further Biochemical Studies of the Human B-Cell Differentiation Antigens B1 and B2," *Hybridoma* 2, no. 1 (1983): 17–28.

21    T. F. Tedder, et. al., "The B Cell Surface Molecule B1 Is Functionally Linked with B Cell Activation and Differentiation," *The Journal of Immunology* 135, no. 2 (1985): 973–79.

22    N. R. Kleinfeld, "Birth of a Health-Care Concern," *The New York Times*, July 11, 1983.

23    L. H. Schloen, "Immortalizing Immunity," *The Sciences* 20, no. 6 (1980): 14–17.

24    Howard Birndorf, interview by M. Shindell, *The San Diego Technology Archive,* April 30, 2008, http://libraries.ucsd.edu/sdta/transcripts/birndorf-howard_20080430.html Web., April 1, 2018.

25    J. A. Ledbetter and E. A. Clark, "Surface Phenotype and Function of Tonsillar Germinal Center and Mantle Zone B Cell Subsets," *Human Immunology* 15, no. 1 (1986): 30–43.

26    I. Hellström, K.E. Hellström, and M. Yeh, "Lymphocyte-Dependent Antibodies to Antigen 3.1, a Cell-Surface Antigen Expressed by a Subgroup of Human Melanomas," *International Journal of Cancer* 27, no. 3 (1981): 281–85.

27    O. W. Press et al., "Monoclonal Antibody 1f5 (Anti-CD20) Serotherapy of Human B Cell Lymphomas," *Blood* 69, no. 2 (1987): 584–91.

28    M. Barinaga, "Biotechnology on the Auction Block," *Science* 247, no. 4,945 (1990): 906–8.

29    A. Y. Liu, et. al., "Production of a Mouse-Human Chimeric Monoclonal Antibody to Cd20 with Potent Fc-Dependent Biologic Activity," *The Journal of Immunology* 139, no. 10 (1987): 3521–26.

30    A. Pollack, "A Biotech King, Dethroned," *The New York Times*, September 5, 2013.

31    Birndorf interview by M. Shindell.

32    F. J. Cummings, "In Memoriam: Mathilda Dodge Wilson (1883–1967)," *Bulletin of the Detroit Institute of Arts* (1975): 4–4.

33    Birndorf interview by M. Shindell.

34    Ibid.

35    Ibid.

36    Ibid.

37    E. K. Wilson, "Biotech Eden," *Chemical and Engineering News* 79, no. 10 (2001): 41–9.

38    K. R. Chi, "The Birth of Biotech-How One Company Helped Seed San Diego's Industry," *The Scientist* 21, no. 12 (2007): 75–77.

39    M. E. Reff, et. al., "Depletion of B Cells in Vivo by a Chimeric Mouse Human Monoclonal Antibody to CD20," *Blood* 83, no. 2 (1994): 435–45.

40    D. G. Maloney et al., "Phase I Clinical Trial Using Escalating Single-Dose Infusion of Chimeric Anti-Cd20 Monoclonal Antibody (Idec-C2b8) in Patients with Recurrent B-Cell Lymphoma," *Blood* 84, no. 8 (1994): 2457–66.

41    A. J. Grillo-López, et. al., "Overview of the clinical development of rituximab," *Seminars in Oncology* 26 (1999): 66–73.

42    D. Fauls and E.M. Sorkin, "Abciximab (C7e3 Fab): A review of its pharmacology and thera-peutic potential in ischemic heart disease," *Drugs* 48 (1994): 583–98.

43    P. Smolewski and T. Robak, "The Preclinical Discovery of Rituximab for the Treatment of Non-Hodgkin's Lymphoma," *Expert Opinion on Drug Discovery* 10, no. 7 (2015): 791–808.

44    M. S. Kinch, "An Overview of FDA-Approved Biologics Medicines," *Drug Discovery Today* 20, no. 4 (2014): 393–8.

45    M. S. Kinch, "An Analysis of FDA-Approved Drugs for Oncology," *Drug Discovery Today* 19, no. 12 (2014): 1831–5.

46    U. Storz, "Rituximab: How Approval History Is Reflected by a Corresponding Patent Filing Strategy," *MAbs* 6, no. 4 (2014): 820–37.

47    R. Lorenzi, "Alexander the Great Killed by Toxic Bacteria?" NBC News, June 16, 2010, http://www.nbcnews.com/id/38282729/ns/technology_and_science-science/t/alexander-great-killed-toxic-bacteria/#.WqK4goJG2ek.

48    J. Lu, F. Jiang, A. Lu, and G. Zhang, "Linkers Having a Crucial Role in Antibody–Drug Conjugates," *International Journal of Molecular Sciences* 17, no. 561.

49    P. Loftus and A. Hufford, "Seattle Genetics Cancer-Drug Trials on Hold after Four Patient Deaths," *The Wall Street Journal*, December 27, 2016.

50    A. Skerra and A. Pluckthun, "Assembly of a Functional Immunoglobulin Fv Fragment in Escherichia Coli," *Science* 240, no. 4,855 (1988): 1038–41.

## 7: DESIGNER DRUGS

1     J. Adams, "The Case of Scirrhous of the Prostate Gland with Corresponding Affliction of the Lymphatic Glands in the Lumbar Region and in the Pelvis," *Lancet* 1, no. 1 (1853): 393–93.

2     W. Lawrence, "Cases of Fungus Haematodes, with Observations, by George Langstaff, Esq. And an Appendix, Containing Two Cases of Analogous Affections," *Medico-Chirurgical Transactions* 8 (1817): 272.

3     D. L. Bilhartz, D. J. Tindall, and J. E. Oesterling, "Prostate-Specific Antigen and Prostatic Acid Phosphatase: Biomolecular and Physiologic Characteristics," *Urology* 38, no. 2 (August 1991): 95–102.

4     A. B. Gutman and E. B. Gutman, "An 'Acid' Phosphatase Occurring in the Serum of Patients with Metastasizing Carcinoma of the Prostate Gland," *The Journal of Clinical Investigation* 17, no. 4 (1938): 473–78.

5     W. Kutscher and H. Wolbergs, "Prostataphosphatase," *Hoppe-Seyler's Zeitschrift für physiologische Chemie* 236, no. 4–6 (1935): 237–40.

6     H. Popper, "Alexander B. Gutman, 1902–1973," *The American Journal of Medicine* 54, no. 6 (1973): 689–93.

7     I. Weise, *Die Berliner Kartoffelrevolution: Eine Fallstudie Zum Sozialen Protest Im Vormärz*, (Berlin: Freien Universität Berlin, 1991).

8     R. Tsuchiya and N. Fujisawa, "On the Etymology of 'Pancreas,'" *International Journal of Gastrointestinal Cancer* 21, no. 3 (1997): 269–72.

9     S. Jolles, "Paul Langerhans," *Journal of Clinical Pathology* 55, no. 4 (2002): 243–43.

10    I. Silberg, "Apposition of Mononuclear Cells to Langerhans Cells in Contact Allergic Reactions. An Ultrastructural Study," *Acta Dermato-Venereologica* 53, no. 1 (1973): 1–12.

11    P. P. Jones and L.A. Herzenberg, "The Early History of Stanford Immunology," *Immunologic Research* 58, no. 2–3 (2014): 164–78.

12    R. Richter, "Research at Blood Center Led to Cancer Vaccine," Stanford Medicine News Center, June 7, 2010, https://med.stanford.edu/news/all-news/2010/06 /research-at-blood-center-led-to-cancer-vaccine.html.

13    S. Markowicz and E. G. Engleman, "Granulocyte-Macrophage Colony-Stimulating Factor Promotes Differentiation and Survival of Human Peripheral Blood Dendritic Cells in Vitro," *The Journal of Clinical Investigation* 85, no. 3 (1990): 955–61.

14    H. Ledford, "Therapeutic Cancer Vaccine Survives Biotech Bust," *Nature* 519, no. 7,541 (2015): 17–18.

15    N. M. Durham and C. G. Drake, "Dendritic Cell Vaccines: Sipuleucel-T and Other Approaches," in *Cancer Immunotherapy, Second Edition* (Toronto, Canada: Elsevier, 2013): 273–86.

16    "The Regulator Disapproves," *Nature Biotechnology* 26, no. 1 (January 2008): 1.

17    R. Baghdadi, "Dendreon Vs Cms: Why the Provenge Coverage Controversy Is Bigger Than Just One Product," *Oncology* 24, no. 10 (2010): 881.

18    G. Lorge, "Closing in on Cancer," *Stanford Alumni Magazine*, January 7, 2016, https://medium.com/@stanfordmag/closing-in-on-cancer-e56cff95af0b.

19    M. Abou-El-Enein, A. Elsanhoury, and P. Reinke, "Overcoming Challenges Facing Advanced Therapies in the Eu Market," *Cell: Stem Cell* 19, no. 3 (2016): 293–97.

20    P. Holko and P. Kawalec, "Economic Evaluation of Sipuleucel-T Immunotherapy in Castration-Resistant Prostate Cancer," *Expert Review of Anticancer Therapy* 14, no. 1 (January 2014): 63–73.

21 S. Reisfeld, "The Story Beind an Israeli Immunologist's Cancer-Fighting Breakthrough," *Haaretz*, November 10, 2017.

22 G. Köhler and C. Milstein, "Continuous Cultures of Fused Cells Secreting Antibody of Pre-defined Specificity," *Nature* 256, no. 5,517 (1975): 495–97.

23 J. Couzin-Frankel, "The Dizzying Journey to a New Cancer Arsenal," *Science* 340, no. 6,140 (2013), 1514–8.

24 G. Gross, T. Waks, and Z. Eshhar, "Expression of Immunoglobulin-T-Cell Receptor Chimeric Molecules as Functional Receptors with Antibody-Type Specificity," *Proceedings of the National Academy of Sciences, USA* 86, no. 24 (December 1989): 10024–8.

25 S. Huler, "Nurturing Science's Young Elite: Westinghouse Talent Search," *Scientist* 5, no. 8 (1991): 20–22.

26 J. Goverman, et. al., "Chimeric Immunoglobulin-T Cell Receptor Proteins Form Functional Receptors: Implications for T Cell Receptor Complex Formation and Activation," *Cell* 60, no. 6 (1990): 929–39.

27 P. S. Linsley and J. A. Ledbetter, "The Role of the Cd28 Receptor During T Cell Responses to Antigen," *Annual Review of Immunology* 11, no. 1 (1993): 191–212.

28 F. L. Locke, et. al., "Clinical and Biologic Covariates of Outcomes in Zuma-1: A Pivotal Trial of Axicabtagene Ciloleucel (Axi-Cel; Kte-C19) in Patients with Refractory Aggressive Non-Hodgkin Lymphoma (R-Nhl)," *Journal of Clinical Oncology* 35, no. 15 (2017): 7512.

29 G. Gross and Z. Eshhar, "Therapeutic Potential of T Cell Chimeric Antigen Receptors (Cars) in Cancer Treatment: Counteracting Off-Tumor Toxicities for Safe Car T Cell Therapy," *Annual Review of Pharmacology and Toxicology* 56 (2016): 59–83.

30 E. Levi-Weinrib, "Israeli Professors Fight for Kite Pharma Sale Spoils," *Globes*, November 5, 2017.

31 N. Holt, *Cured: The People Who Defeated HIV* (New York: Penguin, 2014).

32 C. H. June, "Toward Synthetic Biology with Engineered T Cells: A Long Journey Just Begun," *Human Gene Therapy* 25, no. 9 (2014): 779–84.

33 J. Akst, "Commander of an Immune Flotilla," *Scientist* 28, no. 4 (2014): 56-58.

34 June, "Toward Synthetic Biology with Engineered T Cells: A Long Journey Just Begun" (2014): 779–84.

35 "Doug's Story," PennMedicine.org, accessed May 1, 2018, https://www.pennmedicine.org/cancer/about/patient-stories/cll-doug.

36 Ibid.

37 M. Kalos et al., "T Cells with Chimeric Antigen Receptors Have Potent Antitumor Effects and Can Establish Memory in Patients with Advanced Leukemia," *Science Translational Medicine* 3, no. 95 (2011): 95ra73.

38 H. Auer, "Genetically Modified 'Serial Killer' T Cells Obliterate Tumors in Patients with Chronic Lymphocytic Leukemia, Penn Researchers Report," PennMedicine.org, August 10, 2011, https://www.pennmedicine.org/news/news-releases/2011/august/genetically-modified-serial-ki.

39 S. Barlas, "The White House Launches a Cancer Moonshot: Despite Funding Questions, the Progress Appears Promising," *Pharmacy and Therapeutics* 41, no. 5 (2016): 290.

40 Auer, "Genetically Modified 'Serial Killer' T Cells Obliterate Tumors in Patients with Chronic Lymphocytic Leukemia, Penn Researchers Report."

41 Associated Press, "VP Joe Biden Says Politics Are Impeding Cancer Cure," CBS News, January 15, 2016, https://www.cbsnews.com/news/vice-president-joe-biden-says-politics-are-impeding-cancer-cure/.

42 J. N. Kochenderfer and S. A. Rosenberg, "Chimeric Antigen Receptor–Modified T Cells in Cll," *The New England Journal of Medicine* 365, no. 20 (2011): 1937.

43    A. Zak, "Novartis to Pay June $12.25m+ to Settle Car Patent Lawsuits," Genetic Engineering & Biotechnology News, April 6, 2015, https://www.genengnews.com/gen-news-highlights/novartis-to-pay-juno-12-25m-to-settle-car-patent-lawsuits/81251117/.

44    A. Regalado, "T-Cell Pioneer Carl June Acknowledges Key Ingredient Wasn't His," *MIT Technology Review*, March 14, 2016, https://www.technologyreview.com/s/601027/t-cell-pioneer-carl-june-acknowledges-key-ingredient-wasnt-his/.

## 8: CHECKMATE!

1    "A Few Holes to Fill," *Nature Physics* 4 (2008): 257.

2    "Just Thanck Planck," *The Economist*, December 7, 2000, https://www.economist.com/node/443258.

3    H. Schorle et al., "Development and Function of T Cells in Mice Rendered Interleukin-2 Deficient by Gene Targeting," *Nature* 352, no. 6,336 (1991): 621–4.

4    H. P. Erickson, "Gene Knockouts of C-Src, Transforming Growth Factor Beta 1, and Tenascin Suggest Superfluous, Nonfunctional Expression of Proteins," *The Journal of Cell Biology* 120, no. 5 (1993): 1079–81.

5    B. Sadlack et al., "Ulcerative Colitis-Like Disease in Mice with a Disrupted Interleukin-2 Gene," *Cell* 75, no. 2 (1993): 253–61.

6    D. M. Willerford et al., "Interleukin-2 Receptor A Chain Regulates the Size and Content of the Peripheral Lymphoid Compartment," *Immunity* 3, no. 4 (October 1995): 521–30.

7    W. J. Penhale, A. Farmer, R. P. McKenna, and W. J. Irvine, "Spontaneous Thyroiditis in Thymectomized and Irradiated Wistar Rats," *Clinical and Experimental Immunology* 15, no. 2 (1973): 225.

8    W. J. Penhale et al., "Induction of Diabetes in Pvg/C Strain Rats by Manipulation of the Immune System," *Autoimmunity* 7, no. 2–3 (1990): 169–79.

9    D. Fowell and D. Mason, "Evidence That the T Cell Repertoire of Normal Rats Contains Cells with the Potential to Cause Diabetes. Characterization of the Cd4+ T Cell Subset That Inhibits This Autoimmune Potential," *Journal of Experimental Medicine* 177, no. 3 (1993): 627–36.

10    S. Sakaguchi, K. Fukuma, K. Kuribayashi, and T. Masuda, "Organ-Specific Autoimmune Diseases Induced in Mice by Elimination of T Cell Subset. I. Evidence for the Active Participation of T Cells in Natural Self-Tolerance; Deficit of a T Cell Subset as a Possible Cause of Autoimmune Disease," *Journal of Experimental Medicine* 161, no. 1 (1985): 72–87.

11    S. Sakaguchi, N. Sakaguchi, M. Asano, M. Itoh, and M. Toda, "Immunologic Self-Tolerance Maintained by Activated T Cells Expressing Il-2 Receptor Alpha-Chains (Cd25). Breakdown of a Single Mechanism of Self-Tolerance Causes Various Autoimmune Diseases," *Journal of Immunology* 155, no. 3 (1995): 1151–64.

12    R. Setoguchi, S. Hori, T. Takahashi, and S. Sakaguchi, "Homeostatic Maintenance of Natural Foxp3+ Cd25+ Cd4+ Regulatory T Cells by Interleukin (Il)-2 and Induction of Autoimmune Disease by Il-2 Neutralization," *Journal of Experimental Medicine* 201, no. 5 (2005): 723–35.

13    E. Suri-Payer, A.Z. Amar, A.M. Thornton, and E.M. Shevach, "Cd4+ Cd25+ T Cells Inhibit Both the Induction and Effector Function of Autoreactive T Cells and Represent a Unique Lineage of Immunoregulatory Cells," *The Journal of Immunology* 160, no. 3 (1998): 1212–18.

14    Sakaguchi, "Immunologic Self-Tolerance Maintained by Activated T Cells Expressing Il-2 Receptor Alpha-Chains (Cd25). Breakdown of a Single Mechanism of Self-Tolerance Causes Various Autoimmune Diseases," 1151–64.

15    E. M. Shevach, "Regulatory T Cells in Autoimmmunity," *Annual Review of Immunology* 18, no. 1 (2000): 423–49.

16    C. Sun et al., "Small Intestine Lamina Propria Dendritic Cells Promote De Novo Generation of Foxp3
       T Reg Cells Via Retinoic Acid," *The Journal of Experimental Medicine* 204, no. 8 (2007): 1775–85.

17    D. Mucida et al., "Reciprocal Th17 and Regulatory T Cell Differentiation Mediated by
       Retinoic Acid," *Science* 317, no. 5,835 (2007): 256–60.

18    G. P. Dunn, L.J. Old, and R.D. Schreiber, "The Three Es of Cancer Immunoediting,"
       *Annual Review of Immunology* 22, no. 1 (2004): 329–60.

19    D. Bradford, "Experience: I Ran a Medical Trial That Went Wrong," *The
       Guardian*, April 22, 2016, https://www.theguardian.com/lifeandstyle/2016/apr/22/
       experience-i-ran-medical-trial-that-went-wrong.

20    T. Hünig, "The Storm Has Cleared: Lessons from the Cd28 Superagonist Tgn1412 Trial,"
       *Nature Reviews Immunology* 12, no. 5 (2012): 317–18.

21    M. S. Kinch, *A Prescription for Change* (Chapel Hill, NC: UNC Press, 2016).

22    B. McLaurin, "The Drug Trial: Emergency at the Hospital," BBC2, February 21, 2017,
       http://www.bbc.co.uk/mediacentre/proginfo/2017/08/the-drug-trial.

23    Ibid.

24    Bradford, "Experience: I Ran a Medical Trial That Went Wrong."

25    McLaurin, "The Drug Trial: Emergency at the Hospital."

26    J. Cavallo, "Immunotherapy Research of James P. Allison, Phd, Has Led to a Paradigm
       Shift in the Treatment of Cancer," The ASCO Post, September 15, 2014, http://www
       .ascopost.com/issues/september-15-2014/immunotherapy-research-of-james-p-allison-phd
       -has-led-to-a-paradigm-shift-in-the-treatment-of-cancer/.

27    Ibid.

28    E. Benson, "The Iconoclast," *Texas Monthly*, November 2016, https://www.texasmonthly
       .com/articles/jim-allison-and-the-search-for-the-cure-for-cancer/.

29    A. Piore, "James Allison Has Unfinished Business with Cancer," *Technology Review* 120,
       no. 3 (2017): 78–85.

30    G. J. Freeman et al., "B7, a New Member of the Ig Superfamily with Unique Expression on
       Activated and Neoplastic B Cells," *Journal of Immunology* 143, no. 8 (1989): 2714–22.

31    P. S. Linsley et al., "Binding of the B Cell Activation Antigen B7 to Cd28 Costimulates
       T Cell Proliferation and Interleukin 2 Mrna Accumulation," *The Journal of Experimental
       Medicine* 173, no. 3 (1991): 721–30.

32    *The Big Bang Theory,* season 7, episode 10, "The Discovery Dissipation," directed by
       M. Cendrowski, aired Deember 5, 2013, on CBS.

33    D. R. Leach, M. F. Krummel, and J. P. Allison, "Enhancement of Antitumor Immunity by
       Ctla-4 Blockade," *Science* 271, no. 5,256 (1996): 1734–36.

34    Piore, "James Allison Has Unfinished Business with Cancer," 78–85.

35    Ibid.

36    F. S. Hodi et al., "Improved Survival with Ipilimumab in Patients with Metastatic Mela-
       noma," *New England Journal of Medicine* 363, no. 8 (2010): 711–23.

37    Benson, "The Iconoclast."

38    T. Bakacs, J.N. Mehrishi, and R.W. Moss, "Ipilimumab (Yervoy) and the Tgn1412 Catas-
       trophe," *Immunobiology* 217, no. 6 (2012): 583–9.

39    M. A. Curran, M. K. Callahan, S. K. Subudhi, and J. P. Allison, "Response to 'Ipilimumab
       (Yervoy) and the Tgn1412 Catastrophe,'" *Immunobiology* 217, no. 6 (2012): 590–92.

40    G. Hodgson, *The Colonel: The Life and Wars of Henry Stimson, 1867-1950* (New York:
       Alfred A Knopf Inc, 1990).

41    H. L. Stimson and H. S. Truman, "The Decision to Use the Atomic Bomb," *Bulletin of the
       Atomic Scientists* 3, no. 2 (1947): 37–67.

42    M. Oi, "The Man Who Saved Kyoto from the Atomic Bomb," BBC News, August 9, 2015,
       http://www.bbc.com/news/world-asia-33755182.

43    S. Malloy, "Four Days in May: Henry L. Stimson and the Decision to Use the Atomic Bomb," *The Asia Pacific Journal: Japan Focus* 7, no. 14 (2009).

44    P. Revy et al., "Activation-Induced Cytidine Deaminase (Aid) Deficiency Causes the Autosomal Recessive Form of the Hyper-Igm Syndrome (Higm2)," *Cell* 102, no. 5 (2000): 565–75.

45    Y. Ishida, Y. Agata, K. Shibahara, and T. Honjo, "Induced Expression of Pd-1, a Novel Member of the Immunoglobulin Gene Superfamily, Upon Programmed Cell Death," *The EMBO Journal* 11, no. 11 (1992): 3887–95.

46    Ibid.

47    Y. Agata et al., "Expression of the Pd-1 Antigen on the Surface of Stimulated Mouse T and B Lymphocytes," *International Immunology* 8, no. 5 (1996): 765–72.

48    H. Nishimura, N. Minato, T. Nakano, and T. Honjo, "Immunological Studies on Pd-1 Deficient Mice: Implication of Pd-1 as a Negative Regulator for B Cell Responses," *International immunology* 10, no. 10 (1998): 1563–72.

49    H. Nishimura et al., "Development of Lupus-Like Autoimmune Diseases by Disruption of the Pd-1 Gene Encoding an Itim Motif-Carrying Immunoreceptor," *Immunity* 11, no. 2 (1999): 141–51.

50    H. Dong, G. Zhu, K. Tamada, and L. Chen, "B7-H1, a Third Member of the B7 Family, Co-Stimulates T-Cell Proliferation and Interleukin-10 Secretion," *Nature Medicine* 5, no. 12 (1999): 1365–9.

51    S. Tseng et al., "B7-Dc, a New Dendritic Cell Molecule with Potent Costimulatory Properties for T Cells," *The Journal of Experimental Medicine* 193, no. 7 (2001): 839-46.

52    H. Dong et al., "Tumor-Associated B7-H1 Promotes T-Cell Apoptosis: A Potential Mechanism of Immune Evasion," *Nature Medicine* 8, no. 9 (2002).

53    J. R. Brahmer et al., "Phase I Study of Single-Agent Anti–Programmed Death-1 (Mdx-1106) in Refractory Solid Tumors: Safety, Clinical Activity, Pharmacodynamics, and Immunologic Correlates," *Journal of Clinical Oncology* 28, no. 19 (2010): 3167-75.

54    J. S. Weber et al., "Safety, Efficacy, and Biomarkers of Nivolumab with Vaccine in Ipilimumab-Refractory or -Naive Melanoma," *Journal of Clinical Oncology* 31, no. 34 (2013): 4311–18.

55    D. Berman et al.,"The Development of Immunomodulatory Monoclonal Antibodies as a New Therapeutic Modality for Cancer: The Bristol-Myers Squibb Experience," *Pharmacology and Therapeutics* 148 (2015): 132–53.

56    M. I. Zia, L.L. Siu, G. R. Pond, and E. X. Chen, "Comparison of Outcomes of Phase II Studies and Subsequent Randomized Control Studies Using Identical Chemotherapeutic Regimens," *Journal of Clinical Oncology* 23, no. 28 (2005): 6982–91.

57    S. Koenig, "Positive Phase 3 Data for Opdivo (Nivolumab) in Advanced Melanoma Patients Previously Treated with Yervoy (Ipilimumab) Presented at the Esmo 2014 Congress; First Phase 3 Results Presented for a Pd-1 Immune Checkpoint Inhibitor," Bristol-Myers Squibb, September 29, 2014, https://news.bms.com/press-release/rd-news/positive-phase-3-data-opdivo-nivolumab-advanced-melanoma-patients-previously-t.

58    L. A. Raedler, "Opdivo (Nivolumab): Second Pd-1 Inhibitor Receives Fda Approval for Unresectable or Metastatic Melanoma," *American Health & Drug Benefits* 8 (2015): 180–83.

## 9: THE END OF THE BEGINNING

1    S. P. Kang et al., "Pembrolizumab Keynote-001: An Adaptive Study Leading to Accelerated Approval for Two Indications and a Companion Diagnostic," *Annals of Oncology* 28, no. 6 (2017): 1388–98.

2    D. Shaywitz, "The Startling History Behind Merck's New Cancer Blockbuster," Forbes.com, July 26, 2017, https://www.forbes.com/sites/davidshaywitz/2017/07/26/the-startling-history-behind-mercks-new-cancer-blockbuster/#512ddf0d948d.

3    Kang, "Pembrolizumab Keynote-001: An Adaptive Study Leading to Accelerated Approval for Two Indications and a Companion Diagnostic," 1388–98.

4    J. Rockoff and P. Loftus, "Bristol-Myers Bucks Trend toward Precision Medicine," *The Wall Street Journal*, March 13, 2016.

5    K. Garber, "In a Major Shift, Cancer Drugs Go 'Tissue-Agnostic,'" *Science* 356, no. 6,343 (2017): 1111–2.

6    A. Piore, "James Allison Has Unfinished Business with Cancer," *Technology Review* 120, no. 3 (2017): 78–85.

7    J. Tang, A. Shalabi, and V. M. Hubbard-Lucey, "Comprehensive Analysis of the Clinical Immuno-Oncology Landscape," *Annals of Oncology* 29, no. 1 (2018): 84–91.

8    U. Storz, "Intellectual Property Issues of Immune Checkpoint Inhibitors," *mAbs* no. 8 (2016): 10–26.

9    Ibid.

10   R. Milo, "The Efficacy and Safety of Daclizumab and Its Potential Role in the Treatment of Multiple Sclerosis," *Therapeutic Advances in Neurological Disorders* 7, no. 1 (2014): 7–21.

11   P. Dilokthornsakul, et. al., "Multiple Sclerosis Prevalence in the United States Commercially Insured Population," *Neurology* 86, no. 11 (2016): 1014–21.

12   L. Kappos et al., "Daclizumab Hyp Versus Interferon Beta-1a in Relapsing Multiple Sclerosis," *New England Journal of Medicine* 373, no. 15 (2015): 1418–28.

13   "Nice Says No to Daclizumab (Zinbryta)," Multiple Sclerosis Trust, October 3, 2016, https://www.mstrust.org.uk/news/news-about-ms/nice-says-no-daclizumab-zinbryta.

14   A. J. Rech and R. H. Vonderheide, "Clinical Use of Anti-CD25 Antibody Daclizumab to Enhance Immune Responses to Tumor Antigen Vaccination by Targeting Regulatory T Cells," *Annals of the New York Academy of Sciences* 1,174, no. 1 (2009): 99–106.

# Index